Gastric Cancer

Edited by
Ch. Herfarth and P. Schlag

With 161 Figures and 144 Tables

Springer-Verlag
Berlin Heidelberg New York 1979

Professor Dr. Christian H. Herfarth
Dr. Peter M. Schlag
Department für Chirurgie der Universität
Steinhövelstraße 9, 7900 Ulm
Federal Republic of Germany

Library of Congress Cataloging in Publication Data. Main entry under title: Gastric cancer. 1. Stomach--Cancer. 2. Stomach--Surgery. I. Herfarth, Christian, 1933- II. Schlag, P., 1948- RC280.S8G37 616.9'94'33 79-19624

ISBN-13: 978-3-642-67370-2 e-ISBN-13: 978-3-642-67368-9
DOI: 10.1007/978-3-642-67368-9

Softcover reprint of the hardcover 1st edition 1979

2127/3140-543210

Preface

The problem of gastric cancer, with its multifaceted aspects, offers an example of diversified oncological research, which includes epidemiology, pathogenesis, histomorphology, surgical and conservative therapy in its spectrum. This disease not only constitutes an interesting and important subject for research, but it is also a challenge for the practitioner due to its inordinately poor prognosis.
It therefore appeared a rewarding task to the editors to collect information from individual experts, in order to gain a topical summary of the problems pertaining to gastric cancer, as well as to provide a survey of the progress and the therapeutic possibilities in this field.
This task was particularly enticing, as gastric cancer has lately come to belong to those tumors somewhat relegated to the shadows, although it is, despite its decreased frequency in some western countries, still one of the most prevalent malignant diseases.

This collection should emphasize the need for broadly based knowledge of individual problems as a prerequisite for any satisfactory therapy of an organ tumor. It is therefore the primary concern of this book to furnish anyone with an interest in oncology with this necessary survey.
The editors thank Mrs. Karin Dohmeier and Mrs. Karin Kluge from Springer-Verlag for their cooperation in preparing this monograph. We extend our thanks to Mrs. Susanne Schenk and Mrs. Marga Wild, who contributed so much by her secretarial experience for the success of this volume.

Ulm, September 1979

Ch. Herfarth
P. Schlag

Table of Contents

List of Senior Authors

Beger, H., Professor Dr. med., Chirurgische Universitätsklinik und Poliklinik, Klinikum Westend, Freie Universität Berlin, Spandauer Damm 130, 1000 Berlin 19/FRG

Betzler, M., Dr. med., Abteilung Allgemeine Chirurgie, Department für Chirurgie der Universität Ulm, Steinhövelstr. 9, 7900 Ulm/Donau/FRG

Bittner, R., Dr. med., Chirurgische Universitätsklinik und Poliklinik, Klinikum Westend, Freie Universität Berlin, Spandauer Damm 130, 1000 Berlin 19/FRG

Borchard, F., Professor Dr. med., Pathologisches Institut der Universität Düsseldorf, Moorenstr. 5, 4000 Düsseldorf/FRG

Clémençon, G., Dr. med., Spezialarzt für Innere Medizin, Magen-Darmkrankheiten, Frohheimweg 12, 4600 Olten/Switzerland

Correa, P., Professor Dr. med., Louisiana State University, Medical Center, Department of Pathology, 1542 Tulane Avenue, New Orleans, Louisiana 70112/USA

Dahm, K., Priv. Doz. Dr. med., Abteilung Allgemeinchirurgie der Chirurgischen Universitätsklinik Eppendorf, Martinistr. 52, 2000 Hamburg 20/FRG

Goebell, H., Professor Dr. med., Medizinische Klinik des Universitätsklinikums Essen, Hufelandstr. 55, 4300 Essen 1/FRG

Grundmann, E., Professor Dr. med., Pathologisches Institut der Universität Münster, Westring 17, 4400 Münster/FRG

Hassenstein, E., Dr. med., Department für Radiologie, Abteilung für Strahlentherapie und spezielle Onkologie der Medizinischen Hochschule Hannover, Postfach 610 180, 3000 Hannover/FRG

Herfarth, Ch., Professor Dr. med., Abteilung Allgemeine Chirurgie, Department für Chirurgie der Universität Ulm, Steinhövelstr. 9, 7900 Ulm/Donau/FRG

Hermanek, P., Professor Dr. med., Abteilung für Klinische Pathologie in der Chirurgischen Klinik der Universität Erlangen-Nürnberg, Maximiliansplatz, 8250 Erlangen/FRG

Heymer, B., Professor Dr. med., Abteilung für Pathologie der Universität Ulm, Steinhövelstr. 9, 7900 Ulm/Donau/FRG

Higgins, G. A., Professor Dr. med., Surgical Service, Cancer Chemotherapy Study Group, Veterans Administration Hospital, 50 Irving Street N. W., Washington, D. C. 20422/USA

Hollinger, A., Dr. med., Chirurgische Universitätsklinik A, Kantonsspital Zürich, Rämistrasse 100, 8091 Zürich/Switzerland

Joyeux, H., Dr. med., Unité de Nutrition et Métabolisme, Cliniques Saint-Eloi, 3400 Montpellier/France

Junghanns, K., Professor Dr. med., Chirurgische Klinik der Universität Heidelberg, Im Neuenheimer Feld 110, 6900 Heidelberg 1/FRG

Kummer, D., Professor Dr. med., Chirurgische Klinik und Poliklinik der Eberhard-Karls-Universität Tübingen, 7400 Tübingen/FRG

Lawson, H. H., Professor Dr., Medical School, Department of Surgery, University of Witwatersrand, Hospital Street, Johannesburg 2001/South Africa

Linder, M., Priv. Doz. Dr. med., Chirurgische Klinik im Klinikum Mannheim der Universität Heidelberg, Theodor-Kutzer-Ufer, 6800 Mannheiml/FRG

Mayer, M., Dr. med., Onkologisches Zentrum, Fakultät für Klinische Medizin Mannheim der Universität Heidelberg, Theodor-Kutzer-Ufer, 6800 Mannheim 1/FRG

Meister, H., Dr. med., Abteilung für Pathologie der Universität Ulm, Steinhövelstr. 9, 7900 Ulm/Donau/FRG

Merkle, P., Priv. Doz. Dr. med., Abteilung Allgemeine Chirurgie, Department für Chirurgie der Universität Ulm, Steinhövelstr. 9, 7900 Ulm/Donau/FRG

Meyer, H. J., Dr. med., Klinik f. Abdominal- und Transplantationschirurgie, Department für Chirurgie, Medizinische Hochschule Hannover, Karl-Wiechert-Allee 9, 3000 Hannover/FRG

Nakazato, H., Professor Dr. med., Aichi Cancer Center, 81-1159 Kanokoden, Tashiro-cho, Chikusa-ku; Nagoya 464/Japan

Oehlert, W., Professor Dr. med., Pathologisches Institut, Abt. Experimentelle Pathologie, Klinikum der Albert-Ludwigs-Universität, Albertstr. 19, 7800 Freiburg i. Br./ FRG

Peitsch, W., Dr. med., Klinik u. Poliklinik für Allgemeinchirurgie der Universität Göttingen, Robert-Koch-Str. 40, 3400 Göttingen/FRG

Pfeiffer, C. J., Professor Dr. med., Faculty of Medicine, Memorial University of New Foundland, St. John's New Foundland/Canada

Pichlmayr, R., Professor Dr. med., Klinik für Abdominal- und Transplantationschirurgie, Department für Chirurgie, Medizinische Hochschule Hannover, Karl-Wiechert-Allee 9, 3000 Hannover/FRG

Priesching, A., Professor Dr. med., I. Chirurgische Universitätsklinik, Mariannengasse 28, 1090 Wien/Austria

Rösch, W., Priv. Doz. Dr. med., Medizinische Klinik mit Poliklinik der Universität Erlangen-Nürnberg, Krankenhausstr. 12, 8520 Erlangen/FRG

Saito, T., Dr., med. 2nd Department of Surgery, Kyushu University School of Medicine Fukuoka 812/Japan

Seeger, V., Dr. med., Chirurgische Klinik mit Poliklinik der Universität Erlangen-Nürnberg, Maximiliansplatz, 8520 Erlangen/FRG

Siewert, J. R., Professor Dr. med., Klinik und Poliklinik für Allgemeinchirurgie der Universität Göttingen, Robert-Koch-Str. 40, 3400 Göttingen/FRG

Schachenmayr, W., Priv. Doz. Dr. med., Abteilung für Pathologie der Universität Ulm, Steinhövelstr. 9, 7900 Ulm/Donau/FRG

Schlag, P., Dr. med., Abteilung für Allgemeine Chirurgie, Department für Chirurgie der Universität Ulm, Steinhövelstr. 9, 7900 Ulm/Donau/FRG

Schmähl, D., Professor Dr. med., Institut für Toxikologie und Chemotherapie im Deutschen Krebsforschungszentrum, Im Neuenheimer Feld 280, 6900 Heidelberg/FRG

Schmitz-Moormann, P., Professor Dr. med., Pathologisches Institut der Universität Marburg, Robert-Koch-Str. 5, 3550 Marburg/FRG

Schultis, K., Professor Dr. med., Rudelsweiherstraße 37, 8520 Erlangen/FRG

Troidl, H., Priv. Doz. Dr. med., Abteilung Allgemeine Chirurgie, Chirurgische Universitätsklinik, Hospitalstr. 40, 2300 Kiel/FRG

Winkler, R., Priv. Doz. Dr. med., Abteilung Allgemeinchirurgie, Chirurgische Universitätsklinik Eppendorf, Martinistr. 52, 2000 Hamburg 20/FRG

1 Epidemiology and Pathogenesis

Exogenous Factors in the Epidemiology of Gastric Carcinoma

Carl J. Pfeiffer

Introduction

During the past decade, the great importance of exogenous factors, i.e., environmentally-related factors, has become recognized for cancers of all sites. Although this type of association for cancers of a few sites was considered for many years, there is now a very general recognition that exogenous carcinogenic agents, particularly chemical, but also viral factors, are involved in human cancer etiology, and that other exogenous factors either promote malignant transformations or enhance host susceptibility. The role of exogenous factors in the causation of gastric cancer appear paramount, although this conclusion has been derived by implication, rather than by direct proof of the causative agents. Thus, the demonstration of (a) the lack of importance of hereditary-racial factors generally, (b) the reliable production of gastric cancer in animals by chemical carcinogens, (c) the slowly mounting evidence of specific risk factors in the human environment for gastric cancer, and (d) the massive evidence of carcinogenic-associated exogenous factors for cancers of other sites without any rationale that carcinogenesis in the stomach should be unique, all suggest exogenous carcinogenic factors for gastric carcinoma.

The epidemiologic approach to this problem has already and will continue to contribute much to understanding the early pathogenesis of gastric carcinoma and to identifying risk factors. Although epidemiologic investigation may or may not provide ultimate proof of gastric cancer causation, it will likely clarify the pathogenesis, will lead the way to appropriate laboratory investigations, and should identify control measures which may prevent or decrease the risk of acquiring gastric carcinoma. The criteria for ascertaining the validity of epidemiologic associations relating gastric cancer to exogenous factors are standard criteria, consisting of the strength of statistical association, the presence of a graded or "dose response" relationship, the effectiveness of predictability in prospective studies with human subjects, confirmation in several populations, reconcilation with other types of clinical or laboratory investigations, etc.

The causes of gastric cancer remain unknown and many hypotheses to explain the pathogenesis of this disease, and exogenous agents have been considered. These factors have been reviewed many times previously [5, 11, 21] and will not be discussed exhaustively here. Table 1 outlines a broad array of exogenous factors that have been suggested as being involved in gastric carcinogenesis. The purpose of the present account is (a) to emphasize some of the most important exogenous factors that consistently have been shown to be

Table 1. Sources of exogenous factors associated[a] with increased risk for gastric carcinoma

Environmental	
Acidic or peaty soil	High nitrate content in water
Urban residency	Exposure to environmental talc
Extensive use of nitrate fertilizers	Volcanic rock background
Soft water	Elevated lead or zinc in water
Littoral environment	
Dietary	
Highly salted food	
Smoked foods	
High fat or contaminated oil intake	
Smoking and Drinking	
Cigarette smoking	
Consumption of sake or contaminated whiskey	
Occupational	
Lower socio-economic classes	Agricultural workers
Workers in mines and quarries	Painters
Metal industry workers	Transportation equipment repair and assembly workers
Fishermen	Textile workers
Printers and bookbinders	Ceramic, clay, and stone workers
Construction workers	Clerical workers

[a] In most instances, these factors have been risk-associated in more than one country, but these correlations have not always been confirmed.

associated with gastric carcinoma, (b) to review some of the most recent findings incriminating exogenous factors in gastric carcinogenesis, and (c) to comment briefly on recent data from our own investigations which have suggested the role of exogenous factors in gastric cancer causation.

General Epidemiologic Findings

Epidemiologic data now allow several assumptions to be made about gastric cancer. These include, among other conclusions, the following: (a) more than one carcinogen can likely initiate gastric carcinogenesis, (b) chemical agents, perhaps ingested or formed in vivo, rather than viral agents, are likely inducing agents in most instances, (c) the pathogenesis is very slowly developing, after initial mutagenic changes in gastric stem cells, (d) the diffuse and intestinal types of gastric cancers, which are different diseases, may have different causal factors, (e) the conditions of chronic atrophic gastritis and intestinal metaplasia are closely associated with gastric cancer, thereby facilitating risk analysis and elucidating the pathogenesis, but these conditions are not proven precursor conditions.

Table 1 outlines some of the most frequently confirmed environmental, dietary, or occupational situations which, in several countries, have been risk associated. Some of these factors, such as cigarette smoking and smoked foods contain well-established chemical carcinogens, but others, such as salt (NaCl), are not carcinogenic alone. Thus, ingestion of highly salted food probably creates a promotional condition, such as local osmotic damage to the gastric mucosa, which facilitates action or entry of another agent which is the proximate carcinogen or procarcinogen. As noted, a large number of the high risk occupations are those wherein mineral dust or chemical fumes are inhaled and thus, could also drain into the gastrointestinal tract. It remains unclear precisely what factors in these high risk occupations are operative. The types of foreign agents which might enter the gut in industrialized societies, and their complex interactions and absorption within the gut lumen have recently been reviewed by Pfeiffer [12].

The role of exogenous factors in gastric cancer causation has been supported by several of the classical methods of epidemiologic analysis, including migrant studies, time trend studies, differences in the sex ratio of incidence, dietary, and case control study. Different races residing in high risk zones (Japanese and Caucasians in Japan) or in low risk zones (same races in the United States) have approaching rates, and migration to zones of changed risk imparts changes in incidence similar to the recipient country. A decrease in gastric cancer incidence has been shown almost worldwide, and in both high risk (Japan, Chile) and lower risk countries (United States, Canada, European countries), suggesting life-style changes which alter exposure to exogenous factors. The generally twofold greater susceptibility of males than females is occasionally reversed in local regions, again showing that the inherent sex-related resistance is likely altered by external factors. Dietary studies have long been fraught with difficulties, accuracy and meaningful results, but most items in Table 1 have been well supported. Of particular note also is the accumulating evidence of possibly protective factors in the diet, including milk consumption, and ingestion of fresh vegetables [5, 7], perhaps indicating the protective role of vitamins A or C or other antioxidants, as has been demonstrated as well for cancer of other sites [7] in large scale prospective studies in Japan.

Recent International Findings

During the past 2–3 years, new occupational-risk analyses of gastric cancer patients have shown that rubber workers have a standardized mortality ratio of 183 (age 40–64) for stomach cancer, an elevated risk that was associated with compounding and mixing, milling, cementing, and other processes in this trade [9]. The high risk of stomach cancer for farmers was confirmed by Haenszel et al. [4] and by Hirayama [6] for Japanese farmers. Also, the high risk for fishermen, previously shown in England and Wales, was confirmed in Japan [6] and in Newfoundland, Canada, the triad of fishermen, fish processing plants, and seabirds also being interlinked with enhanced risk [15]. Further, in Japan, the differential patterns among male geographic distributions for gastric cancer versus cerebrovascular disease was confirmed by Nagai [10], with the former disease favoring agricultural workers. Also in 1978 Gaudette et al. [3] reported an elevated gastric cancer incidence in Canadian Hutterites, a religious farming sect.

Reports on dietary factors associated with gastric cancer appearing during the past 3 years have largely confirmed earlier notions. East German case control studies revealed as risk factors, food intolerance, high alcohol consumption, and long use of tobacco [20]. This smoking-related risk, shown in earlier studies, was also associated in 1977 with intestinal metaplasia of the stomach in Hawaiian Japanese [18], and it has been reported that the nornicotine in tobacco smoke can be nitrosated to a small degree in gastric juice of humans to N-nitrosonornicotine [16]. Further, the possible protective effects of dietary milk consumption was supported by data from Chile, and the inverse relationship between gastric cancer mortality and animal protein consumption was shown in Chile and Costa Rica. Fish extracts subjected to nitrosation, but not beef or hot dog extracts were shown to be mutagenic in the Ames test and ascorbic acid prevented this carcinogen formation [8]. Also, recent descriptive epidemiologic reports on gastric cancer from Belgium, contrasting the incidence in Flemish versus Walloon provinces, and a report on gastric carcinoma in Rhodesian Africans [2] have suggested the importance of exogenous factors, such as diet, alcohol, and tobacco consumption.

Gastric Cancer in Newfoundland and Iceland

Iceland has long been characterized as a high incidence island for carcinoma of the stomach, and more recently, the island of Newfoundland has been shown to be the highest risk province in Canada for cancer of this site [15]. As with most countries or regions in the world in which gastric cancer shows a high or moderate incidence, Newfoundland and Iceland demonstrate marked geographic variance in risk throughout the islands. It has been shown in Newfoundland that ethnic differences do not account for the variation in gastric carcinoma mortality, and that environmental factors, such as the geochemical background [15] or occupation are associated with these differences. Analyses of drinking water trace elements in Newfoundland (and Japan) show a positive correlation between gastric cancer and lead content [13], which is of interest because lead is carcinogenic in animals, and was the only element elevated in major river basin water in the United States, as correlated with gastric cancer mortality, according to Berg and Burbank [1]. It has also been demonstrated that lead workers had increased risk of pulmonary carcinoma [19].

A further indication that exogenous factors are involved in gastric cancer is the close parallelism between the Standard Mortality Ratio for this disease in identical occupational groups in both Iceland and Newfoundland (Fig. 1), where the dietary and ethnic factors are different, suggesting common environmental factors.

Fishermen were at greatly enhanced risk in both Iceland and Newfoundland, and it should be noted that fishermen were also at very high risk for cancer of the

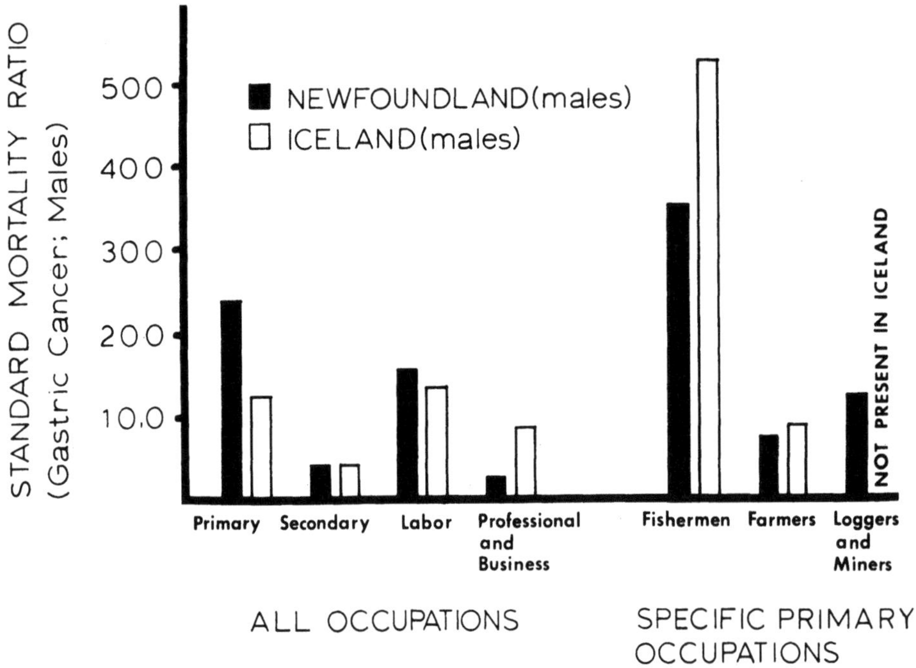

Fig. 1. Data based upon 1960 – 1970 (11 yr) mean death rates, age standardized by world population, and 1961 and 1966 Labor Force Statistics

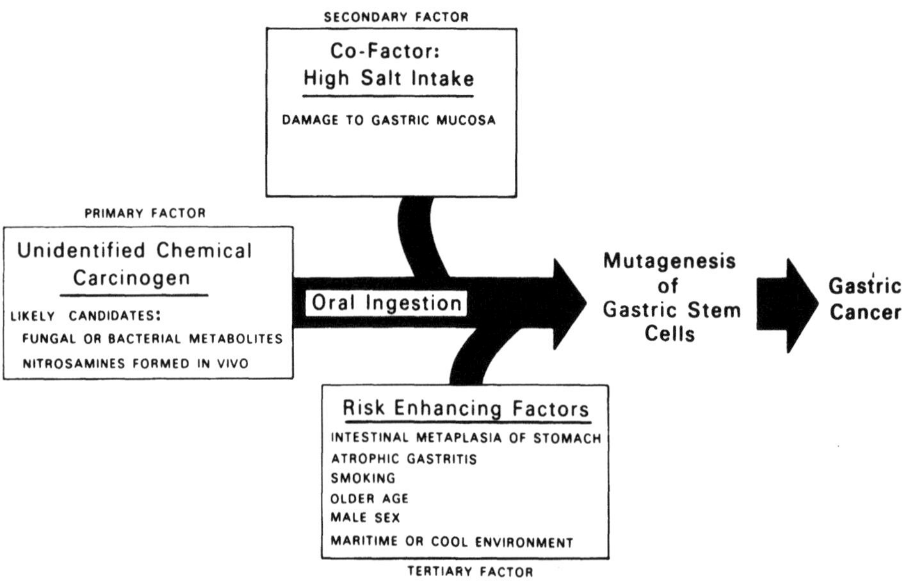

Fig. 2. Hypothesis of stomach cancer etiology

lip in Newfoundland, although the particular carcinogen responsible has not yet been identified [17]. So far, dietary differences have not yet been elucidated that might explain the regional variance in gastric cancer on the island of Newfoundland. To a slight extent, drinking water nitrate was elevated in the high risk zone of Newfoundland, and the NaCl intake throughout the island is high compared to North American standards.

From the foregoing paragraphs, it is evident that exogenous factors, which still remain to be identified, are likely involved in the etiology of gastric cancer. Epidemiologic studies are narrowing down the environmental sources of such carcinogens, and risk-associated occupations, foods, etc. are being identified as possible sources of chemical carcinogens or promoting agents. Figure 2 illustrates a working hypothesis for gastric cancer induction in man, which consolidates the current knowledge based upon both epidemiologic and experimental findings. The ingestion or formation of carcinogenic nitrosamines in the stomach as the carcinogenic agent, and the promotional effect of NaCl and associated conditions of gastritis are shown in this model.

References

1. Berg, J. W., Burbank, F.: Correlations between carcinogenic trace metals in water supplies and cancer mortality. Ann. N.Y. Acad. Sci. *199*, 249–264 (1972)
2. Dent, R. I., Fleming, J. B., Wicks, A. C.: Carcinoma of the stomach in Rhodesian Africans and a comparative review. Clin. Oncol. *3*, 17–26 (1977)
3. Gaudette, L. A., Holmes, T. M., Laing, L. M., Morgan, K., Grace, M. G.: Cancer incidence in a religious isolate of Alberta, Canada, 1953–74. J. Natl. Cancer Inst. *60*, 1233–1238 (1978)
4. Haenszel, W., Kurihara, M., Locke, F. B., Shimuza, K., Segi, M.: Stomach cancer in Japan. J. Natl. Cancer Inst. *56*, 265–274 (1976)
5. Hirayama, T.: Epidemiology of stomach cancer. In: Early Gastric cancer, Murakani, T. (ed.). Gann Monograph on Cancer Res. *11*, 3–19. Baltimore, London, Tokyo: University Park Press 1971
6. Hirayama, T.: Metal-material workers and lung cancer in Japan. Ann. N.Y. Acad. Sci. *271*, 269–272 (1976)
7. Hirayama, T.: A population prospective study on cancer epidemiology in Japan. Proceedings of the Japanese Cancer Association, 36th Annual Meeting, Tokyo, October 1977
8. Marquardt, H., Rufino, F., Weisburger, J. H.: Mutagenic activity of nitrite-treated foods: Human stomach cancer may be related to dietary factors. Science *196*, 1000–1001 (1977)
9. McMichael, A. J., Andjelkovic, D. A., Tyroler, H. A.: Cancer mortality among rubber workers: An epidemiologic study. Ann. N.Y. Acad. Sci. *271*, 125–137 (1976)
10. Nagai, N.: Epidemiological studies on non-infectious chronic diseases in Gunma Prefecture. II. Observations of an area having high risk of malignant neoplasms of the stomach in males. Kitakanto Med. J. *27*, 259–264 (1977)
11. Pfeiffer, C. J.: Epidemiologie des Magenkarzinoms. Leber, Magen, Darm *6*, 59–70 (1976)
12. Pfeiffer, C. J.: Gastroenterologic response to environmental agents – absorption and interactions. In: Handbook of Physiology, Sec. 9, Reaction to Environmental Agents, pp. 349–374, Bethesda: Amer. Physiol. Soc. 1977
13. Pfeiffer, C. J., Fodor, G.: Gastric cancer mortality and water trace elements: International study of Iceland, Newfoundland and Japan. In: Gastric cancer. Pfeiffer, C. J. (ed.), Chapt. 2, Baden-Baden: G. Witzstrock, 1979 (in press)
14. Pfeiffer, C. J., Threlfall, W.: Seabirds – a possible environmental factor in gastric cancer in Newfoundland. Digestion *16*, 1–9 (1977)
15. Pfeiffer, C. J., Fodor, J., Canning, E.: An epidemiologic analysis of mortality and gastric cancer in Newfoundland. J. Can. Med. Assoc. *108*, 1374–1380 (1973)

16. Schweinsberg, F., Sander, J., Schweinsberg, E., Kollat, P.: Nitrosation of nicotine and nornicotine and the formation of N-nitrosonornicotine in the stomach of smokers. Z. Krebsforsch. *84*, 81 – 87 (1975)
17. Spitzer, W. O., Hill, G. B., Chambers, L. W., Helliwell, B. E., Murphy, H. B.: The occupation of fishing as a risk factor in cancer of the lip. N. Engl. J. Med. *293*, 419 – 424 (1975)
18. Stemmermann, G., Haenszel, W., Locke, F.: Epidemiologic pathology of gastric ulcer and gastric carcinoma among Japanese in Hawaii. J. Natl. Cancer Inst. *58*, 13 – 20 (1977)
19. Sunderman, F. W.: Carcinogenic effects of metals. Fed. Proc. *37*, 40 – 46 (1978)
20. Wolff, G., Lauter, J.: On the epidemiology of gastric cancer. Arch. Geschwulstforsch. *46*, 1 – 14 (1976)
21. Wynder, E. L.: On the epidemiology of gastric cancer. In: Racial and geographic factors in tumour incidence. Shivas, A. A. (ed.), pp. 37 – 45. Edinburgh: Univ. Press 1967

Pathogenesis of Gastric Carcinoma: The Role of the Microenvironment*

Pelayo Correa, Carlos Cuello, and Guillermo Montes

Several recent reviews of the epidemiology of gastric cancer are available [3, 4]. One of the salient features brought out is the prolonged latency period of the disease which in most cases is in excess of 30 years. During the prolonged latency period, drastic changes take place in the gastric microenvironment. The purpose of this article is to review briefly our present knowledge concerning the altered microenvironment.

Gastric Mucosa

The progressive changes that take place in the gastric mucosa of persons at high risk to gastric cancer have been well documented in other publications [3, 1]. Of special importance is the development of chronic atrophic gastritis and its frequent complication: intestinal metaplasia. In another section of this monograph, we review our interpretation of the most advanced phases of the precancerous process: the dysplasias.

pH

The gastric juice pH reflects the involvement of the parietal cells by the process of atrophic gastritis. Small foci of gastritis do not result in alteration of pH. Moderate or severe degrees of gastritis are usually associated with an elevated pH, but in some cases the elevated gastrin levels prevent drastic elevations of pH. Achlorhydria may occur in gastric cancer patients, but it is not very frequent because the neoplasia develops before the gastric atrophy progresses to total loss of parietal cells.

Bacteria

Contrary to the normal situation, the gastric juice of populations at high risk contain many viable bacteria. Abnormal presence of *Streptococcus salivarius, Streptococcus viridans, Staphylococci, lactobacilli, veillonellae, bacteroides,* and *bifidobacteria* have been reported. Mixed cultures of these patients have shown marked capacity to reduce nitrate to nitrite [5].

---

* Work supported by contracts NO 1-CP-53521 and NO 1-CP-33286

Nitrate

Nitrate ingestion has been positively correlated with gastric cancer rates in Colombia. Nitrate in the gastric juice is abundant in high-risk populations, but high levels are also found in individuals with normal mucosa as seen in Table 1.

Nitrite

Nitrite is not generally found as such in unprocessed food or drinking water. It is assumed that its presence in human fluids comes principally from reduction of nitrate to nitrite. This has been shown to be accomplished by the flora of the saliva [10]. It probably occurs also in the gastric cavity when reducing bacteria are present. Table 1 shows how patients with atrophic gastritis have a significant excess of nitrite in their gastric juices. Most of these patients have also intestinal metaplasia as a complication of their atrophic gastritis. Figure 1 shows an excellent correlation between pH and nitrite level in the gastric juice. Other investigators have reported a positive correlation of gastric juice nitrite with cancer risk and with atypias of the gastric mucosa [6, 9].

Mutagens

Table 2 presents the results of an assay of 96 samples of gastric juice from Nariño, Colombia tested in the TA100 strain of *Salmonella typhimurium* which detects the mutagen capacity of the gastric juice [8]. It shows how the samples with nitrite have a significantly elevated rate of mutations. This rate is not significantly elevated when S9 mix is added, indicating that most of this activity is direct (not mediated by liver microsomal enzymes).

Table 1. Average values of pH, NO_3 and NO_2 by histologic diagnosis

			Gastric juice					
	Number of cases	Age	pH	(Significance) (T)	NO_3 ppm	(Significance) (T)	NO_2 ppm	(Significance) (T)
Normal + SG[a]	5	36.6	2.3	(0.0001)	74.5	N.S.	0.18	(0.001)
CAG[b] (All)	31	46.8	5.2		85.7		1.70	
pH < 5	18	46.7	2.5		73.2	N.S.	0.25	(0.0003)
pH ≥ 5	18	44.0	7.0		95.2		2.71	

[a] SG = Superficial Gastritis
[b] CAG = Chronic Atrophic Gastritis

Table 2. Number of colony-forming units (CFU) per plate in 96 gastric juice samples. Nariño, Colombia, 1977

S. thyphimurium strain	Background	NO_2 Negative gastric juice	NO_2 Positive gastric juice
TA100	32	31	68
TA100 + S9 mix	42	40	92

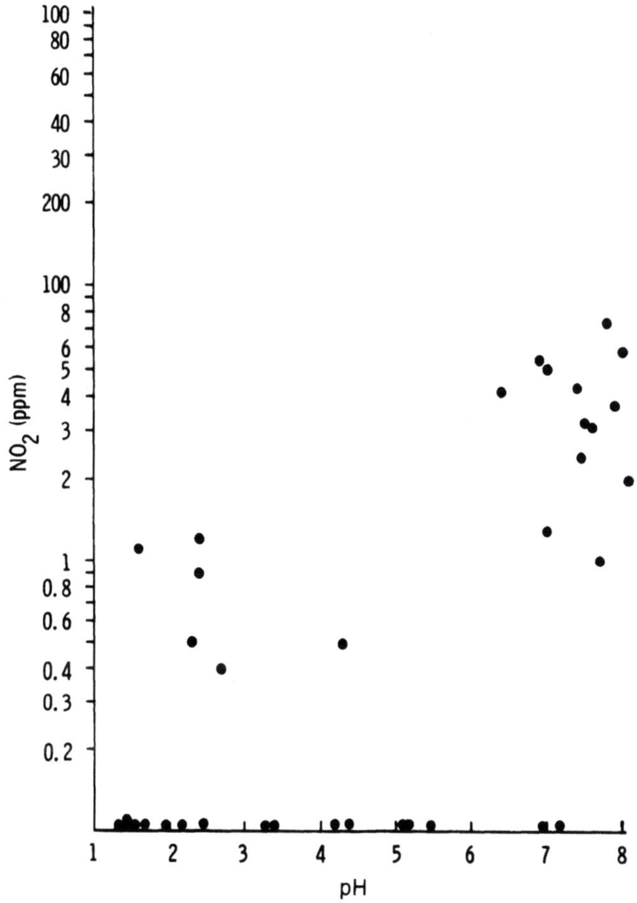

Fig. 1. Correlation between pH and NO_2 in fasting gastric juice

Conclusion

The available information would support our hypothesis that the epidemic type of gastric cancer is the result of a series of mutations probably triggered by nitrosocompounds synthesized in the stomach by the interaction of nitrite and naturally occurring nitrogen compounds [2]. We have recently proposed that nitrosation of spermidine could serve as a model for that reaction [7].

References

1. Correa, P., Cuello, C., Duque, E.: Carcinoma and intestinal metaplasia of the stomach in Colombian migrants. J. Natl. Cancer Inst. *44*, 297 – 306 (1970)
2. Correa, P., Haenszel, W., Cuello, C., Tannenbaum, S., Archer, M.: A model for gastric cancer epidemiology. Lancet *1975 2*, 58
3. Correa, P., Cuello, C., Haenszel, W.: Pathogenese des Magenkarzinoms – Epidemiologische Pathologie vorangehender Lasionen. Leber Magen Darm *6*, 72 – 79 (1976)
4. Correa, P., Cuello, C., Haenszel, W.: Epidemiology of premalignant gastric lesions. In: Pathophysiology of carcinogenesis in digestive organs. Farber, E. et al. (ed.)., pp. 163 – 179. Baltimore: Park Press 1977
5. Hawksworth, G., Hill, M. J., Gordillo, G., Cuello, C.: Possible relationship between nitrates, nitrosamines and gastric cancer in South-West Colombia. In: N-Nitroso compounds in the environment. Vol. 9, pp. 229 – 234. Bogovski, P., Walker, E. A. (eds.). Lyon, France: IARC Scientific Publication 1974
6. Jones, S. M., Davies, P. W., Savage, A.: Gastric juice nitrite and gastric cancer. Lancet *1978 1*, 1355
7. Kokatnur, M., Murray, M., Correa, P.: Mutagenic properties of nitrosated spermidine. Proc. Soc. Exp. Biol. Med. *158*, 85 – 88 (1978)
8. Montes, G., Gordillo, G., Cuello, C., Pelon, W., Johnson, W., Correa, P.: Mutagenic activity of gastric juice. Submitted for publication, Cancer Lett. (1979)
9. Ruddel, W. S. J., Bone, E. S., Hill, M. J., Walter, C. L.: Gastric juice nitrite. A risk factor in the hypochlorhydric stomach? Lancet *1976 2*, 1037 – 1039
10. Tannenbaum, S. R., Archer, M. C., Wishnok, J. S., Correa, P., Cuello, C., Haenszel, W.: Nitrate and the etiology of gastric cancer. In: Origins of human cancer. pp. 1609 – 1625. Cold Spring: Harbor Laboratories 1977

Carcinoma of the Stomach in Urbanized Black South Africans

H. H. Lawson, I. Segal, and L. Ou Tim

This communication is based on experience at Baragwanath Hospital, Johannesburg, South Africa.

The hospital has over 3 000 beds in its numerous clinics and serves a community of about one million Black South Africans.

Some 70 000 general medical and surgical patients are admitted each year and carcinoma of the stomach is not a common condition. By far the most common carcinoma, occurring in almost epidemic proportions, is carcinoma of the esophagus. About 250 new cases of this condition are seen each year.

The number of patients presenting with carcinoma of the stomach are remarkably constant (Fig. 1) – about 20 – 30 cases annually. Benign gastric ulceration is also uncommon, though perhaps it is seen a little more frequently (Fig. 1).

Both conditions affect males more frequently than females – in carcinoma, it is about 78% males and in benign gastric ulceration about 74% (Table 1). The tumor appears to arise in the pyloric antrum in 50% of cases.

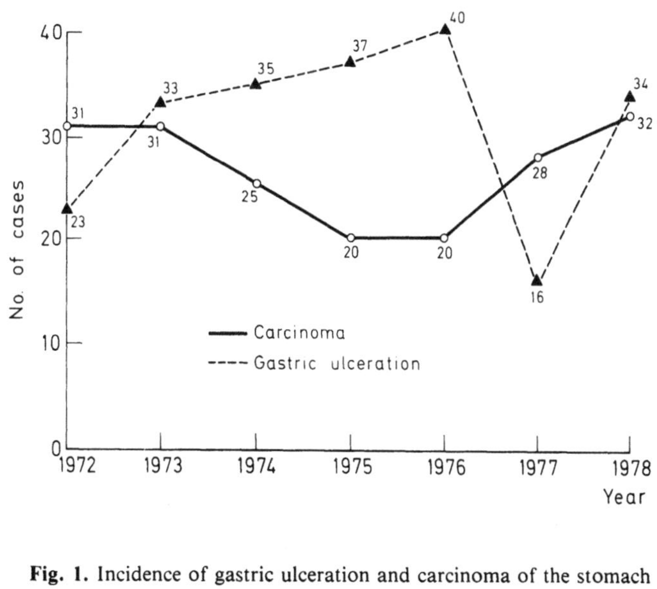

Fig. 1. Incidence of gastric ulceration and carcinoma of the stomach

Table 1. Carcinoma of the stomach in urbanized Black South Africans

Sex incidence	– Males	78%
Site	– Pyloric antrum	50%
Presentation	– Hematemesis of melena	50%
"Curative" surgery	– Less than	5%

The most common presenting features are hematemesis and melena, or abdominal pain.

The disease is always very advanced when the patient presents at the hospital, and less than 5% are suitable for "curative" operative procedures.

It is remarkable that carcinoma should be seen so frequently in the organ above the stomach, that is in the esophagus, and yet be relatively infrequent in the stomach. The duodenum appears to be as resistant to carcinoma in the black South African patient as it is in any other racial group, in spite of the fact that in our black patients, the disease is seen late, and has usually spread to the region lymph glands and the liver.

Figure 2 illustrates a widely infiltrating carcinoma of the pyloric antrum. When the malignant cells approach the duodenum, the cell column narrows rapidly, and the carcinoma is confined to the area below the surface epithelium, but above the antral mucus secreting glands. A total distance of about 2 mm only of duodenal tissue is involved, in spite of the very extensive spread of the tumor within the stomach itself.

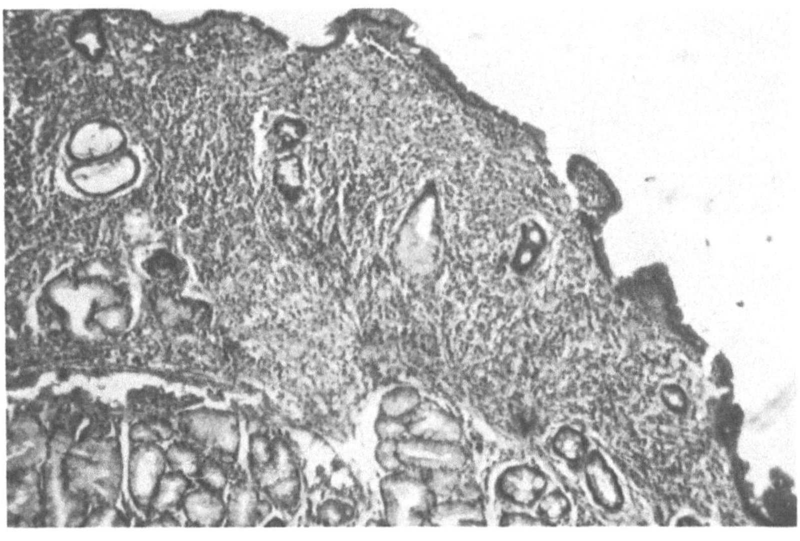

Fig. 2. Carcinoma of the pyloric antrum with very limited spread into the duodenum

Carcinogenic Substances and Carcinogenesis – Their Clinical Significance

D. Schmähl

Introduction

Up to now, the etiology of human gastric cancer has been unknown to a large extent. Speculations are made about dietetic influences as well as about the influence of exogenous chemical factors which may, for instance, be taken in by food. From epidemiologic and geographic pathology, we know that there is an excessive incidence of gastric cancer in, e.g., Japan, Chile, or Venezuela, whereas this type of tumor only occurs very rarely or even shows a decreasing tendency in other countries, e.g., the United States or in the Federal Republic of Germany [13]. These well-known facts from epidemiology as well as immigrant studies [1, 3] have shown us that exogenous factors obviously play the decisive role, even though they are unknown to a large extent.

Chemical carcinogens can be divided into at least two groups regarding their mechanism of action: *locally* acting carcinogens which induce a tumor at the site of application and *systemic* carcinogens which lead to tumors in certain organs after absorption, e.g., via the bloodstream, i.e., they have a certain specific organotropism of action. In the case of gastric carcinomas, it has to be considered that this type of tumor may be induced predominantly by locally acting carcinogens which reach the stomach, for instance, by the diet.

Benzopyrene

If one regards the chemical carcinogens known up to now, it should be taken into consideration that carcinogenic hydrocarbons of the type of 3,4-benzopyrene possibly play a role for carcinogenesis in the human stomach. In favor of this assumption are epidemiologic studies indicating that the incidence of gastric cancer is high within populations who eat great amounts of smoked food. These studies, however, are not uniform. Animal experiments in rats fed with excessive amounts of smoked food in order to induce cancer were not positive [10]. However, the possibility should be considered and appropriate preventive measures should be taken (e.g., by fixing a maximum limit for 3,4-benzopyrene in smoked food). The *Deutsche Forschungsgemeinschaft* (German Research Council) has already started some efforts in this direction.

Nitrostilbene

One of the well-known chemical carcinogens which induce a high yield of gastric cancer in animal experiments is 4-nitrostilbene which was already described as carcinogenic in rats after oral application in 1955 [2]. It is assumed that this compound is transformed in the stomach into the respective amine. Therefore, it can be assumed that in principle, aromatic amines may be regarded as potential carcinogens for the stomach, even though in human pathology they have been known and described only as carcinogens of the bladder (e. g., β-naphthylamine, benzidine) (ref. in [8]).

N-Nitrosocompounds

Very important for carcinogenesis are results proving that *N*-nitrosocompounds can induce cancer in a great number of animal species (ref. in [9]). Therefore, it is highly probable that these compounds can also act carcinogenic in man. Extensive studies carried out by a number of working groups have shown that many N-nitrosocompounds can lead to gastric cancer in various animal species (e.g., *N*-methyl-*N'*-nitro-Nitrosoguanidine [12] or acetoxymethyl-methylnitrosamine (AMMN) [14]). Whereas the former compound induces predominantly carcinomas of the glandular stomach in different animal species, the latter substance causes nearly a 100% yield of carcinomas of the forestomach after a very short induction time.

Studies with AMMN carried out in our institute by K. Reusch with rats [5] have shown a complete waste of the epithelium with ulcerations and bleedings after application of AMMN by gavage; these studies were in acordance with Japanese studies in dogs [6] regarding the histogenesis and the cytokinetics of the tumors.

The regeneration of the epithelium in the first week is followed by a lymphocytic infiltration with vascularization, extension of the epithelium, and increase of the proliferating area which may lead to hyperkeratosis. From a cytogenetic point of view, a complete loss of DNA-synthesizing cells is observed, which lasts approximately 24 hours. This is followed by a reparation of the proliferating layer until about 1 week after treatment, and then by an increase of the proliferating cells. From the 2nd to the 5th week, the multilayered proliferating cells increase. Apparently, the DNA-synthesis is accelerated at that time. Principally, similar changes can be observed in the glandular stomach; however, they do not develop cancer in this model. Furthermore, a circumscribed damaging of the mucosa with a decrease of the height of the mucosa, ulcerations as well as mucous and submucous bleedings are observed. Here, too, the ulcus heals up within 1 week and the same changes as in the forestomach can be observed. Finally, there is a circumscribed hyperplasia (from the 6th week on) which rarely changes into an adenoma. On a cellular level, a loss of divisable cells is observed, i.e., an inhibition of the DNA-synthesis up to 10 hours after application. A regeneration phase lasts up to 24 hours after application, and from the 2nd to the 8th week undifferentiated cells are observed which may reach up to the top of the crypts (Table 1).

Table 1. Reactions of the rat stomach after application of carcinogen (AMMN, 70 mg/kg perorally)

	Forestomach (Keratinizing squamous epithelioma)		Glandular stomach (mucosa)	
	Changes		Changes	
Reactions	Histological	Cell-kinetic	Histological	Cell-kinetic
Damage	Waste of epithelium	Loss of divisable cells Inhibition of DNA-synthesis up to 24 h	Ulcerations Bleedings	Loss of proliferating cells Inhibition of DNA-synthesis up to 24 h
Regeneration in the 1st week	Reparation of epithelium, lymphocyte infiltration, formation of connective tissue, vascularization	Regeneration of the proliferating compartment (1st week)	Formation of mucosa lymphocyte infiltration, formation of connective tissue vascularization	Regeneration of the proliferating compartment within 24 h
Hyperplasia starting in the 2nd week	Swelling of epithelium, increase of proliferating growth, hyperkeratosis	Increase of proliferating cells (2–3 layers), accelerated DNA-synthesis	Undifferentiated cells up to the top of the crypts, intramucous lymphocyte infiltration	Proliferating cells up to the tops of the crypts
Starting in the 6th week	Profilerations of the epithelium, cell atypia, papillomas (8/9)	Increase of proliferating cells (multilayered) normalization of DNA-synthesis	Circumscribed hyperplasia, adenoma (1/9)	Normalization of proliferation activity

Starting out from the well-known fact that human cancer never develops in a healthy mucosa, but shows more or less characteristic preliminary stages, it could be discussed whether there is a similar procedure in the human stomach as observed in animals, e.g., as a consequence of contact with carcinogenic substances. In this context, *N*-nitrosocompounds seem to be of special importance [9]. Human beings do not only contact these substances by exogenous access, e.g., via food; the stomach acts as a "synthetic laboratory" for the endogenous formation of these substances whenever amines meet nitrites in the acid environment of the stomach. Therefore, *N*-nitrosocompounds can be formed in the stomach "in statu nascendi" and act on the mucosa of the stomach. So far, the concentrations obtained can only be estimated. In all probability, they are relatively low. Based on a lifetime of 60 years, however, the amount of these substances that are not only taken in but also formed endogenously in the stomach should not be underestimated.

Conclusion

In the previous chapters, I deliberately put some provocative theses up for discussion. Up to now, there is no proof for the allegation that the food is "carcinogenic" for the stomach, and there is also no scientific proof for the assumption that the diet per se has to be regarded as a carcinogenic factor. It is rather probable that carcinogens in the diet or their precursors might play a role for the cancerization of the stomach. Experimental studies which are designed to elucidate this problem have only just been started in a series of laboratories and will be evaluated later. It is, however, highly probable that the gastric carcinoma is a tumor that is caused by exogenous influences and provoked mainly by locally acting carcinogens.

Accordingly, famous specialists in gastric surgery claim that progress in the problem of gastric cancer can only be made by the prevention of this disease and by elimination of the carcinogens causing this type of tumor [4].

References

1. Dunn, J. E.: Cancer epidemiology in populations of the United States with emphasis on Hawaii and California and Japan. Cancer Res. *35*, 3240–3245 (1975)
2. Druckrey, H., Schmähl, D., Mecke, R.: Erzeugung von Magenkrebs an Ratten durch 4-Nitrostilben. Naturwissenschaften *42*, 215–216 (1955)
3. Haenszel, W., Kurikara, M.: Studies of Japanese migrants. J. Natl. Cancer Inst. *51*, 1765–1779 (1973)
4. Longmire, N. P., jr.: Gewandelte Aspekte des Magenkarzinoms. Münch. Med. Wochenschr. *119*, 613–616 (1977)
5. Reusch, K., Frank, N., Wiessler, M.: Morphological and autoradiographical investigations on carcinogenesis with acetoxymethyl-methylnitrosamine (AMMN) in the stomach of rats. Z. Krebsforsch. in press
6. Saito, T., Sasaki, O., Tamada, R., Iwamatsu, M., Matsukuchi, T., Inokuchi, K.: Follow-up studies of experimental stomach cancer in dogs. Proc. 7th Int. Symp. of Princess Takamatsu Cancer Res. Fund, Tokyo 1977
7. Schmähl, D.: Entstehung, Wachstum und Chemotherapie maligner Tumoren. Aulendorf: Editio Cantor 1970
8. Schmähl, D.: Nitrosamines and gastric cancer, Editorial. Acta Hepatogastroenterol. (Stuttg.) *25*, 333–335 (1978)
9. Schmähl, D., Habs, M.: Carcinogenesis of N-nitrosodiethylamine (DENA) in different animal species – New results in chickens and domestic rats. Int. J. Cancer in press
10. Schmähl, D., Reiter, A.: Prüfung von Räuchereiprodukten auf krebserzeugende Wirkung. Z. Krebsforsch. *59*, 397–401 (1953)
11. Sugimura, T., Kawadi, T.: Experimental stomach carcinogenesis. Natl. Cancer Res. Inst. Tokyo: Plen. Publ. 1978
12. Sugimura, T., Fujimura, S. T., Kosuge, T., Baba, T., Saito, T., Nagao, M., Hosoi, H., Simosato, Y., Yokoshima, T.: Production of adenocarcinomas in glandular stomach of experimental animals by N-methyl-N-nitro-N-nitrosoguanidine. Gan. *8*, 157–196 (1969)
13. Waterhouse, J., Muir, C., Correa, P. Powell, J.: Cancer incidence in five continents. IARC Sci. Publ. *15*, (1976)
14. Wiessler, M., Schmähl, D.: Zur carcinogenen Wirkung von N-Nitroso-Verbindungen. 5. Mittlg. Acetoxymethylmethylnitrosamin. Z. Krebsforsch. *85*, 47–49 (1976)

Summary: Epidemiology and Pathogenesis of Gastric Cancer

Although the exact cause of gastric cancer in humans is still unknown, a number of risk-associated factors has been determined in the environment and in the diet. Gastric cancer is certainly based on a multifactorial pathogenesis. Bedding this in catchword phrases, we can say that gastric cancer develops through the simultaneous presence of initiating factors in predisposed individuals under conditions favoring its growth. The epidemiological studies warrant the conclusion that environmental factors are of decisive import. Apart from the socioeconomic details, contact with chemical carcinogens and cocarcinogens plays a determining part. The type of food conservation (smoking or pickling), composition of drinking water (concentration of nitrates and trace elements) are of the utmost importance in the pathogenesis of gastric cancer. Preexisting alterations of the gastric mucosa promote exogenous carcinogenesis, whereby the carcinogens themselves can damage the gastric mucosa. The probability of succumbing to gastric cancer becomes the greater, the longer and the more intense the contact with various exogenous carcinogens and cocarcinogens has been during a period of increased susceptibility and vulnerability. The prominent epidemiological feature of stomach cancer is the overriding influence of exposures during the first decades of life, which apparently determines the succeeding course of events. It remains to be considered, that a part of the patients potentially endangered by gastric cancer does not "experience" the carcinoma due to other causes of death.

In contrast to this mostly epidemic type of gastric cancer, which is often preceded by a lengthy process of gastric mucosal atrophy, there is the endemic type of gastric cancer, whose occurrence is largely independent of exogenous factors. The predisposition for this type is linked to heredity. This form of gastric cancer cannot be significantly influenced even by possible protective procedures and preventive abstention from the environmental factors initially described.

2 Experimental Gastric Cancer

Experimental Gastric Cancer: Pathogenesis and Clinico-Histopathologic Correlation

Takao Saito, Osamu Sasaki, Tadakuni Matsukuchi, Masayoshi Iwamatsu, and Kiyoshi Inokuchi

Introduction

Studies of experimental gastric cancer have markedly progressed over the last 10 years. Sugimura and Fujimura [10] first produced gastric cancer in rats by treatment of *N*-methyl-*N*′-nitro-*N*-nitrosoguanidine (MNNG). Subsequently, similar gastric cancers were produced in hamsters [2] and dogs [12] by MNNG. *N*-ethyl-*N*′-nitro-*N*-nitrosoguanidine (ENNG), the homologue of MNNG, was also found to be effective in producing gastric cancer in the same species [11, 3]. Experimental gastric cancer of dogs showed histologic features quite similar to those of human gastric cancer, metastasized to regional lymph nodes or other organs and was transplantable to nude mice [13].

The morphological changes in the stomach during carcinogenesis were sequentially investigated in rats [7] and hamsters [2] to elucidate precursors of gastric carcinoma. Dogs were more suitable for this study because prolonged observation by repeated endoscopy and biopsy were possible in the same animal.

We have performed long-term sequential studies of MNNG- and ENNG-induced carcinogenesis in the stomach of dogs by endoscopy and biopsy [8]. In the present paper, we wish to focus attention on correlation between experimental gastric cancer and its preceding lesions from a clinico-histopathologic viewpoint.

Gastric Cancer and its Preceding Lesions in the Stomach of Dogs

Material and Methods

MNNG and ENNG were administered to 23 male beagle dogs, 7 – 9 months of age. Fifteen dogs received MNNG at the concentration of 50 – 83 μl/ml with or without 4 mg/ml Tween 60 in drinking water for 35 – 63 weeks. Eight dogs received ENNG at the concentration of 150 μg/ml with or without Tween 60, either in a dog food mixture or in drinking water, for 52 weeks. The stomach of all dogs were endoscopically examined and biopsied every 5 – 10 weeks. The longest period of sequential studies was 216 weeks. Three of the ENNG-treated dogs are still under observation. The remaining 20 dogs were necropsied and 18 stomachs were histologically examined by making multiple step-sections of the entire stomach. The histologic studies have not been completed in two stomachs.

Initial Changes

Cancer was produced in the angulus and/or the fundus of the stomach by both MNNG and ENNG. Additional cancer was produced in the antrum by ENNG (Fig. 1). Before the development of gastric cancer, several lesions had been serially observed at these predilection sites in the stomach, which are summarized in Fig. 2.

Following the initiation of the carcinogen administration, superficial erosive changes first appeared diffusely in the wide regions of the stomach mucosa, including the predilection sites of cancer in all cases (Fig. 3). This lesion was endoscopically seen als hyperemia or discoloration of the mucosa with multiple punctuate hemorrhages. Histologically, it showed destruction of foveolar epithelium and prominent proliferation of immature regenerative epithelium at the superficial or deep levels of the mucosa. The pyloric or fundic glands were absent or reduced in number in the deeper layers of the mucosa with infiltration of small round cells. Then, multiple localized erosions appeared at the center of the superficial erosive changes in the angulus and fundus. These changes were not commonly observed in the antrum. The erosion gradually progressed to become ulceration in the angulus in most of MNNG- and ENNG-treated dogs and in the fundus in most of ENNG-treated dogs. The ulcer did not develop in the fundus in most cases of ENNG-treated dogs. Atypical glands were usually found in immature regenerative epithelium of ulcer and erosion.

After the carcinogenic agents were discontinued, the ulcer rapidly healed and changed into an ulcer scar. The healing of both erosion and superficial erosive

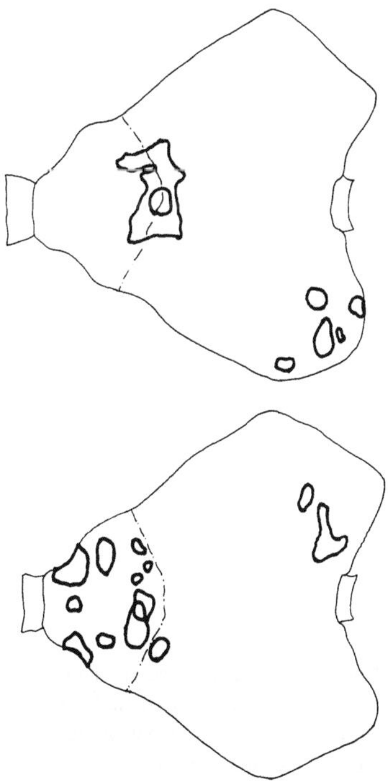

Fig. 1. Predilection sites of experimental gastric cancer in dogs produced by MNNG (*top*) and ENNG (*bottom*)

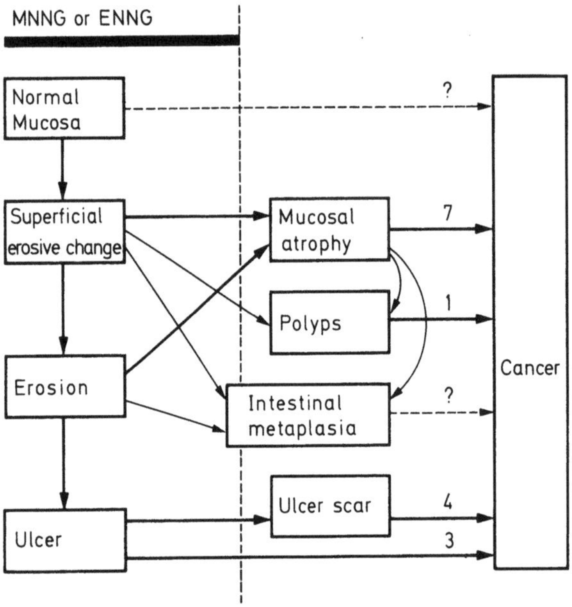

Fig. 2. Correlation between initial lesions and cancer in the stomach of dogs induced by MNNG and ENNG

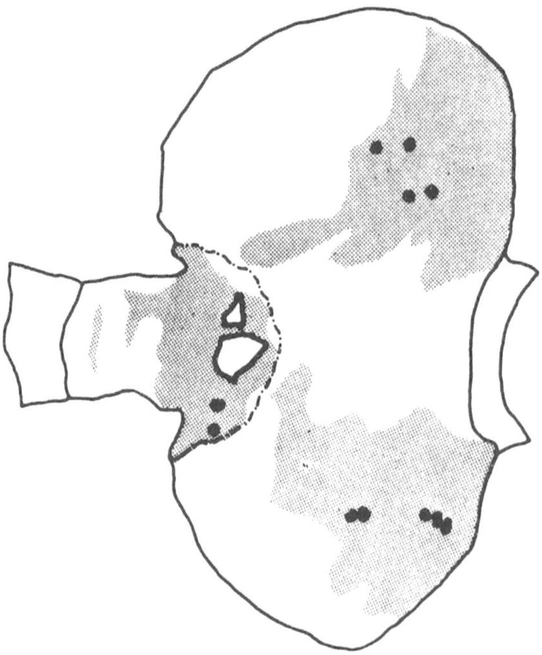

Fig. 3. The sites of superficial erosive change (screened areas), erosion, and ulcer (panelled areas) in the stomach of a dog (No. 11, the 44th experimental week), which died during MNNG administration

change left atrophic mucosa by reparative regeneration. Hyperplasia of foveolar epithelium was common in mature regenerative epithelium of those two healed lesions. The development of one or more polyps in the atrophic mucosa of the antrum and fundus were observed in several animals after the cessation of carcinogen administration. Histologic examination of specimens obtained by biopsy or necropsy showed that they were benign hyperplastic polyps. Intestinal metaplastic glands were observed only in a small number of cases as scattered islands either in mature regenerative epithelium of superficial erosive change and erosion during carcinogen administrations or of atrophic mucosa after the termination of carcinogens.

Preceding Lesions of Cancer

Combined endoscopy and biopsy studies clearly showed the preceding lesions from which at least 15 cancers developed. Seven of these 15 cancers were diagnosed by specimens obtained by both biopsy and necropsy. The diagnosis of the remaining ones was made by biopsy alone since the dogs bearing these cancers are still under observation or necropsy examinations are still incomplete. Figure 2 shows the relation between cancer and its preceding lesions. Four cancers arose from a healed ulcer (Figs. 4, 5, and 6), while three cancers developed directly from an active ulcer (Figs. 7 and 8). The average duration from the onset of the experiment to the diagnosis of cancer by biopsy was 106 weeks in the former and 76 weeks in the latter. Since the latter cancers developed soon after the cessation of carcinogen administration (24 weeks average), it seemed that the ulcers did not have time to heal. Seven cancers originating from active or healed ulcers were located in the angulus.

Another seven cancers arose from atrophic mucosa which was the end result of erosion or superficial erosive change. Two of them were located in the angulus, while four and one were present in the fundus and the antrum, respectively. Average period required for the diagnosis of those seven cancers originating from mucosal atrophy was 109 weeks. The remaining one cancer originated from polyp (Figs. 9 and 10). This polyp appeared at the superficial erosive changes in the antrum in the 58th week and showed macroscopic characteristics of a benign polyp. Repeated biopsy of the lesion had consistently shown hyperplasia of foveolar epithelium until the 145th week, when adenocarcinoma was found in the biopsy specimens. Then, the tumor suddenly started to grow rapidly. The development of cancer from intestinalized mucosa and normal mucosa was not recognized by endoscopy and biopsy.

The location of cancers and associated lesions in necropsied stomachs were extensively investigated. All cancers were present in either atrophic mucosa or ulcer scar, but not in intestinalized mucosa or normal mucosa.

Changes from Early Cancer to Advanced Cancer

The 15 cancers described above were, or have been, endoscopically followed up to 120 weeks. All but one cancer grew to a larger mass. One case showed spontaneous early regression. Growth of the experimental cancers from the early

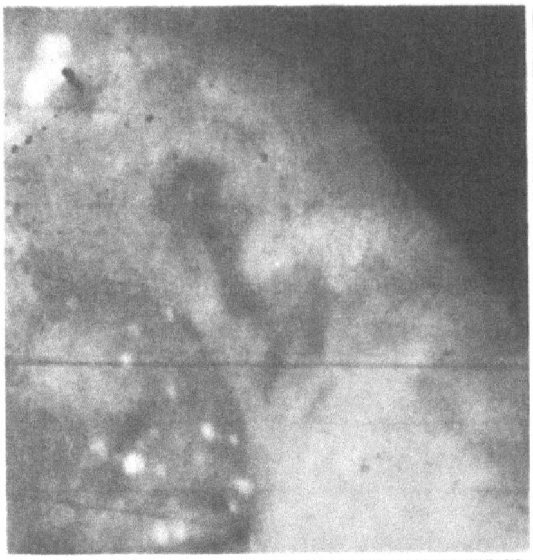

Fig. 4

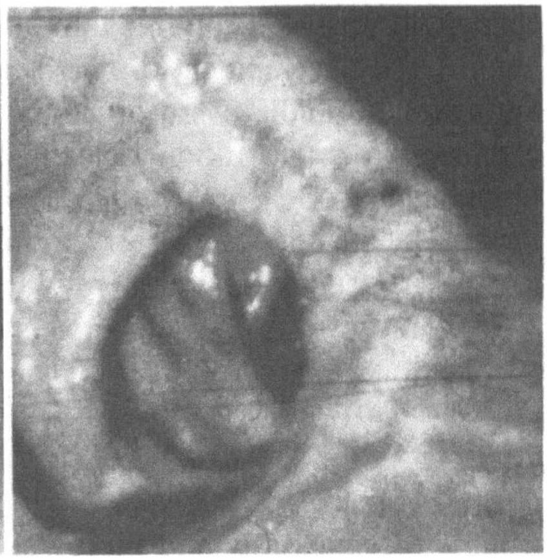

Fig. 5

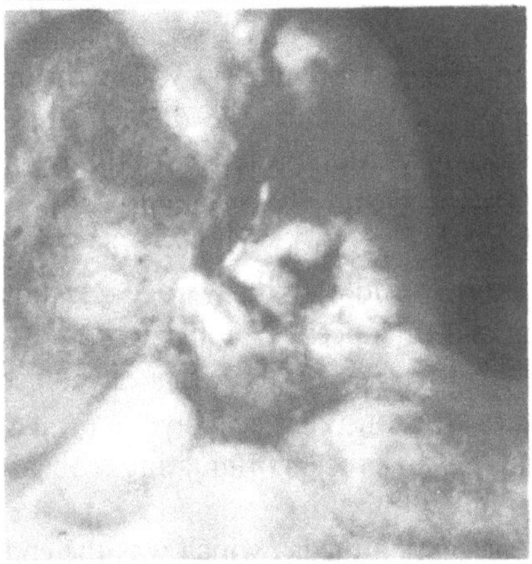

Fig. 6

Fig. 4. Active ulcer at the angulus in the stomach of a dog (No. 3) at the 44th week
Fig. 5. Ulcer scar at the 64th week which resulted from the active ulcer shown in Fig. 4
Fig. 6. Cancer at the 102nd week which developed from the ulcer scar shown in Fig. 5

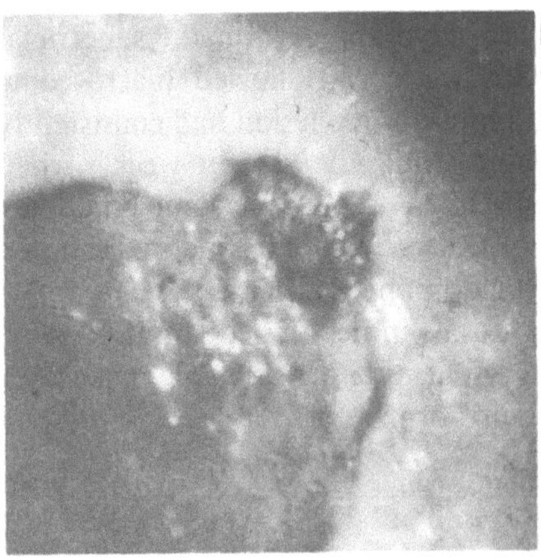

Fig. 7

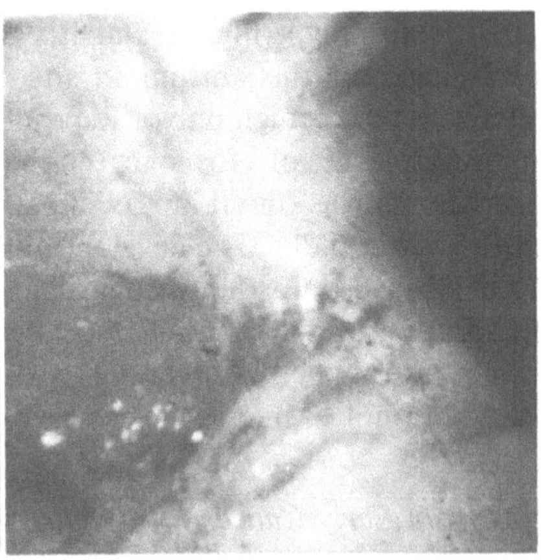

Fig. 8

Fig. 7. Active ulcer at the angulus in the stomach of a dog (No. 25) at the 25th week
Fig. 8. Cancer at the 59th week which developed from the active ulcer shown in Fig. 7

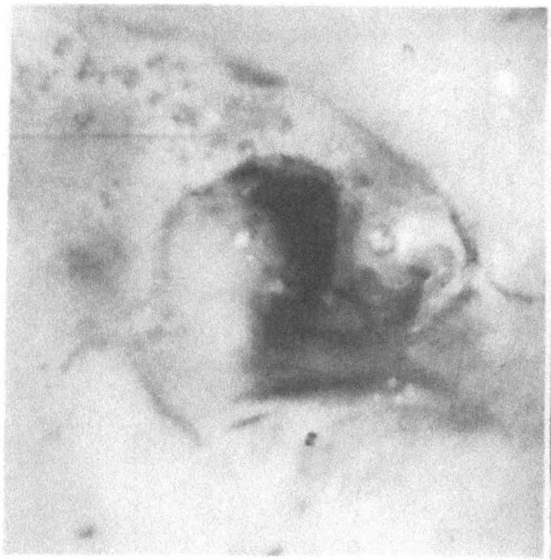

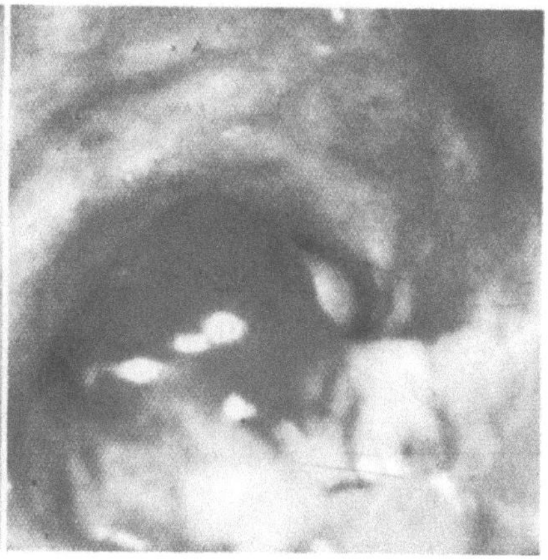

Fig. 9 Fig. 10

Fig. 9. Polyp at the antrum in the stomach of a dog (No. 21) at the 78th week
Fig. 10. Cancer at the 176th week which developed in the polyp shown in Fig. 9

stage to the advance stage was analyzed based on macroscopic characteristics observed by endoscopy examination. Figure 11 summarizes the patterns of growth from early cancer to advanced cancer in the 15 cases. Macroscopic classification of early cancer was based on the criteria established by the Japanese Gastroenterological Endoscopy Society. Advanced cancer was classified according to Borrmann's definition.

The initial gross changes of early cancer which had been found by endoscopy and biopsy included the following three types; slightly elevated lesion (type IIa), slightly depressed lesion (type IIc), and depressed lesion (type III). Six of 15 cancers were type IIa, mainly locating in the fundus or the antrum, while eight and one were type IIc and type III, respectively, and present in the angulus.

Early cancer of type IIa changed to type IIa + IIc or grew to type I. We are still in the process of investigating the transformation of early cancer of type IIa + IIc and type I to advanced cancer. Early cancer of type IIc changed to type IIc + IIa by elevation of the margin of the lesion. The type IIc + IIa cancer, however, became ulcerated and seemingly returned to the previous type, IIc by desquamation of the elevated margin, followed by repeated transformation to IIc + IIa again. Covering of ulcerated cancerous tissues with regenerative epithelium was observed from the surrounding mucosa. This phenomenon, called "malignant cycle" [6] in human gastric cancer, was found in two cases in which the cancer of type IIc + IIa, ultimately grew to advanced cancer of Borrmann's type 2. One of two of Borrmann's type 2 cancers further grew and changed to Borrmann's type 3. This case died in the 216th week, when metastasis of gastric cancer to paracoeliac lymph nodes was found. Early cancer of type III developed at the active ulcer of the angulus and grew to Borrmann's type 2 cancer. Early cancer of type IIb and advanced cancer of Borrmann's type 1 and 4 have not been observed.

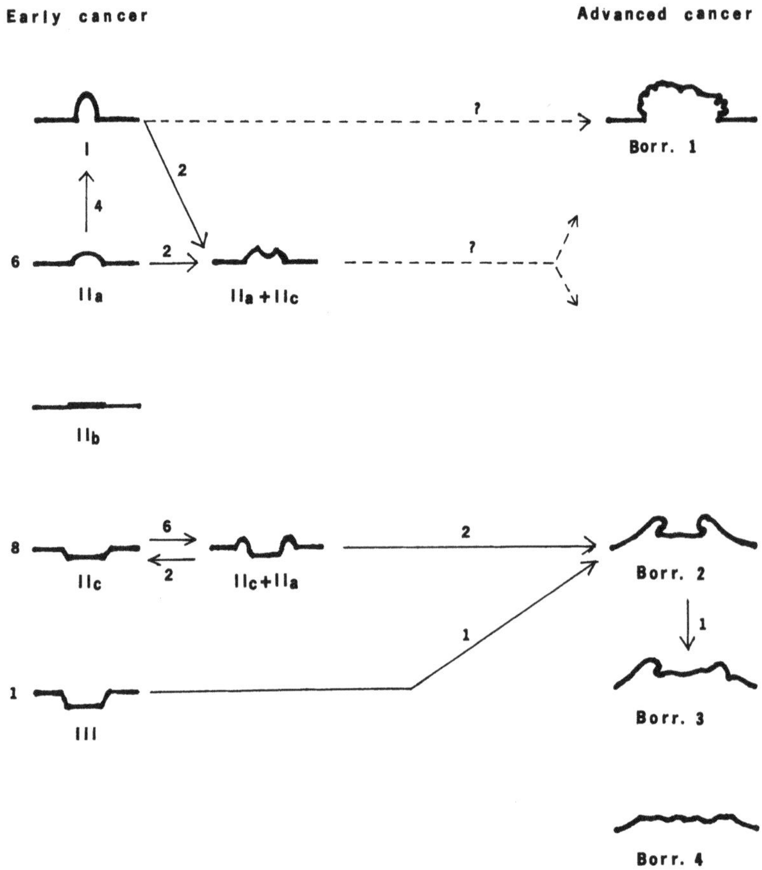

Fig. 11. The scheme on the changes from early cancer to advanced cancer which were observed endoscopically in the stomach of dogs

Susceptibility of Experimental Chronic Gastric Ulcer in Rats to MNNG

Superficial erosive change, erosion, and ulcer as main initial changes were produced at the predilection areas of cancer in the stomach of dogs by the administration of MNNG or ENNG. Erosion was also observed as an initial lesion in the antrum, the predilection site of cancer, of rats [7] and hamsters [2]. On the contrary, erosion was scarcely found in the stomach of mice and guinea pigs (unpublished data), which are resistant to production of gastric cancer by MNNG [11]. Therefore, it appears that superficial erosive change and erosion are initial changes required in gastric carcinogenesis induced by MNNG and ENNG.

Since superficial erosive change and erosion were observed only within the period of continuous administration of carcinogenic agents, the mucosa with repeated or continuous regeneration, as in erosions, appears to be more susceptible to carcinogens than the normal mucosa. In order to test this hypothesis, we attempted to find out whether or not experimental chronic ulcer as a source of regeneration is more susceptible to MNNG.

Using rats, five different techniques to produce chronic gastric ulcer were compared. Following extensive experiments, we have chosen the formalin-injection method as the best technique to obtain long-lasting chronic ulcer. When 0.05 ml of 100% formalin (40% formaldehyde) was injected into the anterior wall of the glandular stomach of male Wistar rats, active ulcer extending deep to the serosa was usually produced in all cases. Open ulcer which is histologically not covered with regenerative epithelium, was found in 10 of 10 cases 4 weeks after the injection and in 8 of 12 cases 54 weeks after.

Male Wistar rats (average body weight 140 g) were injected with 100% formalin into the anterior wall of the corpus of the glandular stomach, where induction of cancer by MNNG is known to be negligible. Four weeks after formalin injection, the rats received MNNG solution at the concentration of 83 µg/ml for 30 weeks and then tap water for 20 weeks before sacrifice. Chronic ulcer was macroscopically and histologically found in the anterior wall of the corpus of the stomach in 128 cases, 49 of which had open ulcer and 44 of which had ulcer extended to the serosa. Cancer, coexisting with experimental chronic ulcer, was found in two cases. The ulcer of those two cases extended to the serosa and the surface of the ulcer was covered by a single layer of immature regenerative epithelium (low grade healing). Adenocarcinoma in these two rats invaded cicatric tissues of the ulcer involving all layers of gastric wall and adhered to the liver. One cancer was found in an additional rat at the region of the corpus where ulcer was not found. No cancer was found in the corpus of the 20 control rats without formalin injection. Unexpectedly, incidence of cancer was very low in the antrum of the formalin-injected group.

The result of this experiment strongly suggested that the experimentally induced gastric ulcer is more susceptible to MNNG than normal mucosa.

Conclusion

The following similarities between experimental gastric cancer and human gastric cancer were found in the present studies:

1) Gastric cancer in humans is found in some pathological mucosa, such as mucosal atrophy, intestinalization, mucosal hyperplasia, ulcer (ulcer scar), and polyps [5]. It is supposed that those associated lesions may be precursors of gastric cancer [9, 1]. The studies of experimental gastric cancer of dogs showed that all cancers observed did not develop from the normal mucosa, but from the abnormal mucosa with mucosal atrophy, ulcer, ulcer scar, or polyps. The preceding lesions of cancer in dogs coincide with four of the six associated lesions of cancer in humans. Close similarity is seen between the associated lesions of cancer in humans and the preceding lesions of cancer in dogs. Experimental studies suggest that gastric cancer may develop from the associated lesions in humans.

2) Gross types of experimental gastric cancer were able to be classified according to the criteria used in human gastric cancer. The types of I, IIa, IIa + IIc, IIc, IIc + IIa and III were found in early cancer, while Borrmann's type 2 and 3 were observed in advanced cancer in dogs. Several types of growth patterns

from early cancer to advanced cancer were demonstrated in gastric cancer of dogs. The findings obtained in dogs do not contradict clinical findings in humans which have been found occasionally. Information collected from this kind of study would be useful in understanding human gastric cancer, especially the characteristics of early cancer.

3) The malignant cycle is found in early gastric cancer in humans. Our studies showed that the malignant cycle occurs in early gastric cancer of slightly depressed type in dogs.

4) It has been argued that chronic gastric cancer may transfrom to cancer in humans. Our studies strongly suggest that the experimentally-induced gastric chronic ulcer in rats is more susceptible to MNNG than the normal mucosa.

On the other hand, dissimilarities were found as follows:

1) The development of cancer was not observed from intestinalization and hyperplastic mucosa in our experiment. Focal scattered islands of intestinal metaplastic glands were found in some dogs. However, we were unable to show the development of cancer from metaplastic glands. There is a possibility that cancer may develop from intestinalization [4] or mucosal hyperplasia by the modification of carcinogen administration schedule.

2) Early cancer of type IIb and advanced cancer of Borrmann's type 1 and 4 were not observed in experimental gastric cancer of dogs. There is also a possibility that further studies may show those types.

References

1. Correa, P., Cuello, C., Duque, E., Burbano, L. C., Garcia, F. T., Bolanos, O., Brown, C., Haenszel, W.: Gastric cancer in Columbia. III. Natural History of precursor lesions. J. Natl. Cancer Inst. *57*, 1027–1035 (1976)
2. Kogure, K., Sasadaira, H., Kawachi, T., Shimosato, Y., Tokunaga, A., Fujimura, S., Sugimura, T.: Further studies on induction of stomach cancer in hamsters by N-methyl-N'-nitro-N-nitrosoguanidine. Br. J. Cancer *29*, 132–142 (1974)
3. Kurihara, M., Sirakabe, H., Murakami, T., Yasui, A., Izumi, T., Sumida, M., Igarashi, A.: A new method for producing adenocarcinomas in the stomach of dogs with N-ethyl-N'-nitro-N-nitrosoguanidine. Gan. *65*, 163–177 (1974)
4. Matsukura, N., Kawachi, T., Sasajima, K., Sano, T., Sugimura, T., Hirota, T.: Induction of intestinal metaplasia in the stomachs of rats by N-methyl-N'-nitro-N-nitrosoguanidine. J. Natl. Cancer Inst. *61*, 141–144 (1978)
5. Ming, S.: Tumor of the esophagus and stomach. Atlas Tumor Pathol. *7*, 115–213 (1973)
6. Sakita, T., Oguro, Y.: Endoscopic diagnosis of early gastric cancer. In: Gastrointestinal panendoscopy. Berry, L. H. (ed.), pp. 278–294. Illinois: Thomas 1974
7. Saito, T., Inokuchi, K., Takayama, S., Sugimura, T.: Sequential morphological changes in N-methyl-N'-nitro-N-nitrosoguanidine carcinogenesis in the glandular stomach of rats. J. Natl. Cancer Inst. *44*, 769–783 (1970)
8. Saito, T., Sasaki, O., Tamada, R., Iwamatsu, M., Inokuchi, K.: Sequential studies of development of gastric carcinoma in dogs induced by N-methyl-N'-nitro-N-nitrosoguanidine. Cancer *42*, 1246–1254 (1978)
9. Siurala, M., Seppälä, K.: Atrophic gastritis as a possible precursor of gastric carcinoma and pernicious anemia. Acta Med. Scand. *166*, 455–474 (1959)
10. Sugimura, T., Fujimura, S.: Tumor production in glandular stomach of rats by N-methyl-N'-nitro-N-nitrosoguanidine. Nature *216*, 943–944 (1967)
11. Sugimura, T., Kawachi, T.: Experimental stomach cancer. Methods Cancer Res. *7*, 245–308 (1973)

12. Sugimura, T., Tanaka, N., Kawachi, T., Kogure, K., Fujimura, S., Shimosato, Y.: Production of stomach cancer in dogs by N-methyl-N′-nitro-N-nitrosoguanidine. Gan. *62,* 67 – 68 (1971)
13. Taguchi, T., Fujita, M., Usugane, M.: Heterotransplantation of a canine gastric cancer induced by N-methyl-N′-nitro-N-nitrosoguanidine into nude mice. Biken J. *18*, 175 – 177 (1975)

Epithelium at the Gastroenteral Borderline – Comparison of Animal Experiments and Clinical-Pathological Investigations

H. Meister and P. Schlag

Introduction

For some time now, clinical and autopsy findings have indicated an increased incidence of gastric cancer after resective ulcer therapy [3, 5, 11, 13, 15, 16]. The risk of primary cancer development in a gastric stump is twice as high (8% – 10%) than for a comparable control group of patients with healthy stomachs, for whom the rate of cancer morbidity is 5% [5, 10, 13, 26, 29]. Numerous factors are under discussion regarding the pathogenesis of cancer in the operated stomach, although none can be singled out as having a clearly predisposing significance. It is therefore not yet ascertained, whether the incidence of gastric stump cancer depends on the type of the ulcer necessitating the primary operation [8, 10, 11, 24, 26, 34], nor are there any conclusive statements concerning the incidence of cancer related to the surgical procedure originally chosen [3, 5, 10, 11, 16, 23, 29, 33].

Inflammatory atrophic or metaplastic lesions of the gastric mucosa and epithelial shifts at the gastrointestinal borderline with succeeding polypoid-cystic epithelial proliferation [1, 10, 23, 26, 27, 37] are supposed to support cancerogenesis in the operated stomach. Under the influence of the carcinogen *N*-methyl-*N'*-nitro-*N*-nitrosoguanidine (MNNG), indications of cancer predisposition of the gastroenteroanastomosis in the resected stomach were obtained in animal experiments [4]. As in man, changes in the environment and inflammatory metaplastic processes at the epithelial borderline are postulated, resulting, among other things, from a reflux of bile and pancreatic secretions [4, 6, 7, 17, 32]. Some authors, on the other hand, reject the thesis of an altering influence of bile reflux on the gastric mucosa [18, 31, 38]. It was the purpose of the present investigation on animals to test by means of various surgical procedures, whether the enterogastric reflux, in combination with application of a carcinogen (MNNG), has any influence on proliferative changes of the epithelium at the gastrointestinal borderline in the nonresected rat stomach. The localization and the extent of demonstrable lesions of the gastric mucosa of patients, on whom a gastroenterostomy without stomach resection had been performed 20 – 25 years before in treatment of a benign stricture of gastric passage, were compared with those of the experimentally-induced mucosal lesions.

Material and Methods

Patients

The stomachs of ten patients with an average age of 60 years were examined, on whom a retrocolic gastroenterostomy without gastric resection had been performed

20 – 25 years before due to a benign stricture of the gastric passage. The resection samples were prepared histologically according to a standardized procedure [21], and those regions of the wall close to the anastomosis were exhaustively examined. Microscopically and histologically determined changes were recorded in diagrams.

Animal Experiments

Male SPF-Wistar rats, body weight 180 – 200 g (bred by Thomae, Biberach, West-Germany), were not fed 24 h before surgery and were placed on wide-mesh metal grids to prevent coprophagy.

Surgical Procedures

The following surgical procedures were performed under Nembutal narcosis and the following groups of animals were formed:

a) Gastrotomy
A 1 cm incision was made at the greater curvature of the stomachs of the experimental animals and again closed with 5 – 6 single sutures (Mersilene 6/0) stitched through all layers. This group of animals served as a control.

b) Antecolic Gastroenterostomy without Enteroanastomosis
The small intestine of the experimental animals was antecolically drawn upward 2 cm aboral to the ligament of Treitz and anastomosed to the stomach at the greater curvature for a length of 1 cm with 6 – 8 single sutures (Mersilene 6/0) stitched through all layers. This results in an obligatory enterogastric reflux.

c) Y-Gastroenteroanastomosis according to Roux
The small intestine of the experimental animals was severed 2 cm aboral to the ligament of Treitz. The aboral portion of the small intestine was anastomosed to the greater curvature of the stomach with 6 – 8 single sutures stitched through all layers, the oral portion of the severed intestinal loop was appended terminolaterally to the efferent small intestine 3 cm aboral to the gastroenteroanastomosis. An enterogastric reflux was prevented by interrupting the continuity of stomach and duodenum in the pyloric region and closing their lumen with single sutures.

d) Gastrotomy and Pyloroplasty
Experimental animals, on which an operation to increase the caliber of the pyloric opening had been performed in addition to gastrotomy, were to show how much alteration of the gastric mucosa is induced by altered pyloric function.

e) Truncal Vagotomy
In order to examine the consequences of altered secretory and tonic nervous stimulation on the gastric epithelium, the experimental animals were subjected to a truncal vagotomy only. To further determine whether additional surgical treat-

ment has any modifying influence in this case, equal numbers of animals from groups a – d were also vagotomized.

f) Implantation of a Small Intestinal Patch
In order to examine the influence of the immediate proximity of intestinal and gastric mucosa on changes of the epithelium regardless of anastomosis conditions, a "patch" was implanted in the stomach. To do this, a 1 cm section of the upper jejunal wall was isolated with its mesenterial vascular trunk, and opened at the side opposite to the mesenterial attachment. The patch thus formed was implanted under maintained circulation into the opened anterior wall of the stomach of the experimental animals with single sutures (Mersilene 6/0). The separated jejunal loop was anastomosed terminoterminally.

Application of Carcinogen

The experimental animals were given as much water as they wanted 12 h postoperatively, food was withheld for 48 h, whereafter the animals received a standard diet (Fuko-Futter, Fa. Fundel, Ulm, West Germany). *N*-methyl-*N*-nitro-*N*-nitrosoguanidine (MNNG) was given to half of the animals of various groups 5 weeks after surgery according to a procedure specified by Dahm et al. [4].

Morphological Examinations

All animals of the experimental group in question were sacrificed in a carbon dioxide atmosphere 35 – 36 weeks after surgery; surgical samples were prepared immediately thereafter. Safeguarding the anastomoses, the stomachs were opened at the greater curvature, spread on cork plates and fixed in 4% buffered formalin solution. Fifteen to 17 wall segments were usually excised. Step-wise sections 4 – 6 μm thick were cut from the blocks and stained with HE. In the histological evaluation, regenerative hyperplastic and proliferating mucosal alterations in the sense of adenomatous epithelial lesions were considered with reference to specifications by Saito [30] and Bralow [2] and catalogued according to their degree of severity. Carcinomas were recorded without graduation. The findings in 15 animals each for the various gastric surgeries with or without carcinogen treatment were compared in this manner.

Results

Patients

All of the stomachs examined exhibited chronic atrophic gastritis, some with intestinal metaplasia, which was localized particularly in that portion of the stomach close to the anastomosis. Various stages of epithelial dysplasias were also found here [12, 25]. Four patients had a cancer at the anastomosal site. Histologically one of them proved to be an early intestinal-type cancer. Two of them were moderately differentiated adenocancers, the fourth was a signet ring cell carcinoma.

Coinciding with the increase in inflammatory and proliferating mucosal lesions, dilated glands appeared in the tunica mucosa, infiltrating the frequently hypertrophied and frayed regions of the lamina muscularis mucosae and extending further into the tela submucosa. The epithelial coating of these cysts, which macroscopically appeared as polypoid lesions, turned out to be mucoid-differentiated cylindrical epithelium comparable to the epithelium of the foveolae gastricae and the stomach surface (Fig. 1).

Experimental Animals

The changes of the mucosa experimentally induced with MNNG in rat stomachs were also localized mostly in the stomach region close to the anastomosis or near

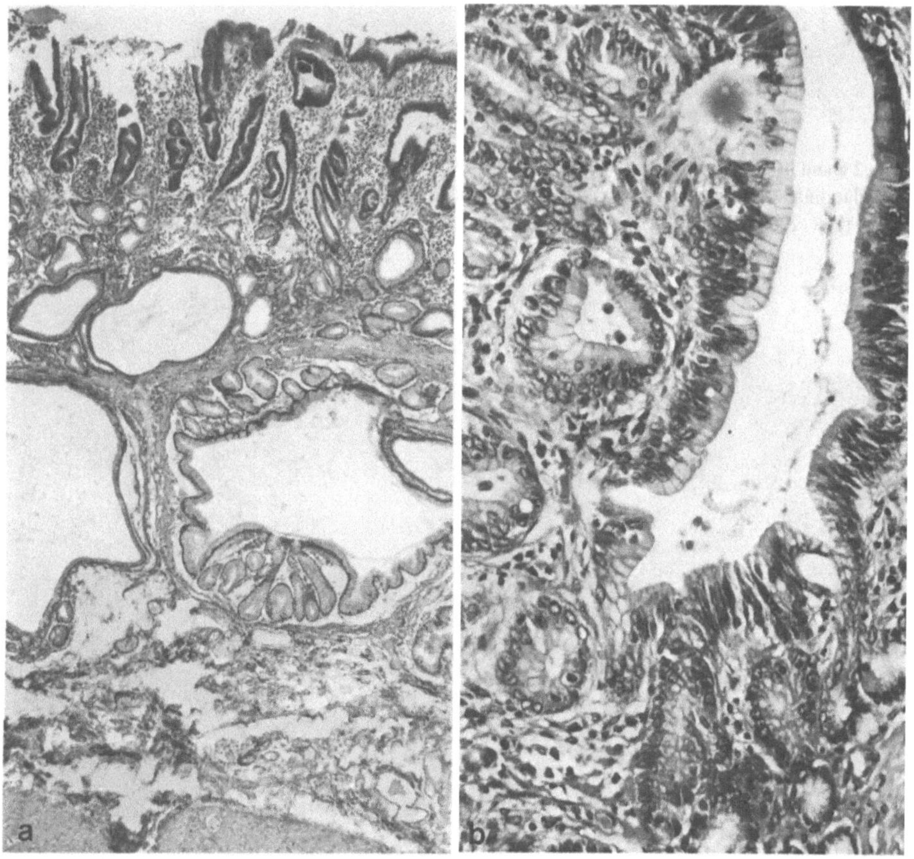

Fig. 1. a) Gastroenterostomy of a patient 23 years after the operation: numerous, cystically dilated glands in the tunica mucosa infiltrating the lamina muscularis mucosae and extending further into the tela submucosa. b) The cysts are coated with prismatic, muciparous epithelium similar to the epithelium on the gastric surface. (a × 54; b × 350; HE)

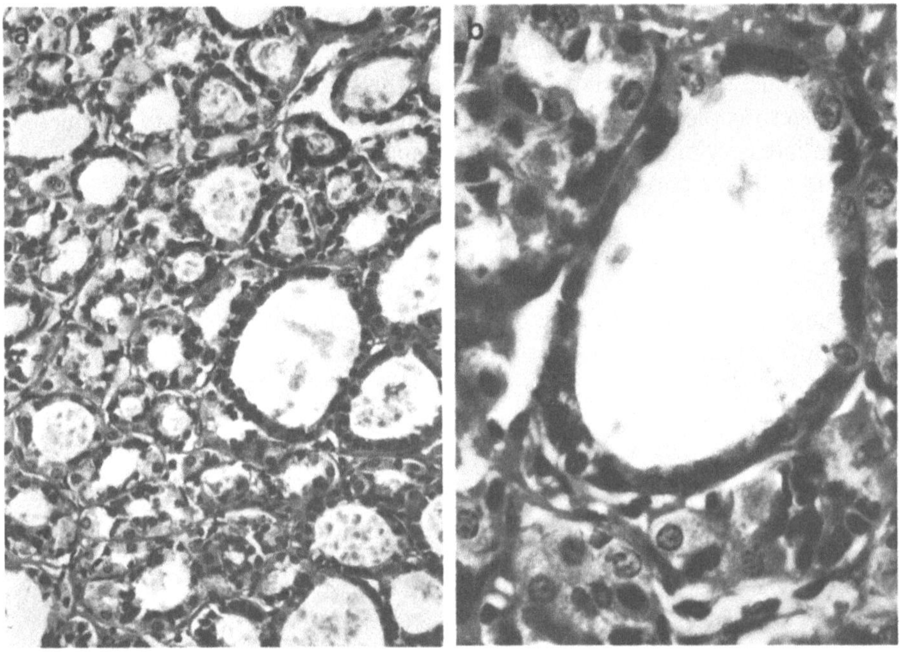

Fig. 2 a and b. Gastroenterostomy of a rat treated with MNNG; numerous distended corpus glands in the glandular portion of the stomach morphologically reminiscent of cysts of the glandular body in man. (a × 220; b × 437; HE)

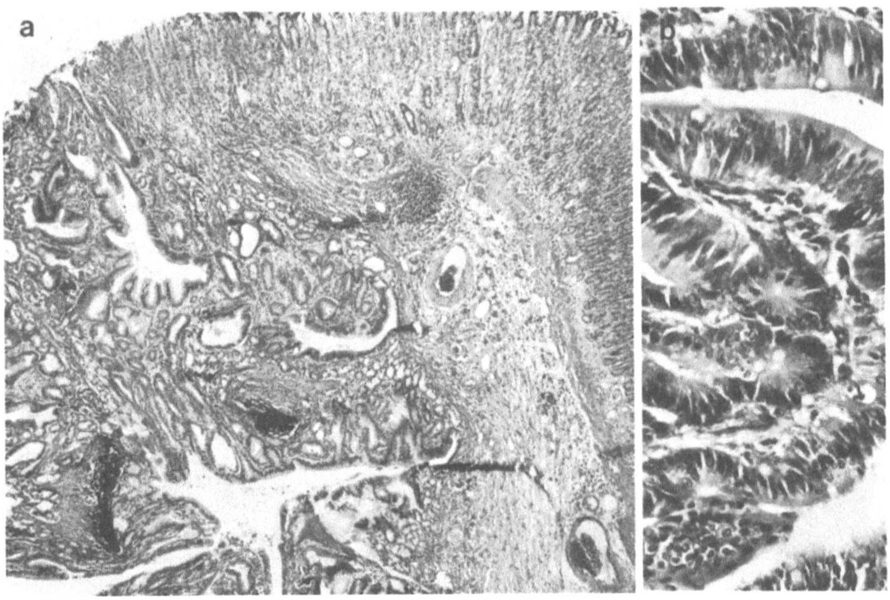

Fig. 3 a and b. Gastroenterostomy of a rat treated with MNNG: adenomatous proliferation (a) with cystically distended, in parts mucoid differentiated, in parts atypical glandular formations (b). (a × 54; b × 350; HE)

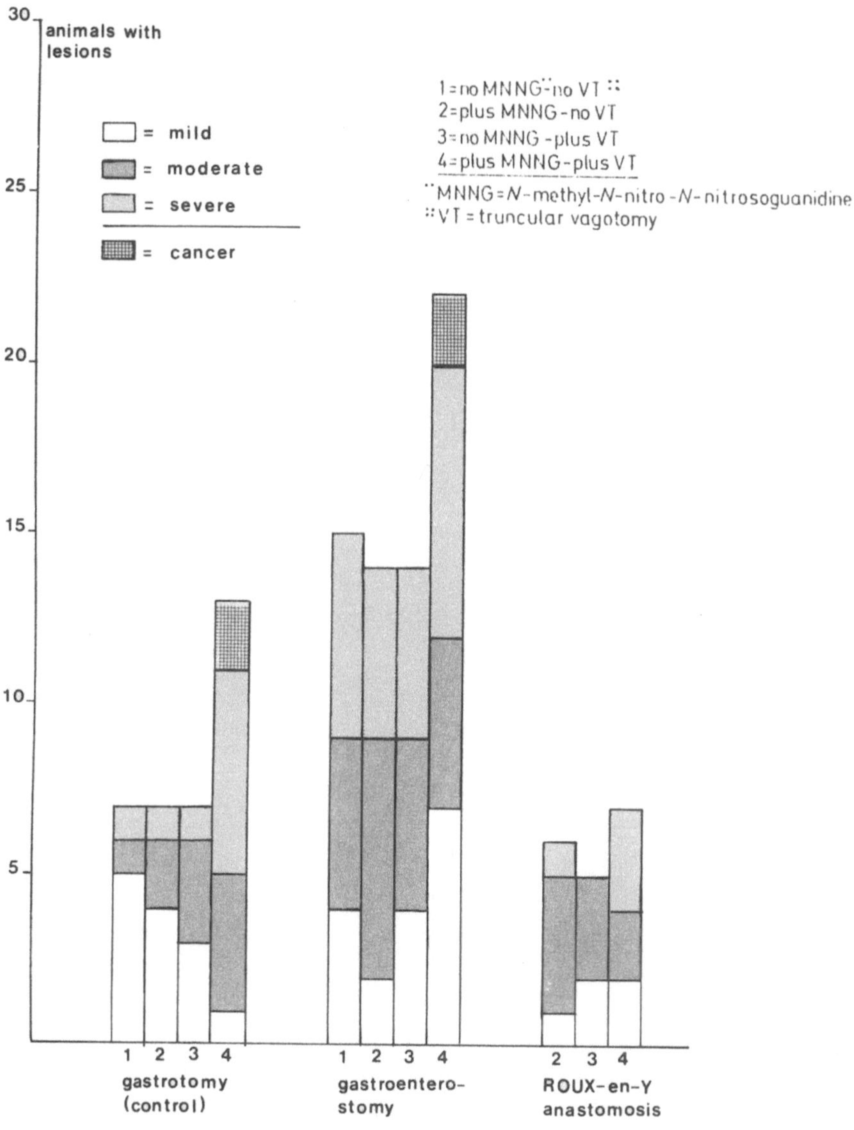

Fig. 4. Incidence of adenoma-like epithelial lesions and cancer in rats

gastrotomy or the enteral patch. Cystic glandular formations were found in the tunica mucosa, reminiscent in their structure – without any accompanying inflammatory reactions – of cysts of the glandular body [9] as they are known in man (Fig. 2).

Once inflammatory infiltration and fibrosis had occurred, the number of distended glands increased, extending beyond the lamina muscularis mucosae into the tela submucosa with increasing cystic dilatation and epithelial dedifferentiation (Fig. 3).

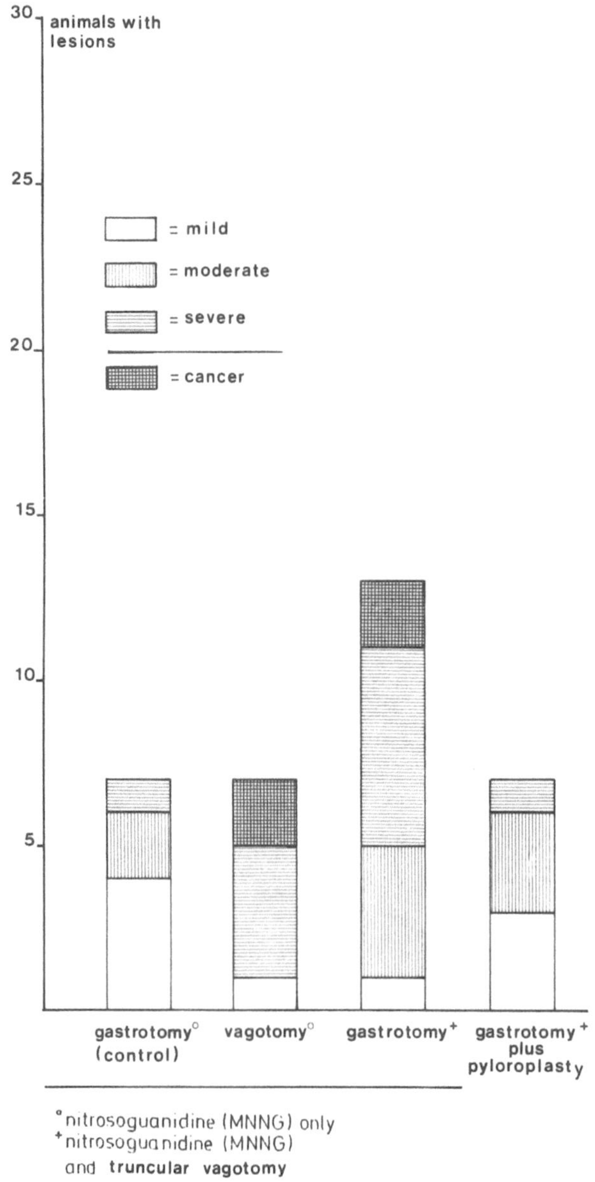

Fig. 5. Incidence of adenoma-like epithelial lesions and cancer in rats

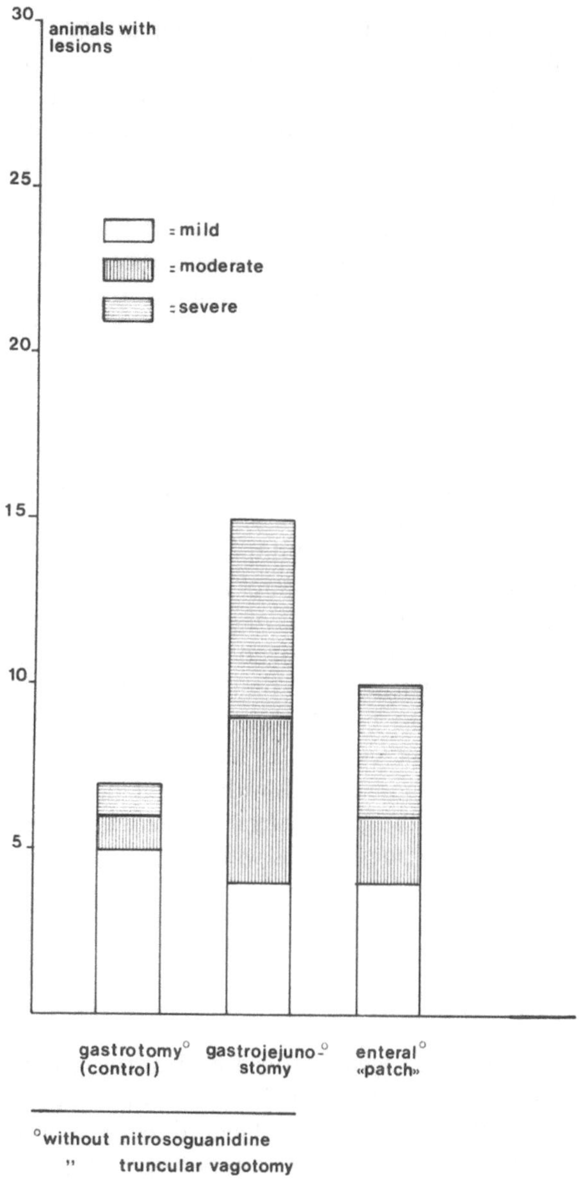

Fig. 6. Incidence of adenoma-like epithelial lesions and cancer in rats

Adenomatous epithelial proliferation had already been found in those animals exclusively gastrotomized (group a). Additional application of carcinogen (MNNG) or vagotomy in itself has only a slight augmenting influence on epithelial proliferation, which is, however, significantly increased if MNNG is combined with truncal vagotomy. Carcinomas were demonstrated in two animals of this group (Fig. 4, left column). Adenomatous proliferation was more frequent and more impressive for the group with the obligatory enterogastric reflux (group b). It was also evident here, that carcinogenic treatment only caused increased mucosal proliferation in combination with the truncal vagotomy. Two experimental animals treated in this manner had developed a carcinoma (Table 4, center column). Such severe epithelial changes could not be determined for rats after gastroenterostomy according to Roux (group c) (Fig. 4, right column).

The enhancing influence of truncal vagotomy on proliferative changes in the epithelium in combination with carcinogen treatment (MNNG) is made clear by the fact that those animals, on which only a vagotomy had been performed (group e), also developed distinct adenomatous lesions of the mucosa as well as carcinomas, unlike the control group (Fig. 5). Compared to the vagotomized and carcinogen-treated animals of group a, pyloroplasty of similarly treated animals (group d) resulted in a significant decrease of epithelial proliferation despite vagotomy, matching the results obtained for the control group exposed to carcinogen. The neighborhood of gastric and intestinal mucosa without any other treatment caused an increased cellular proliferation at the epithelial borderline in those animals with a small intestine patch. Compared with this, the epithelium of the gastroenteral borderline showed an even greater proliferative tendency after anastomosis with obligatory enterogastric reflux (Fig. 6).

Discussion

With the carcinogenic influence of nitrosoguanidine (MNNG) cancer can be induced in rats with partially resected stomachs [4]. The present investigation showed that with otherwise standardized experimental conditions, no carcinomas initially developed near the anastomosis after gastroenterostomy *without* stomach resection. The most severe mucosal lesion found was an adenomatous proliferation with considerable epithelial atypicalities in parts. There was no graduated difference of these epithelial alterations in animals exposed and not exposed to carcinogen. The cause of this may be that – compared to the results obtained for resected rat stomachs – a lesser local concentration of carcinogenic substance per area of stomach surface was active in the nonresected stomach. It is also feasible that the carcinogen was more highly activated in the alkaline environment established by the resective procedure and the concomitant reduction of HCl-producing mucosa [20]. The lack of the trophic effect of gastrin can possibly play a part after partial stomach resection, making the mucosa more vulnerable.

Although no increased cancer risk is known for vagotomized patients to date [5], experiments indicated alterations of the mucosa after vagotomy to be a disposing factor for carcinogenesis [14, 22]. The present results also show that severe adenomatous epithelial lesions and carcinomas can be induced in various groups of experimental animals by truncal vagotomy, though only in combination with nitrosoguanidine (MNNG). Altered secretory and tonic nervous effects with their consequences to the gastric epithelium must play a decisive role. The fact that significantly less epithelial proliferation occurs after pyloroplasty despite carcinogen treatment and vagotomy may be due to an accelerated passage of stomach contents and a reduced time of contact with the carcinogen. The proximity of gastric and intestinal mucosa without carcinogenic influence or vagotomy already resulted in a greater epithelial proliferation at the epithelial borderline than did the simple gastrotomy under equal experimental conditions.

The most significant result of the present investigation was that the proliferative changes described in the mucosa occur to a considerably greater extent after gastroenterostomy without enteroanastomosis independent of exposition to carcinogen or truncal vagotomy, whereas they were distinctly rarer and milder after gastroenterostomy according to Roux. This is obviously based on the fact that a chronic enterogastric reflux along the epithelium at the gastroenteral borderline is prevented by the gastroenterostomy according to Roux.

The comparison of experimentally induced mucosal changes with those in old gastroenterostomies in humans yields certain morphological parallels. The cystic-glandular and adenomatous hyperplasias frequently observed in the tela submucosa are an expression of an increased proliferation of gastric epithelium in man and experimental animal, although they should not be given the significance of malignant neoplasias on the basis of their localization alone. These epithelia could possibly be displacements caused by the surgery, which have gone on proliferating in deeper layers of the wall. Glandular proliferation similar to neoplasia below the threshhold of infiltrating tumors in man is known as gastritis cystica polyposa [19]. There is experimental [1] and clinical-pathological proof that carcinoma can develop from these kind of lesions [27].

Conclusion

Establishing a gastroenterostomy without enteroanastomosis in experimental animals favors the development of adenomatous epithelial lesions at the gastroenteral borderline independent of exposition to MNNG. Comparable changes in the mucosa can also be determined in humans with old gastroenterostomies. The extent of such changes in the mucosa can be modified by vagotomy, pyloroplasty, or the prevention of an obligatory duodenogastric reflux (Roux-en-Y-method), whereby the vagotomy has the effect of increasing proliferation. A comparison of the mucosal changes at the gastroenteral anastomosis exhibited by man and animal indicates that a multitude of factors is obviously in a position to cause environmental changes at the gastroenteral borderline, stimulating epithelial proliferation to the point of cancer. Today it does not appear justified to give any single factor, such as intestinal reflux, a carcinogen, or different surgical techniques, the sole priority in this process.

References

1. Borchard, F., Rumpf, P., Schacht, U., Palomba, P.: Formale Genese des chemisch induzierten Magenkarzinoms der Ratte nach Vagotomie und Gastroenterostomie. Verh. Dtsch. Ges. Pathol. *60*, 452 (1976)
2. Bralow, S. P.: Experimental gastric carcinogenesis. Digestion *5*, 290 (1972)
3. Clémencon, G., Baumgartner, R., Leuthold, E., Miller, G., Neiger, A.: Das Karzinom im operierten Magen. Dtsch. Med. Wochenschr. *101*, 1015 (1976)
4. Dahm, K., Werner, B.: Experimentelles Anastomosencarcinom. Ein Beitrag zur Pathogenese des Magenstumpfkarzinoms. Langenbecks Arch. Chir. *333*, 211 (1973)
5. Dahm, K., Werner, B.: Das Karzinom im operierten Magen. Dtsch. Med. Wochenschr. *100*, 1073 (1975)
6. Dahm, K., Eichen, R., Werner, B., Kozuschek, W.: Gastroenterale Anastomosen und Karzinom im operierten Magen. Chirurg *47*, 494 (1976)
7. Dahm, K., Schreiber, H. W., Werner, B., Knipper, A., Mitschke, H.: Zur Bedeutung des duodenogastrischen Refluxes für die Karzinomentstehung im Resektionsmagen. Innere Med. *4*, 297 (1977)
8. Domellöf, L., Eriksson, S., Jamiger, K. G.: Carcinoma and possible precancerous changes of the gastric stump after Billroth II resection. Gastroenterology *73*, 462 (1977)
9. Elster, K., Eidt, H., Ottenjann, R., Rösch, W., Seifert, E.: Drüsenkörperzysten, eine polypoide Läsion der Magenschleimhaut. Dtsch. Med. Wochenschr. *102*, 183 (1977)
10. Gerstenberg, E., Albrecht, A., Kreutz, K., Voth, H.: Das Magenstumpfkarzinom: eine Spätkomplikation des operierten Magens? Dtsch. Med. Wochenschr. *90*, 2185 (1965)
11. Griesser, G., Schmidt, H.: Statistische Erhebungen über die Häufigkeit des Karzinoms nach Magenoperationen wegen eines Geschwürleidens. Med. Welt *35*, 1836 (1964)
12. Grundmann, E.: Histologic types and possible initial stages in early gastric carcinoma. Beitr. Pathol. *154*, 256 (1975)
13. Hilbe, G., Salzer, G. M., Hussl, H., Kutschera, H.: Die Carcinomgefährdung des Resektionsmagens. Langenbecks Arch. Klin. Chir. *323*, 142 (1968)
14. Kowalowski, K.: Relationship between vagotomy, peptic ulcer and gastric adenocarcinoma in rats fed 2.7-diacetylaminofluorene. Can. J. Surg. *16*, 210 (1973)
15. Krause, V.: Late prognosis after partial gastrectomy for ulcer. A follow-up study of 361 patients operated upon from 1902 to 1933. Acta Chir. Scand. *114*, 341 (1957)
16. Kühlmayer, R., Rokitansky, O.: Das Magenstumpfcarcinom als Spätproblem der Ulcuschirurgie. Langenbecks Arch. Klin. Chir. *278*, 361 (1954)
17. Lawson, H. H.: Effect of duodenal contents on the gastric mucosa under experimental conditions. Lancet *1964 1*, 469
18. Lechner, H. J.: Untersuchungen zum Zusammenhang zwischen Gallereflux und Magenerkrankungen. Med. Welt *26*, 72 (1975)
19. Littler, E. R., Gleiberman, E.: Gastritis cystica polyposa. Cancer *29*, 205 (1972)
20. McCalla, D. R.: Reaction of N-Methyl-N'-Nitro-N-Nitrosoguanidine and N-Methyl-N'-Nitroso-p-Toluenesulfonamide with DNA in vitro. Biochem. Biophys. Acta *1955*, 114 (1968)
21. Meister, H., Holubarsch, Ch., Haferkamp, O., Schlag, P., Herfarth, Ch.: Gastritis, Intestinal Metaplasia and Dysplasia versus Benign Ulcer in stomach and duodenum and Gastric Carcinoma – A Histotopographical Study. Path. Res. Pract. *164*, 259 (1979)
22. Morgenstern, L.: Vagotomy, gastroenterostomy and experimental gastric cancer. Arch. Surg. *96*, 920 (1968)
23. Morgenstern, L., Yamakawa, T., Seltzer, D.: Carcinoma of the gastric stump. Am. J. Surg. *125*, 29 (1973)
24. Nicholls, J. C.: Carcinoma of the stomach following partial gastrectomy for benign gastroduodenal lesions. Br. J. Surg. *61*, 244 (1974)

25. Oehlers, W., Keller, P., Hentze, M., Strauch, M.: Die Dysplasien der Magenschleimhaut. Dtsch. Med. Wochenschr. *100,* 1950 (1975)
26. Peitsch, W., Burkhardt, K.: Zur Pathogenese und Klinik des Magenstumpfcarcinoms. Langenbecks Arch. Chir. *341*, 195 (1976)
27. Qizilbash, A. H.: Gastritis cystica and carcinoma arising in old gastrojejunostomy stoma. CMA Journal *112*, 1432 (1975)
28. Reynolds, K. W., Johnson, A. G., Fox, B.: Is intestinal metaplasia of the gastric mucosa a premalignant lesion? Clin. Oncol. *1,* 101 (1975)
29. Saegesser, F., Jämes, D.: Cancer of the gastric stump after partial gastrectomy for ulcer. Cancer *29*, 1150 (1972)
30. Saito, T., Inokvci, Takayama, S., Sugimusa, T.: Sequential morphological changes in N-Methyl-N-Nitro-N-Nitrosoguanidine carcinogenesis in the glandular stomach of rats. J. Natl. Cancer Inst. *44*, 769 (1970)
31. Sander, S., Myren, J., Helsingen, N.: The effect of Bile reflux on the gastric mucosa. Gastroenterologica *101*, 3 (1964)
32. Schlag, P., Meister, H., Feyerabend, G., Merkle, P.: Der Einfluß des duodenogastrischen Refluxes auf das Epithel an der gastroenteralen Anastomose. Eine experimentelle Untersuchung. Langenbecks Arch. Chir. *344*, 207 (1977)
33. Schreiber, H. W., Farthmann, E., Schumpelick, V., Kortmann, K. B.: Umwandlungsoperationen nach Magenoperationen wegen Ulkus (Gastrojejunostomie, BII) in Gastroduodenostomie (Billroth I). Dtsch. Med. Wochenschr. *101*, 1392 (1976)
34. Schrumpf, E., Serck-Hanssen, A., Stadaas, J., Aune, S., Myren, J., Osner, M.: Mucosal changes in the gastric stump 20 – 25 years after partial gastrectomy. Lancet *1977 3,* 467
35. Siurala, M., Varis, K., Wiljaselo, M.: Studies of patients with atrophic gastritis: A 10 – 15 year follow up. Scand. J. Gastroenterol. *1,* 40 (1966)
36. Skinner, J. M., Heenan, P. J., Whitehead, R.: Atrophic gastritis in gastrectomy specimens. Br. J. Surg. *62*, 23 (1975)
37. Taksdal, S., Stalsberg, H.: Histology of gastric carcinoma occurring after gastric surgery for benign conditions. Cancer *32*, 162 (1973)
38. Wickbom, G., Bushkin, F. L., Linares, C., Dragstedt, L. R.: On the corrosive properties of bile and pancreatic juice on living tissue in dogs. Arch. Surg. *108*, 680 (1974)
39. Willems, G., Vansteenkiste, J., Limbosch, J. M.: Stimulating effect of gastrin on cell proliferation kinetics in canine fundic mucosa. Gastroenterology *62*, 583 (1972)

Experimental Cancer of the Gastric Stump

K. Dahm, B. Werner, R. Eichen, and H. Mitschke

During the last 5 years, carcinoma of the gastric stump has become a well-known clinical entity. It refers to a carcinoma occurring in the gastric remnant after partial resection for benign disease. To rule out the presence of an occult carcinoma at the time of the original resection, a time interval of at least 5 years should have elapsed since operation. The available data indicate that, when 20 – 25 years have passed since resection, the risk of development of a stump carcinoma is increased and steadily increasing [1, 6, 19, 20]. Therefore, the threat of this late complication of a stomach resection has influenced substantially the trends of modern gastric surgery promoting the breakthrough of more conservative procedures, such as vagotomy, in the treatment of peptic ulcer.

When starting our experimental work in 1971, we were impressed by the autopsy studies of Kühlmayer & Rokitansky [11] as well as of Hilbe et al. [10] which showed that patients with stomach resections are about two times more susceptible to cancer development in the gastric remnant than nonoperated controls. Later on, we learned more details about the characteristic features of the gastric stump carcinoma, one of which is the localization of the tumor near the gastroenteral anastomosis [9] (Fig. 1). Another point of interest is that gastric stump carcinomas are found predominantly in patients operated on according to the Billroth II procedure with short loop gastroenteric anastomosis (Table 1). When a Billroth II procedure with short loop gastroenteric anastomosis (Polya type) is performed, the duodenogastric reflux passes unavoidably through the gastric remnant. In such cases, the reflux containing bile as well as duodenal juices may contribute via atrophic gastritis to the development of a stump carcinoma [6].

Bearing these observations in mind, we looked for an experimental model in order to answer the following questions:

1) Is the resected stomach really more susceptible to cancer development than the intact one?

2) Is there any influence of chronic duodenogastric reflux on cancer development in the operated stomach?

Material and Methods

Animals

Experimental studies were carried out on male Wistar rats, 3 – 4 months of age. Using ether anesthesia, the abdomen was opened through a midline incision. After ligating the main gastric artery, the resection of the glandular part of the

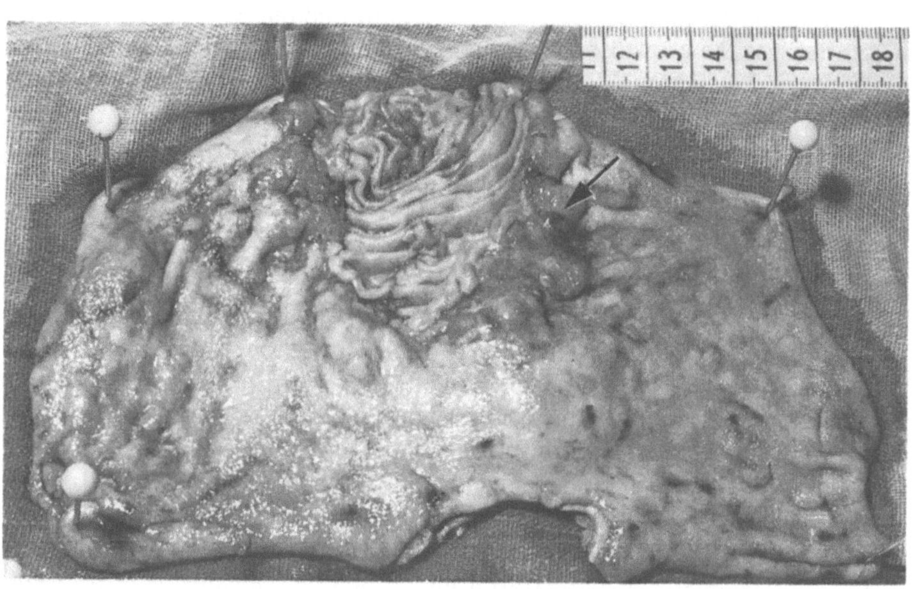

Fig. 1. Carcinoma of the gastric stump of a male patient, 23 years after partial resection for ulcer disease. The stomach mounted, showing the gastric mucosa, the GE, and the jejunal pleats. The tumor arises from the margin of the GE (*arrow*)

Table 1. Frequency of the gastric stump carcinoma after different types of gastroenteric anastomoses (Billroth I and Billroth II)

Anastomosis	Reflux	Stump carcinoma
Billroth I	small	3
Billroth II		
retrocolic (Polya)	large	79
antecolic (Braun)	small	9
various	small	2
		n = 93

stomach, including the antrum and the pylorus, was performed by incising the stomach wall 4 – 5 mm distal of the limiting ridge which separates the forestomach from the glandular stomach. By this procedure, sufficient glandular tissue remained to be observed for malignant change.

After adapting the diameter of the gastric remnant to the diameter of the small intestine by 4 – 5 narrowing sutures, the anastomosis was made either with the duodenum according to Billroth I or with the proximal jejunum according to Billroth II using all-layer single stitches (silk, 6 – 0). Details of feeding the animals before and after surgery have been described elsewhere [4]. The rats were arranged in the following groups (first series):

Billroth I group: Resection and gastroduodenostomy (37 rats).

Billroth II group: Resection and gastrojejunostomy (29 rats).

Control group: Resection and gastroduodenostomy or gastrojejunostomy (20 rats).

Control group: Intact animals (44 rats).

In a second series of experiments, we tried to find out whether the reflux of bile influences the growth of carcinomas in the gastric stump. Therefore, the gastroenteric anastomosis (GE) was made either as short loop GE (Polya type), thus supplying a continuous duodenogastric reflux, or as Y-shaped GE (Roux type). By the latter technique, bile and duodenal secretions are derived quantitatively into the jejunum without coming into contact with the remaining part of the stomach (Fig. 2). Particulars have been published by Dahm et al. [5].

Administration of the Carcinogen

N-Methyl-*N′*-nitro-*N*-nitrosoguanidine (MNNG) was purchased from Aldrich Chemical Co., Milwaukee, Wisconsin (United States), or from EGA Chemie, Steinheim, W. Germany. A stock solution of MNNG (2 g/l) was prepared every 4 days and appropriately diluted with demineralized water to obtain a final concentration of 120 mg/l. The instructions of handling MNNG containing solutions were observed [17, 22]. Five weeks after operation, the animals were exposed to the carcinogen, with the exception of the control rats with stomach resection. The drinking bottles were refilled with fresh solution of MNNG every 3 – 4 days. The rats were allowed to drink ad libitum. Operated controls were kept on normal tap water.

Autopsy and Histological Evaluations

Autopsy was performed on all experimental animals when they died or were killed. All organs were carefully examined. The stomach was opened along the greater curvature, cleaned, and spread out on a small cork plate. The histological

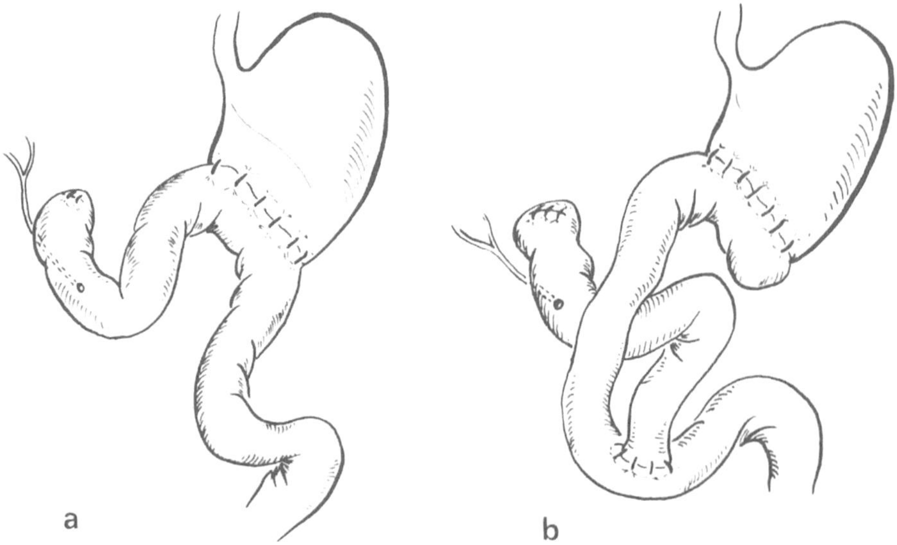

Fig. 2. Surgical procedures suitable to induce or to avoid reflux. **a** Partially resected stomach with short loop GE undergoing continuous reflux (Billroth II group). **b** Same item with Y-shaped GE (Roux group). Bile and duodenal juices are diverted into the jejunum

evaluations were on serial sections of 7 μ thickness from the tissue fixed by Bouin-solution and embedded in parafine. The histological diagnosis of the lesions with marked atypical growth in the glandular stomach was based on the criteria described in the literature [17, 22].

Autopsies of the second experimental series have been evaluated using histological criteria similar to those in human pathology [8, 14, 15]. The following definitions have been used: dysplasia (grade I – III), erosion, glandular proliferation, borderline lesion, early carcinoma, advanced carcinoma. Dysplasia of the epithelium has been defined according to the terms of Oehlert et al. [15], comprising cytological as well as structural irregularities of the glandular epithelium. Erosions have been divided into acute erosions and into healing ones. The latter are characterized by a little dysplasia of the epithelium as well as by proliferations of well-differentiated glands into the surroundings of the erosion. Proliferations of glands, limited to the mucosa, have been designated as glandular proliferations (with or without dysplasia). The infiltration of glands showing little atypical structures into the submucosa is described as borderline lesion (Fig. 3). This alteration corresponds approximately to the term "downwards adenomatous growth" described by Saito et al. [17]. The diagnosis of an early gastric cancer was made when glands with marked cellular and structural atypia, invading the mucosa or the submucosa, were seen. Advanced cancer is defined as malignant infiltration of the tunica muscularis propria (P_3) or the serosa (P_4).

Most of the MNNG-induced carcinomas of the rat can be classified as intestinal types according to Laurén [12], whereas only a few tumors were diagnosed

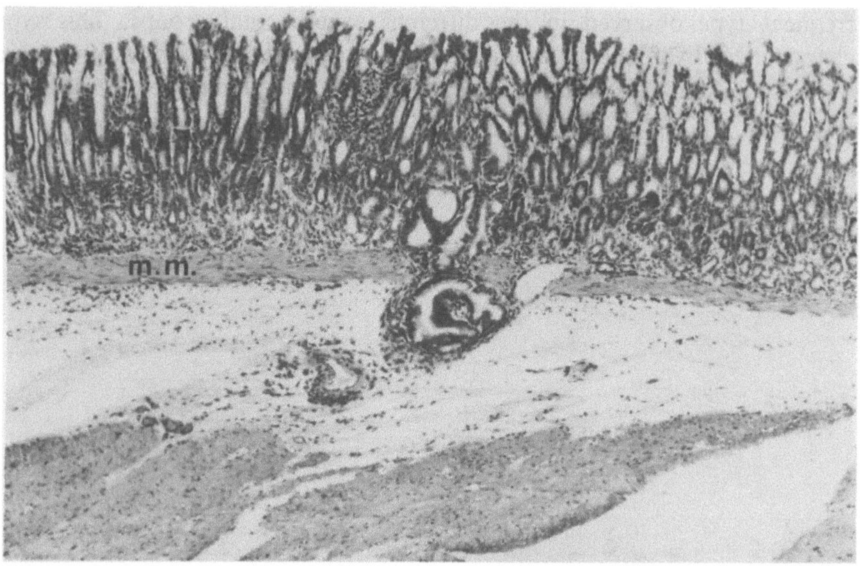

Fig. 3. Infiltration of glands, showing little atypical structures, into the submucosa of the intact stomach of the rat 26 weeks after daily oral administration of MNNG (borderline lesion) (*m. m.* = muscularis mucosae)

showing the diffuse type with signet-ring cells. The time-dependent histological alterations taking place in the stomach of the rat after administration of MNNG, are summarized in Figure 4. Based on the criteria of Saito et al. [17] as well as on our own definitions, no difficulties have arisen in diagnosing an experimental cancer of the stomach. Therefore, all quantitative statements concerning the different experimental groups are confined to the diagnosis of carcinoma. Precancerous changes, including the borderline lesions, were not considered.

Results

Autopsy Findings

The operated animals (Billroth I group and Billroth II group) as well as 24 rats of the intact control group were sacrificed 31 weeks after starting the daily feeding of MNNG. The remaining 20 rats of this group were killed after 41 weeks. Of 66 operated animals, 25 rats developed gastric stump carcinomas of various size and localization (Figs. 5 and 6). Most of the tumors, i.e., 12 of the Billroth I group and 10 of the Billroth II group, were localized in the vicinity of the gastroenteric anastomosis. The malignant alterations appeared macroscopically as ulcers, irregular nodules, mural thickening, or globular masses varying from several millimeters to more than one centimeter in diameter. Ulcerous defects of the mucosal relief of the gastric remnant were detected in a few selected animals by X-ray studies (Fig. 7).

Microscopic Findings

The intestinal type of carcinoma, as described by Laurén [12], was the most frequent type observed in the different experimental groups. This type is characterized by atypically branched glands infiltrating the tunica submucosa as well as the tunica muscularis propria (Fig. 8). The glands were lined by cells

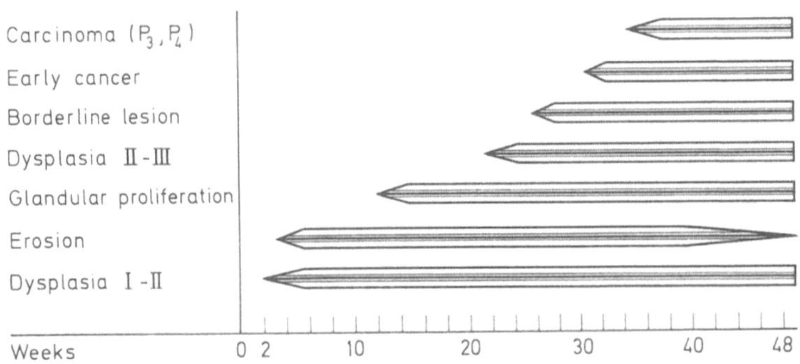

Fig. 4. Histological alterations taking place in the stomach of the rat dependent on time of MNNG exposure

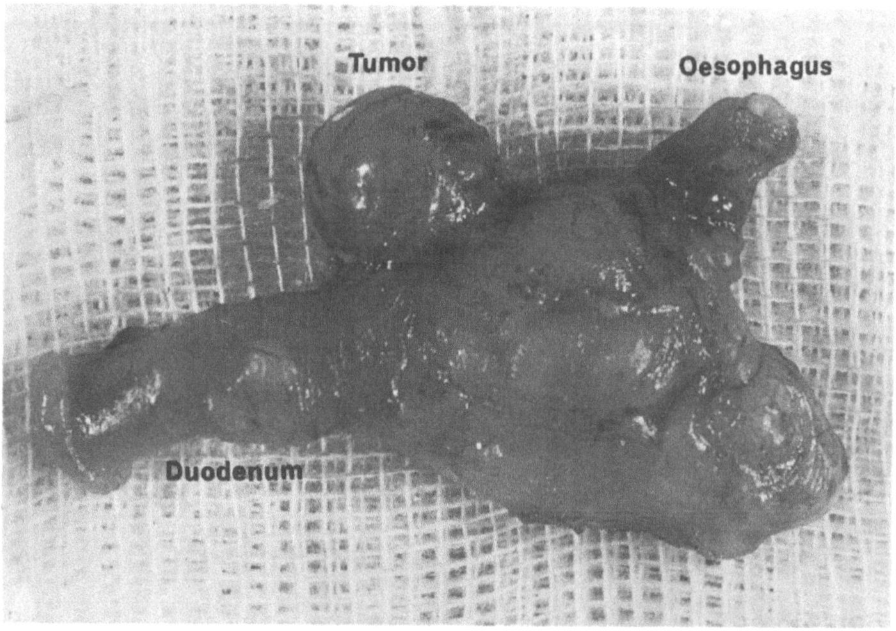

Fig. 5. Carcinoma of the gastric stump of a rat, 31 weeks after daily administration of MNNG. The tumor starts from the lesser curvature near the gastroduodenostomy (Billroth I group). From [4]

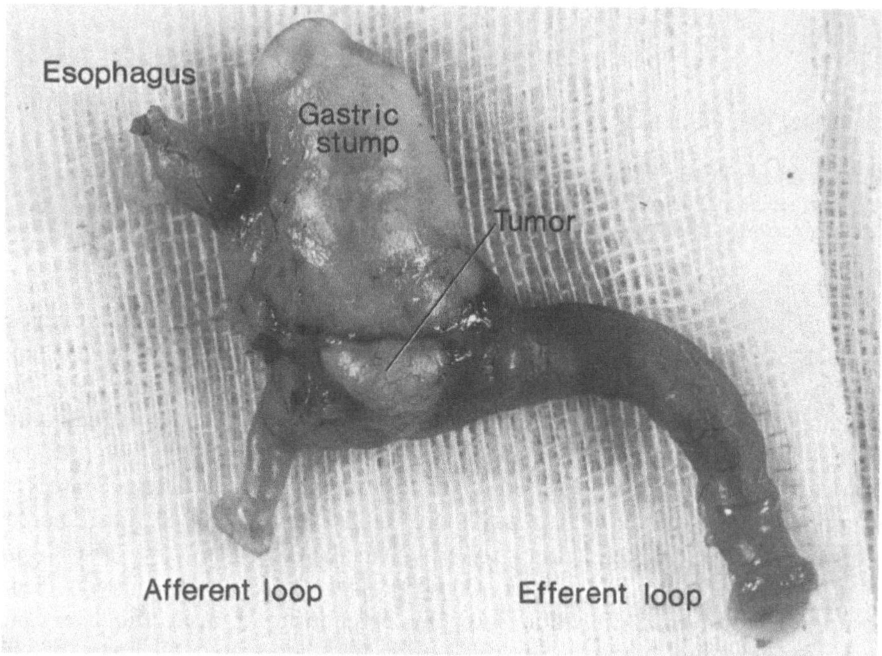

Fig. 6. Carcinoma of the gastric stump, arising from the gastrojejunal anastomosis of a rat, 31 weeks after daily oral administration of MNNG (Billroth II group). From [4]

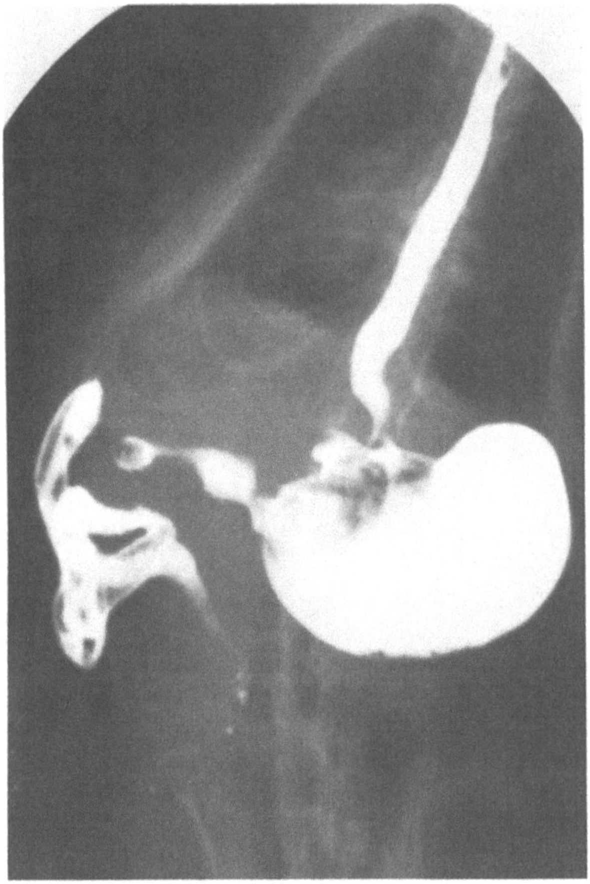

Fig. 7. X-ray study of the resected stomach of a rat, 31 weeks after daily oral administration of MNNG, showing an ulcerous defect at the lesser curvature (Billroth I group). From [4]

showing the distinguishing marks of malignancy, such as hyperchromasia, irregular shape of the nucleus, shifting of the size relation between nucleus and plasma, and increased mitotic figures (Fig. 9). In the advanced state, the malignant cell growth formed large cyst-adenoidal proliferations and, finally, invaded all the coats of the resected stomach, including the serosa, thus fulfilling Stewart's criteria (Fig. 10). The stroma of the tumors showed various degrees of inflammation. In the gastric stump of three animals, a diffuse type of carcinoma, exhibiting the typical signet-ring cells, was detected (Fig. 11).

Metastasis, be it hematogenous or by the lymphatic system, has not been observed. However, infiltration into the neighborhood, i.e., the liver and pancreas, occurred often, when the tumor had penetrated all coats of the stomach. The MNNG-induced carcinogenesis is not limited to the stomach. Apart from the malignant alterations of the gastric stump, we found four adenocarcinomas and three sarcomas of the small intestine.

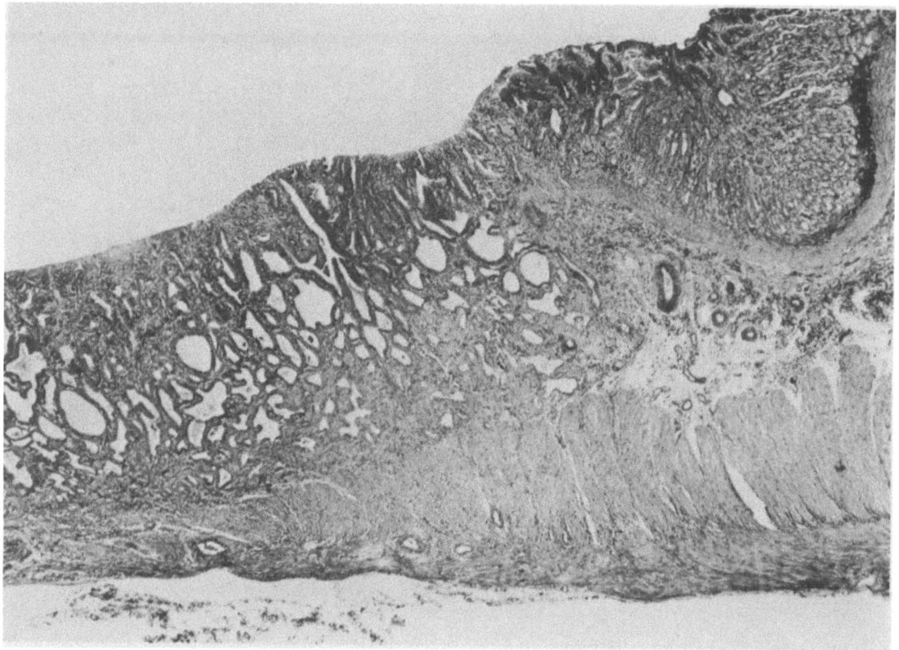

Fig. 8. Histological section of an intestinal type of cancer of the gastric stump, 31 weeks after daily oral administration of MNNG. The tumor infiltrates the tunica muscularis propria and the tunica submucosa. (PAS, × 80)

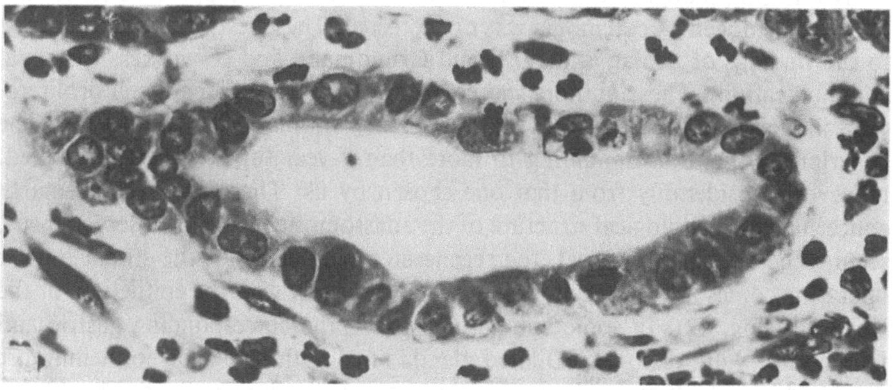

Fig. 9. Cross section of a gland of an intestinal type of carcinoma at higher magnification, showing hyperchromasia, pleomorphic nuclei, increased mitotic figures and a shift of the size relation between nuclei and plasma. (HE, × 360)

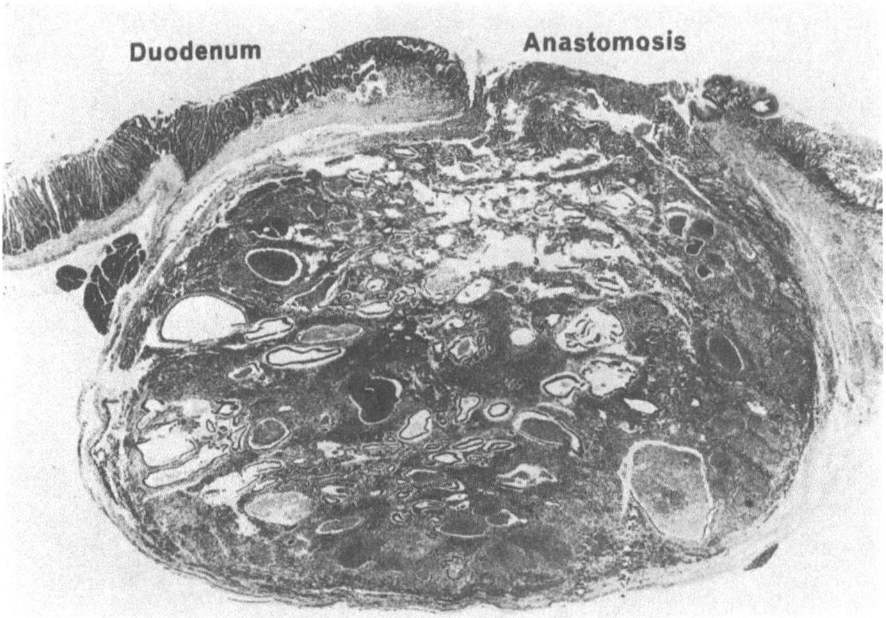

Fig. 10. Cancer of the gastric stump of a rat, 31 weeks after daily oral administration of MNNG. The intestinal type of carcinoma located at the gastroduodenostomy has penetrated all coats including the serosa. (HE, × 6)

Cancerous and precancerous lesions in the intact stomachs of nonoperated control rats were similar to those described in the literature [17, 22]. A detailed description is therefore omitted here.

No striking changes were seen in the rats which had been operated on but not fed the carcinogen. A carcinoma was not detected. These results stand in contrast to the findings of Schlag et al. [18] and Grundmann and co-workers (personal communication). These authors succeeded in detecting malignant cell proliferations in the anastomotic region of rats kept under normal diet and tap water. The experimental period, amounting to more than a year (up to 2 years) differed, however, considerably from that one chosen by us. Therefore, some remarks concerning the histological structure of the anastomotic region as observed by us, seem to be useful. In general, the regenerated epithelium of the stomach after operation comes into connection tightly and steplessly with the epithelium of the small gut (Fig. 12). In some animals, however, the corresponding gastric and jejunal layers are distorted. Dilated glands lined with a regular epithelium are displaced into the tunica submucosa, the tunica muscularis propria (Fig. 13), or into layers which consist of connective tissue with scattered muscle fibers. It should be pointed out that, based on cytological as well as structural criteria, these alterations can be clearly distinguished from the respective malignant changes.

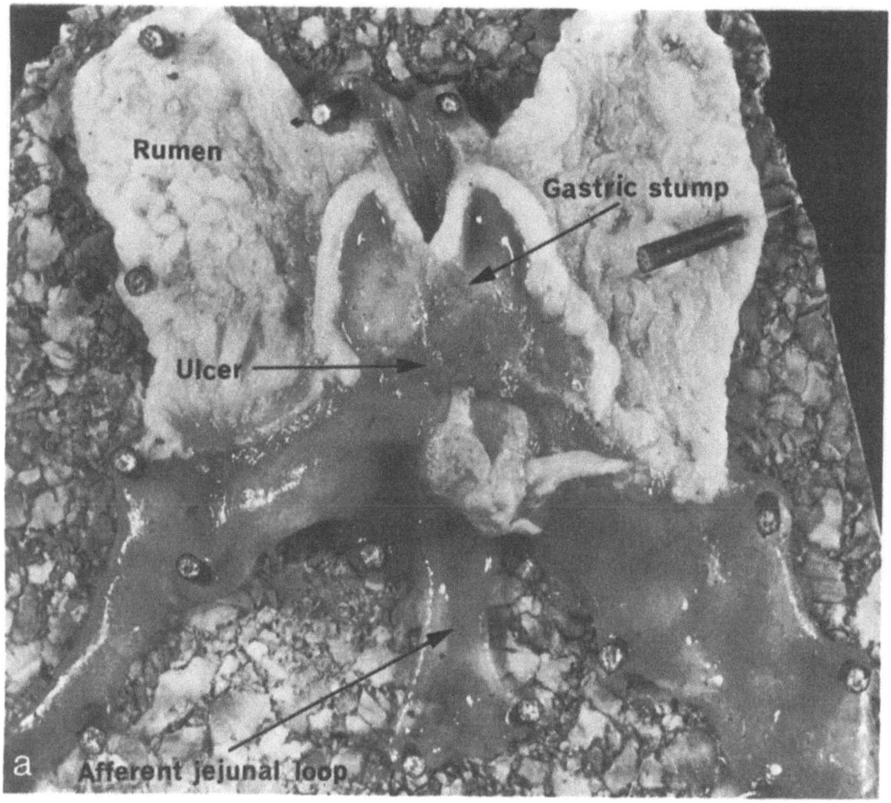

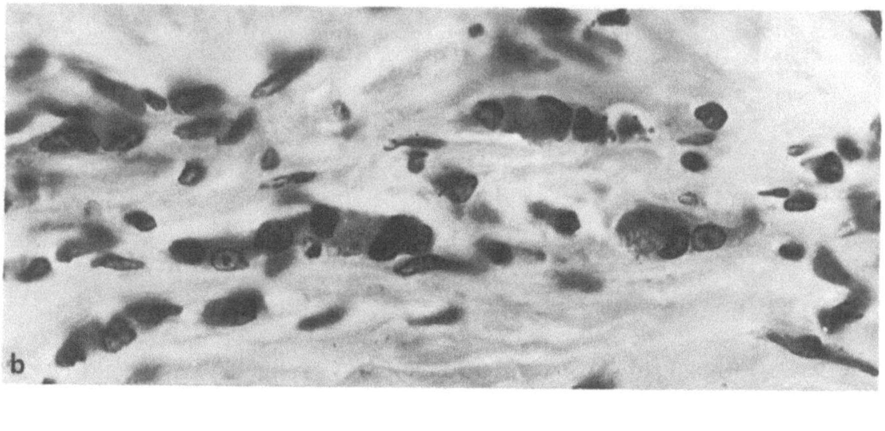

Fig. 11. Carcinoma of the gastric stump of a rat imitating an ulcer at the gastroenteric anastomosis, 31 weeks after daily oral administration of MNNG (Billroth II group). **a** Aspect of the B II specimen opened through the afferent loop. A mucous secretion adheres to the center of the ulcer. **b** Histological examination shows a signet ring cell type of carcinoma. (HE, × 360). From [4]

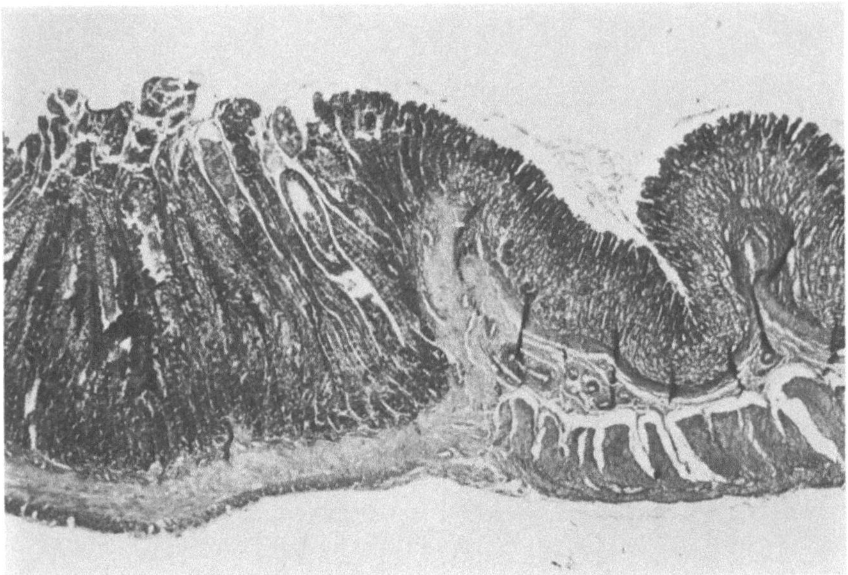

Fig. 12. Histological section of the gastrojejunostomy of a rat, 36 weeks after stomach resection (operated control group; no MNNG feeding). At the anastomosis, the corresponding layers of the gastric and jejunal walls are healed without scars and distortions. (PAS, × 80)

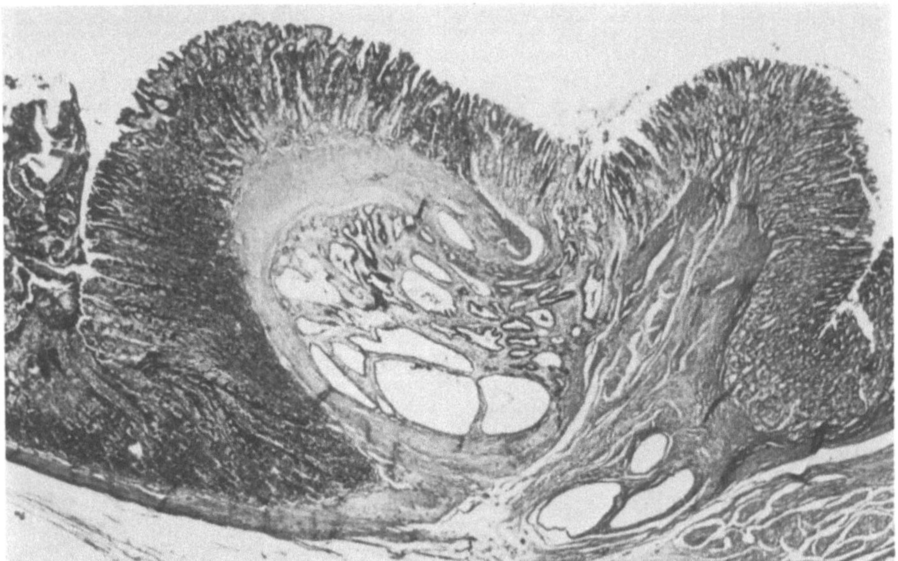

Fig. 13. Histological section of the gastrojejunostomy of a rat, 36 weeks after stomach resection (operated control group; no MNNG feeding). The corresponding layers of the stomach and jejunum are interrupted. At the anastomosis, dilated glands are displaced into the tunica submucosa and the tunica muscularis propria. However, signs of malignant cell growth are not observed

Susceptibility of the Resected Stomach to Experimental Carcinogenesis

Summing up, the rats of the Billroth I group and those of the Billroth II group, 25 of 66 rats developed adenocarcinomas of the gastric stump. As can be seen from Fig. 14, only one borderline lesion was observed in the corresponding control group with intact stomachs killed together with the operated animals 31 weeks after feeding the carcinogen. However, when the remaining 20 rats of this group were sacrificed after 41 weeks, gastric carcinomas were found in 11 rats. These findings demonstrate that the partially resected stomach of the rat is very susceptible to malignant cell growth. In the majority of the operated animals, the induction and development of gastric cancer is finished about 2 months earlier as compared to rats with intact stomachs. Probability evaluations indicate a statistically significant difference between these two groups. On the other hand, no statistically significant difference was found between animals of the Billroth I group and those of the Billroth II group.

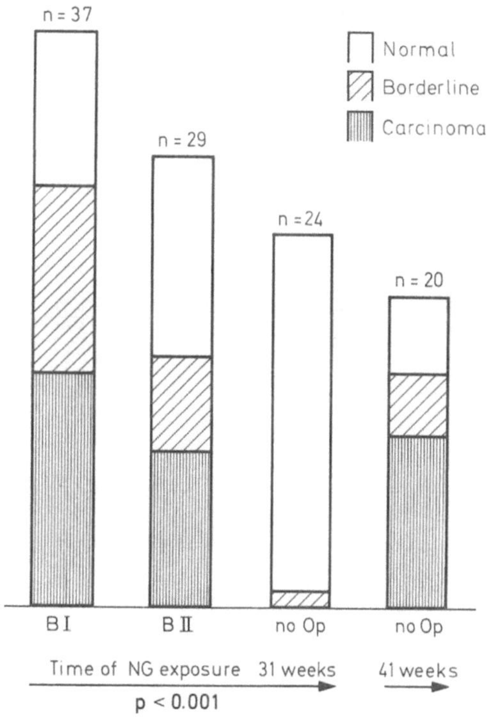

Fig. 14. Frequency of carcinomas and borderline lesions found in 110 rats undergoing various experimental procedures

Influence of the Duodenogastric Reflux on Cancer Development in the Gastric Remnant

Why is the operated stomach more susceptible to cancer development than the intact one? In a second series of experiments, we tried to investigate some of the reasons which might be causal for the accelerated formation of carcinomas in the gastric stump.

Clinical observations have pointed to the dominant role of the duodenogastric reflux occurring in the gastric stump due to certain types of gastroenteric anastomoses [3]. Carcinomas of the gastric stump are found predominantly in patients with the Polya type GE inundating the gastric mucosa with bile acids and duodenal secretions (Fig. 2a). Therefore, the following experimental approach was used [3]: male Wistar rats (n = 72) were subjected to partial stomach resection. The GE was made either as short loop GE, thus providing a continuous duodenogastric reflux, or GE according to Roux. Due to the Y-shaped GE of Roux, the duodenogastric reflux is avoided by quantitative derivation of bile and duodenal secretions into the jejunum. At autopsy, most of the carcinomas were found in operated rats undergoing continuous reflux (Billroth II group). The incidence of carcinomas of the gastric stump was significantly lower in animals without reflux (Roux group; Fig. 15).

Discussion

The results of our experiments demonstrate that the partially resected stomach of the rat is more susceptible to induction of cancer than the intact one. Twenty-

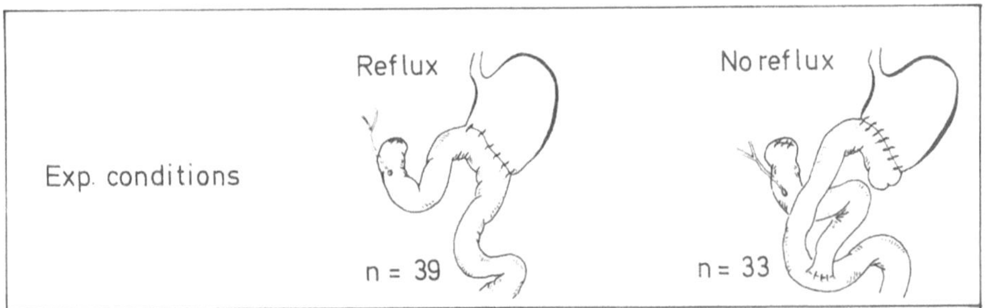

	Reflux	No reflux
Killed at the end of exp.	22	21
Cancer of the gastric stump	7	1
Sarcoma of the gastric stump	2	0

Fig. 15. Effect of duodenogastric reflux on cancer incidence of the gastric stump of 72 rats, 33 weeks after daily oral administration of MNNG. From [5]

five of 66 rats subjected to stomach resection according to Billroth I or Billroth II and fed MNNG daily, developed carcinomas in the gastric remnant. The process of tumor formation in the resected stomach was completed within a lifespan of 17 – 31 weeks, thus showing a very short time of induction of experimental gastric cancer. In contrast to these findings, the development of cancer in the intact stomach of Wistar rats requires an average of more than 41 weeks of continuous oral administration of MNNG [17, 22]. The results of our first experimental series suggest that the gastroenteric anastomosis has an accelerating influence on cancer formation of the stomach. These findings were confirmed by Rumpf et al. [16] in similar studies in the rat.

The second series of experiments was undertaken in order to detect factors or conditions which might favor the malignant cell growth near the gastroenteric anastomosis. The results demonstrate that, in rats, the duodenogastric reflux contributes substantially to the development of carcinomas of the gastric stump. Bile and duodenal secretions are known to act as detergents, thereby damaging the mucosal barrier of the stomach. These substances are, as numerous clinical studies have shown [6, 23], responsible for the transformation of a normal gastric mucosa into an atrophic one. The atrophic gastritis, arising as a consequence of this transformation, is thought to be the main risk factor for the development of gastric carcinoma.

The specificity of MNNG in producing stomach cancer in the experimental animal may be explained by its chemical property of interacting with the DNA of the cells. MNNG leads to partial methylation of DNA; the main products being formed are 7-methylguanine and 3-methyladenine [2]. The extent of methylation increases when an alkaline milieu is prevailing [13], a condition which is given near the gastroenteric anastomosis.

Many questions concerning the pathogenesis of cancer in the stomach resected for benign disease are not resolved. The presented findings suggest a causal relationship between stomach resection and cancer development in the gastric stump under defined experimental conditions. Whether this assumption holds true as far as the respective cancer in man is concerned remains the aim of further investigations.

Summary and Conclusion

In this work, an experimental model of cancer of the gastric stump is presented, imitating some of the peculiarities, and thus suitable for studying the pathophysiology of this disease. In a first series of experiments, 66 male Wistar rats were subjected to partial stomach resection according to the Billroth I or the Billroth II procedure. These rats, as well as control animals, were fed the carcinogen *N*-methyl-*N'*-nitro-*N*-nitrosoguanidine (MNNG). Of 66 rats, 25 developed carcinomas in the gastric remnant. The tumors were characterized histologically as adenocarcinomas. Mostly, the carcinomas were localized near the gastroenteric anastomosis. The process of tumor development in the resected stomach of the rat was completed within 17 – 31 weeks on continuous feeding of

MNNG in a concentration of 120 mg/l in the drinking water[1]. In contrast to these findings, the formation of cancer in the intact stomach required an average of 41 weeks under the same experimental conditions. With regard to the incidence of malignant changes, no significant difference was observed between animals undergoing the Billroth I method and those undergoing the Billroth II method. The results suggest that the resected stomach of the rat is more susceptible to induction of cancer than the intact one. Exposure of the resected stomach to an oral carcinogen induces carcinogenesis predominantly in the anastomotic region.

In a second series, we tried to answer the question whether the duodenogastric reflux has any influence on the malignant cell growth in the gastric stump, especially at the anastomosis. Seventy-two male Wistar rats were subjected to partial stomach resection. The gastroenteric anastomosis (GE) was performed either as short loop anastomosis (Billroth II; n = 39), thus providing a continuous duodenogastric reflux, or as Y-shaped GE (according to Roux; n = 33). By the latter technique, bile and pancreatic juices are diverted into the jejunum without coming into contact with the remaining part of the stomach. All animals, including a control group with intact stomachs, were fed MNNG in the drinking water. At autopsy, most of the tumors were found in the animal group subjected to chronic duodenogastric reflux (Billroth II group). In contrast to these findings, the incidence of carcinomas was significantly lower in rats without reflux (Roux group or intact control animals). The results of our experiments demonstrate that, in rats, the duodenogastric reflux contributes substantially to the development of carcinomas of the gastric stump.

References

1. Clémencon, G., Baumgartner, R., Leuthold, E., Miller, G., Neiger, A.: Das Karzinom des operierten Magens. Dtsch. Med. Wochenschr. *101,* 1015–1020 (1976)
2. Craddock, V. M.: The reaction of N-methyl-N'-nitro-N-nitrosoguanidine with deoxyribonucleic acid. Biochem. J. *106,* 921–922 (1968)
3. Dahm, K., deHeer, K.: Cancer risk of the stomach resected for ulcer: The role of duodenogastric reflux. Z. Krebsforsch. *87*, 343–344 (1976)
4. Dahm, K., Werner, B.: Experimentelles Anastomosencarcinom. Ein Beitrag zur Pathogenese des Magenstumpfcarcinoms. Langenbecks Arch. Chir. *333*, 211–236 (1973)
5. Dahm, K., Eichen, R., Mitschke, H.: Das Krebsrisiko im Resektionsmagen. Zur Bedeutung des duodenogastrischen Refluxes bei verschiedenen gastroenteralen Anastomosen. Langenbecks Arch. Chir. *344*, 71–82 (1977)
6. Domellöf, L., Januger, K.-G.: The risk for gastric carcinoma after partial gastrectomy. Am. J. Surg. *134*, 581–584 (1977)
7. Domellöf, Eriksson, S., Januger, K.-G.: Carcinoma and possible precancerous changes of the gastric stump after Billroth II resection. Gastroenterology *73*, 462–468 (1977)
8. Grundmann, E.: Histologic types and possible initial stages in early gastric carcinoma. Beitr. Pathol. *154,* 256–280 (1975)
9. Hammar, E.: The localization of precancerous changes and carcinoma after previous gastric operation for benign condition. Acta Pathol. Microbiol. Scand. (A) *84,* 495–507 (1976)
10. Hilbe, G., Salzer, G. M., Hussl, H., Kutschera, H.: Die Carcinomgefährdung des Resektionsmagens. Langenbecks Arch. Klin. Chir. *323*, 142–153 (1968)

[1] Control animals either with intact stomachs treated with the carcinogen or operated and kept under normal diet and tap water showed no cancer formation up to the 31st week.

11. Kühlmayer, R., Rokitansky, O.: Das Magenstumpfcarcinom als Spätproblem der Ulcuschirurgie. Langenbecks Arch. Klin. Chir. *278*, 361–375 (1954)
12. Laurén, P.: The two histological main types of gastric carcinoma: diffuse and so-called intestinal-type carcinoma. An attempt at a histo-clinical classification. Acta Pathol. Microbiol. Scand. *64*, 31–49 (1965)
13. McCalla, D. R.: Reaction of N-methyl-N′-nitro-N-nitroguanidine and N-methyl-N′-nitroso-p-toluenesulfonamide with DNA in vitro. Biochim. Biophys. Acta *155*, 114–120 (1968)
14. Mitschke, H.: Pathologisch-anatomische Grundlagen der Krebsrisikoerkrankungen und des Frühcarcinoms des Magens. Chirurg *49*, 465–472 (1978)
15. Oehlert, W., Keller, P., Henke, M., Strauch, M.: Die Dysplasien der Magenschleimhaut. Das Problem ihrer klinischen Bedeutung. Dtsch. Med. Wochenschr. *100,* 1950–1956 (1975)
16. Rumpf, P., Schacht, U., Palomba, P., Kremer, K., Schmitz, H., Borchard, F.: Chemisch induzierte Karzinogenese des Rattenmagens nach Vagotomie und Resektion. Z. Gastroenterol. *16*, 85–94 (1978)
17. Saito, T., Inokuchi, K., Takayama, S., Sugimura, T.: Sequential morphological changes in N-methyl-N′-nitro-N-nitrosoguanidine carcinogenesis in the glandular stomach of rats. J. Natl. Cancer Inst. *44*, 769–783 (1970)
18. Schlag, P., Meister, H., Feyerabend, G., Merkle, P.: Der Einfluß des duodenogastrischen Refluxes auf das Epithel an der gastroenteralen Anastomose. Eine experimentelle Untersuchung. Langenbecks Arch. Chir. *344*, 207–217 (1977)
19. Schmid, E., Vollmer, R., Adlung, J., Blaich, E., Goebell, H., Heinkel, K., Kimmig, J.-M., Probst, M.: Zur endoskopischen Diagnostik des Karzinoms im operierten Magen. Z. Gastroenterol. *14*, 521–530 (1976)
20. Stalsberg, H., Taksdal, S.: Stomach cancer following gastric surgery for benign conditions. Lancet *1971 II,* 1175–1177
21. Stewart, H. L., Snell, K. C., Morris, H. P., Wagner, B. P., Ray, F. E.: Carcinoma of the glandular stomach of rats ingesting N,N′-2,7-fluorenylenebisacetamide. Nat. Cancer Inst. Monogr. *5,* 105–139 (1961)
22. Sugimura, T., Fujimura, S., Baba, T.: Tumor production in the glandular stomach and alimentary tract of the rat by N-methyl-N′-nitro-N′-nitrosoguanidine. Cancer Res. *30*, 455–465 (1970)
23. Werner, B., Leppin, A., Seiler, I., Mitschke, H., Soehendra, N., Farthmann, E., Rehner, M., Dahm, K.: Duodenaler Reflux und Gastritis im Billroth I Magen. Dtsch. Med. Wochenschr. *100,* 2385–2388 (1975)

Formal Pathogenesis of Chemically-Induced Cancers After Gastric Operation

F. Borchard

The chemical carcinogen, *N*-methyl-*N'*-nitro-*N*-nitrosoguanidine (MNNG), was added in two doses (30 and 100 mg/liter/day) to the drinking water of different groups of rats: one control group of 80 rats was not subject to any operation, 50 rats were operated according to the method Billroth-II, and 50 additional rats were vagotomized with a pyloroplasty. Twenty-five rats, each of the latter two groups received the high dose and the low dose, respectively. Details of the experiment [10] and preliminary morphological findings concerning carcinogenesis [1] have been described already.

After 480 days of exposure, the incidence of carcinoma was significantly higher in the experimental groups with the high dose of the carcinogen. There was also a significantly higher incidence of cancers after gastric resection than in the control group and the group with vagotomy (cf. Table 1; for details see Rumpf et al., 1978).

The cancers exclusively occurred in the antral region in the control group and after vagotomy, although this group exhibited more tumours along the line of the pyloroplasty. After Billroth-II resection, the cancers developed, almost exclusively, along the anastomosal suture. Diffuse atrophic changes of the gastric mucosa were found in many animals of the high dose group, especially in rats with vagotomy. In the fundic mucosa, spotty cystic changes of the glands were also found, which corresponded to the *Drüsenkörperzysten* (body gland cysts) recently described by Elster et al. [4]. In such mucosal cysts, changes in cell turnover have been found [5]. Only a few glands with intestinal metaplasia were seen, which corresponds to the extreme rarity of signet-ring cell carcinoma in this experiment.

The carcinogenesis in the control rats mainly followed the scheme given by Saito et al. [11] with the development of erosions followed by nodular superficial regenerative proliferations. These proliferations apparently developed into

Table 1. Incidence of cancer after resection or vagotomy and pyloroplasty in comparison to control group

	Control		Vagotomy and pyloroplasty		Billroth-II resection	
MNNG (mg/l/d)	30	100	30	100	30	100
	6/40	21/40	2/22	11/21	8/16	15/18
	(15%)	(52.5%)	(9.1%)	(52.4%)	(50%)	(83.3%)

superficial adenomas from which carcinoma could arise. We also saw a deep regenerative proliferation that turned into adenoma, ending up in invasive carcinoma (cf. Fig. 1).

The second type of carcinogenesis via dysplasia had been proposed by Borchard et al. [1] and Uchida et al. [13], and was recently confirmed by Kunze et al. [8].

The third type of carcinogenesis was found in the anastomosal region. It is connected with the misplacement of gastric or intestinal glands into the submucosa or muscularis, which could be traced by nonabsorbable suture threads. Already, very early after operation, retention cysts appeared from these misplaced glands. These cysts sometimes bulged the anastomosal side to form polyps, which have been mistaken for carcinoma when absorbable suture threads were used [3]. It is worth mentioning that carcinoma in the resected stomach could not be induced according to the method of these authors by Schlag et al. [12]. The fate of these retention cysts depends on the type of misplaced mucosa: we never saw the development of adenomas from enteral mucosa. Mucosa from the gastric fundus usually showed pseudopyloric metaplasia in these retention cysts, and the development of carcinoma may occasionally take place. Several deep adenomas with various degrees of dysplasia arose from misplaced antral mucosa. In rare cases, the development of carcinoma out from misplaced glands could also be traced.

Usually, the development of carcinoma in the gastric stump involves different types of carcinogenesis. One has to assume that the mucosa on top of the retention cysts is subject not only to the action of the carcinogen, but also to increased mechanical injury, bile reflux, and bacterial contamination, thus causing erosions and proliferative changes. We found superficial regenerative nodules and adenomas growing into the retention cysts or initial deep adenomas arising in these misplaced glands. The development of cystic changes [9, 6] with the increased risk of malignant potential has also been described in the human stomach [7]. In advanced carcinomas, these processes could not be traced back to the initial stage (cf. Fig. 1).

The complex experimental carcinogenesis in the gastric stump after antrectomy and after vagotomy cannot entirely be compared to the carcinogenesis in the human stomach. The main differences are the facts that [1] the human anastomosis is not continuously subject to high doses of carcinogens, and [2] the dislocation of gastric glands into deeper layers of the gastric wall does not occur as often as in the rat stomach, because single suture technique is usually not applied in operations of the human stomach. Another factor which seems to be important for the etiology of these lesions may be bile reflux, not only potentiating the effects of the carcinogen by the alkaline pH of this fluid, but also causing increased cell turnover by damage to the superficial epithelium. Schlag (cf. p. 120) has also pointed out the importance of bacteria to the genesis of nitrosamines. Although there is the impression of an increase of carcinoma in the human gastric stump, the incidence of precancerous lesions still has to be defined [2].

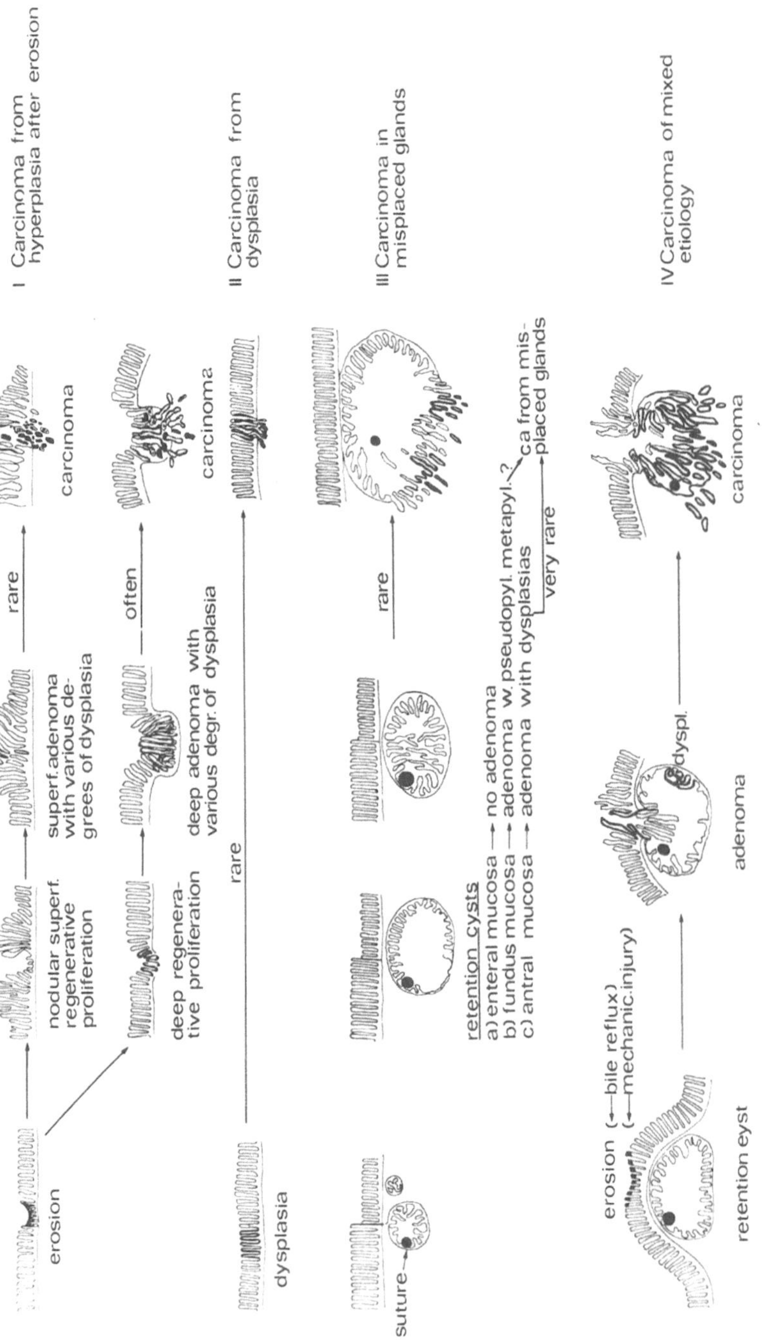

Fig. 1. Hypothesis of the formal carcinogenesis in the operated stomach

References

1. Borchard, F., Rumpf, P., Schacht, U., Palomba, P.: Formale Pathogenese des chemisch induzierten Magenkarzinoms der Ratte nach Vagotomie und Gastroenterostomie. Verh. Dtsch. Ges. Pathol. *60*, 452 (1976)
2. Borchard, F., Mittelstaedt, A., Kieker, R.: Incidence of epithelial dysplasia after partial gastric resection. Pathology (Research and Practice) in press
3. Dahm, K., Werner, B.: Experimentelles Anastomosencarcinom. Langenbecks Arch. Chir. *333*, 211 – 236 (1973)
4. Elster, K., Eidt, H., Ottenjann, R., Rösch, W., Seifert, E.: Drüsenkörperzysten, eine polypoide Läsion der Magenschleimhaut. Dtsch. Med. Wochenschr. *102*, 183 – 187 (1977)
5. Fujita, S., Hattori, T.: Cell proliferation, differentiation, and migration in the gastric mucosa: A study on the background of carcinogenesis. In: Pathophysiology of carcinogenesis in digestive organs. Farber, E. et al. (eds.), pp. 21 – 34. University Park Press 1977
6. Griffel, B., Engleberg, M., Reiss, R., Saba, K.: Multiple polypoid cystic gastritis in old gastroenteric stoma. Arch. Pathol. *97*, 316 – 318 (1974)
7. Iwanaga, T., Koyama, H., Takahashi, Y., Taniguchi, H., Wada, A.: Diffuse submucosal cysts and carcinoma of the stomach. Cancer *36*, 606 – 614 (1975)
8. Kunze, E., Schauer, A., Seefeldt, C.: Bedeutung der Dysplasie für die Entwicklung des Magenkarzinoms. Verh. Dtsch. Ges. Pathol. in press
9. Littler, E. R., Gleibermann, E.: Gastritis cystica polyposa. Cancer *29*, 205 – 209 (1972)
10. Rumpf, P., Schacht, U., Palomba, P., Kremer, K., Schmitz, H., Borchard, F.: Chemisch induzierte Karzinogenese des Rattenmagens nach Vagotomie und Resektion. Z. Gastroenterol. *16*, 85 – 94 (1978)
11. Saito, T., Inokuchi, K., Takayama, S., Sugimura, T.: Sequential morphological changes in N-methyl-N′-nitro-N-nitrosoguanidine carcinogenesis in the glandular stomach in rats. J. Natl. Cancer Inst. *44*, 769 – 783 (1970)
12. Schlag, P., Meister, H. Feyerabend, G., Merkle, P.: Der Einfluß des duodenogastrischen Refluxes auf das Epithel an der gastroenteralen Anastomose. Eine experimentelle Untersuchung. Langenbecks Arch. Chir. *344*, 207 – 217 (1977)
13. Uchida, Y., Schlake, W., Roessner, A., Rühland, D., Themann, H., Grundmann, E.: Development of tumors in the glandular stomach of rats after oral administration of carcinogens. Z. Krebsforsch. *87*, 199 – 212 (1976)

Vagotomy and Gastric Cancer

K. Junghanns, S. Ivankovic, R. M. Seufert, and L. von Gerstenbergk

The most popular treatment in Germany for peptic disease of the stomach and duodenum is still resection. Vagotomy is slowly increasing in popularity among the younger surgeons. One of the many reasons mentioned against resection is the alarming number of cancers found in the gastric remnant 20–25 years following gastrectomy. Long standing chronic mucosal atrophy and biliary reflux could be the basis for the neoplastic changes.

Since vagotomy has only recently been introduced, there is no long-term follow-up of these patients and the state of their gastric mucosa. In the experimental animal, it was possible to show that on oral administration of carcinogens [3], the number of tumors increased in the resected stomach [1, 2]. This close relationship to human pathology suggested trying the use of carcinogens in vagotomized rats to see whether there is a higher incidence of gastric cancer than in controls.

Material and Methods

Fifty-eight Wistar rats had a truncular vagotomy and Heineke von Mikulicz pyloroplasty. They were fed 4 mg/day *N*-methyl-*N'*-nitro-*N*-nitrosoguanidine (MNNG) diluted in their daily ration of water. Twenty-seven animals died before the first developed a palpable tumor after 377 days. Sixty-five served as unoperated controls, receiving the same amount of carcinogen. Sixteen died before the first developed a tumor after 476 days.

Results

Of the vagotomized animals 29 of 31 were tumor positive after a median time of $430\ {}^{+80}_{-35}$ days elapsed. They had received between 1016 and 2040 mg of MNNG. The mean dose was 1.8 g/animal. Once a tumor was palpable, the animals were sacrificed. They showed adenocarcinomas of the glandular part of the stomach, two had metastases. Other findings were liver cysts and a colon cancer. The effect of the vagotomy was examined by pH measurements 3 months after vagotomy showing pH values between 7 and 8.

In the control group, 37 of 49 surviving rats showed tumors after a minimal induction time of 476 days. They had received 2.2 g/animal for a mean time of $562 \begin{smallmatrix} +70 \\ -50 \end{smallmatrix}$ days. The maximal induction time was 695 days (Tables 1 and 2).

In the control group, more tumors showed in the duodenum and jejunum. There was no statistically significant difference in the distribution between the two groups.

Discussion

Vagotomy and pyloroplasty do not increase the number of gastric cancers after orally administered MNNG in the Wistar rat. Previous experiments by Kowalewski [6, 7, 8] show a higher number of cancers after using 2.7 diacetylaminofluorene in the vagotomized rat. Since he did not add a pyloroplasty, stasis could be an important factor. In our experiments, we ruled this out by radiological examinations.

Rumpf [9], using a similar experimental model as we used, found no increase in gastric cancer after vagotomy, but a higher incidence following gastric-resection.

Conclusion

These experiments may suggest that there is probably no danger of an increasing amount of gastric cancer following vagotomy and pyloroplasty. If this is applicable to man too, the fatal hazard of resection as operative treatment for peptic ulcer disease is ruled out by using vagotomy.

Table 1. Gastrointestinal tumors after MNNG

	Tumor	No tumor	%	t 50	D 50
Vagotomy + Pyloroplasty + MNNG	29	2	93.5	$430 \begin{smallmatrix} +80 \\ -35 \end{smallmatrix}$	$1.8\text{ g} \begin{smallmatrix} +0.2 \\ -0.1 \end{smallmatrix}$
MNNG (controls)	37	12	75.5	$562 \begin{smallmatrix} +70 \\ -50 \end{smallmatrix}$	$2.2\text{ g} \begin{smallmatrix} +0.2 \\ -0.1 \end{smallmatrix}$

Table 2. Distribution of gastrointestinal tumors after MNNG

	Glandular stomach Pylorus	Duodenum	Jejunum
Vagotomy + Pyloroplasty + MNNG	19 (54.3%)	13 (37.1%)	3 (8.6%)
MNNG (controls)	21 (48.8%)	16 (37.2%)	6 (13.9%)

References

1. Dahm, K., Werner, B.: Experimentelles Anastomosencarcinom. Ein Beitrag zur Pathogenese des Magenstumpfcarcinoms. Langenbecks Arch. Klin. Chir. *333,* 211 – 236 (1973)
2. Dahm, K., Werner, B.: Anastomosencarcinom im resezierten Magen der Ratte nach Gabe von N-Methyl-N′-nitro-N-nitrosoguanidin. Dtsch. Med. Wochenschr. *98*, 2486 – 2487 (1973)
3. Ivankovic, S.: Praenatale Carcinogenese. In: Handbuch d. allg. Pathologie. Berlin, Heidelberg, New York: Springer 1975
4. Junghanns, K.: Magenkrebs und Dünndarmtumoren. In: Standardisierte Krebsbehandlung. Berlin, Heidelberg, New York: Springer 1974
5. Junghanns, K.: Long-term survival in gastric carcinomia. In: Digestive surgery. Padova: Piccin Medical Books 1972
6. Kowalewski, K.: Relationship between vagotomy peptic ulcer and gastric adenocarcinoma in rats fed 2,7-Diacetylaminofluorene. Can. J. Surg. *16*, 210 – 217 (1973)
7. Morgenstern, L.: Vagotomy, gastroenterostomy and experimental gastric cancer. Arch. Surg. *96*, 920 – 923 (1968)
8. Morgenstern, L., Yamakawa, I. V., Seltzer, D.: Carcinoma of the gastric stump. Am. J. Surg. *125*, 29 – 38 (1973)
9. Rumpf, P., Schacht, U., Palomba, P., Kremer, K., Schmitz, H., Borchard, F.: Chemisch induzierte Karzinogenese des Rattenmagens nach Vagotomie und Resektion. Z. Gastroenterol. *16*, 85 – 94 (1970)

Susceptibility to Experimental Gastric Ulcer – Experimental Gastric Cancer, and Gastric Region

C. J. Pfeiffer

For many years, the relationship between gastric ulcer in humans and gastric cancer in humans, and the determinants which create susceptibility to ulcer or cancer have been debated. Although it is now generally recognized that most gastric carcinomas probably do not arise from previous chronic gastric ulcers, the common denominator frequently seen of intestinal metaplasia of the stomach, chronic atrophic gastritis, frequent localization in the distal stomach, parallel high incidence in some countries, etc. still present an intriguing question of association of these diseases. Since good animal models for both experimental gastric carcinoma [11], by means of chronic administration of *N*-methyl-*N'*-nitro-*N*-nitrosoguanidine (MNNG), and for chronic gastric ulcer now are available, this relationship soon may be elucidated. Furthermore, it has recently been demonstrated [7] that intestinal metaplasia of the animal stomach can now be reliably induced by at least one chemical carcinogen, thereby providing us with the tools to explore these important relationships.

The clinical experience of gastric anastomoses being susceptible, after many years, to gastric cancer [1, 4, 14], and analogous data on chemically induced esophageal strictures or chronic ulcerative disease of the large intestine, eventually undergoing malignant change, suggest that healed mucosal tissue is labile to such change. Experiments in rats [2] showing gastric anastomoses, especially of the Billroth Type II, as being susceptible to chemical carcinogens also support this concept. We have demonstrated in our laboratory that the margin of healing chronic gastric ulcers in rats induced by acetic acid contains cystic dilated glands similar to those shown in various premalignant conditions [9]. Japanese workers have shown similar results with other ulcer models. Kowalewski and his associates have shown in Canada [5] the enhancement of malignant transformation in rats of thermocautery-induced ulcer by 2,7 diacetylaminofluorene (2,7-DAAF). Vagotomy increased 2,7-DAAF tumors in the rat stomach in the Canadian study, and vagotomy increased 20-methylcholanthrene-induced adenocarcinomas in the rat stomach in American reports [6]. Other workers [13] in Japan (Ito and Nagayo) found that indometacine caused ulcers in the rat fundus, and the MNNG-induced tumors mostly in the antrum, but when these agents were given concurrently, adenocarcinomas appeared in the fundus. We are presently conducting experiments in Kyoto, Japan on the relationship of chronic antral ulcers and of chronic fundic ulcers in the rat, as induced by acetic acid, with MNNG-induced tumor development, and the role of hormones and NaCl ingestion [8]. Hopefully, these results will soon indicate the relationship between ulcer site versus susceptibility to malignant transformation. The fact that Takahashi et al.

[12] demonstrated that restraint-water immersion stress in rats promoted MNNG-induced stomach tumors in rats, and that surgery itself (especially, laparotomy) enhanced tumorigenicity of 3,4,9,10-dibenzpyrene in mice [3], suggests that many remote factors may alter the course of gastric cancer induction. Further, salt intake has been shown in humans to be a common factor in gastric ulcer, metaplasia, and gastric cancer [10]. It can therefore be anticipated that experimental manipulation of experimental ulcer and metaplasia will clarify gastric cancer pathogenesis. It will be useful if nonrodents are applied in such experiments as well as rats.

References

1. Dahm, K., DeHeer, K.: Cancer risk of the stomach resected for ulcer: The role of duodenogastric reflux. Z. Krebsforsch. *87*, 343 – 344 (1977)
2. Domellöf, L., Janunger, K. G.: The risk for gastric carcinoma after partial gastrectomy. Am. J. Surg. *134*, 581 – 584 (1977)
3. Gottfried, B., Molomut, N., Patti, J.: Effect of repeated surgical trauma on chemical carcinogenesis. Cancer Res. *21*, 658 – 660 (1961)
4. Hammer, E.: The localization of precancerous changes and carcinoma after previous gastric operation for benign condition. Acta Pathol. Microbiol. Scand. [A] *84*, 495 – 507 (1976)
5. Kowalewski, K., Todd, E. F.: Carcinogenic action of 2,7-diacetylaminofluorene on the stomach of rats with experimental gastric ulcer. Scand. J. Gastroenterol. *6*, 323 – 328 (1971)
6. Kowalewski, K.: Relationship between vagotomy, peptic ulcer and gastric adenocarcinoma in rats fed 2,7-diacetylaminofluorene. Can. J. Surg. *16*, 210 – 217 (1973)
7. Matsukura, N., Kawachi, T., Sasagima, K., Sano, T., Sugimura, T., Hirota, T.: Induction of intestinal metaplasia in the stomachs of rats by N-methyl-N′-nitro-N-nitrosoguanidine. J. Natl. Cancer Inst. *61*, 141 – 144 (1978)
8. Nagai, T., Tobe, T., Fujimura, M., Pfeiffer, C. J.: Effects of MNNG, cocarcinogenic factor sodium chloride, and gastrin on gastric ulcers induced by acetic acid: Observations on the healing processes of antral and fundic ulcers. Annual Meeting of Japanese Experimental Ulcer Conference, Kyoto, Dec. 1978
9. Okabe, S., Pfeiffer, C. J., Roth, J. L. A.: A method of producing penetrating gastric and duodenal ulcers in rats. Am. J. Dig. Dis. *16*, 277 – 284 (1971)
10. Stemmermann, G., Haenszel, W., Locke, F.: Epidemiologic pathology of gastric ulcer and gastric carcinoma among Japanese in Hawaii. J. Natl. Cancer Inst. *58*, 13 – 20 (1977)
11. Sugimura, T., Kawachi, T.: Experimental stomach cancer. Methods Cancer Res. *7*, 245 – 308 (1973)
12. Takahashi, A., Onoda, K., Kawashima, K., Kato, R., Omiro, Y., Ishidate, M.: Effect of stress on formation of stomach tumor in rats by N-methyl-N′-nitro-N-nitrosoguanidine. Gan. *61*, 295 – 296 (1970)
13. Takahashi, M., Shirai, T., Fukushima, S., Hahanouchi, M., Hirose, M., Ito, N.: Effect of fundic ulcers induced by iodoacetamide on development of gastric tumors in rats treated with N-methyl-N′-nitro-N-nitrosoguandine. Gan. *67*, 47 – 54 (1976)
14. Terjesen, T., Erichsen, H. G.: Carcinoma of the gastric stump after operation for benign gastroduodenal ulcer. Acta Chir. Scand. *142*, 256 – 260 (1976)

Summary: Experimental Gastric Cancer

The possibility of inducing gastric cancer in animals under suitable conditions with oral application of *N*-methyl-*N'*-nitro-*N*-nitrosoguanidine marks a decisive advance in experimental research. Carcinogenesis generally proceeds along ulcerous or adenomatous alterations of the gastric mucosa in this case. Most of the carcinomas thus induced are of the intestinal type. In accord with clinical findings, these cancers also do not develop from normal mucosa in experiments with animals. Experimental research leads to presume, that in this case, the gastric carcinoma also develops from associated mucosal lesions known in man. Chronic atrophic gastritis and epithelial dysplasias are considered to be preliminary stages. The chronic gastric ulcer induced in animal experiments is also more prone to malign transformation. The carcinogenesis can be accelerated by various alterations of the gastric mucosa. This indicates that carcinogenesis proceeds in two stages. Chronic damage to the gastric mucosa, even if it is not induced by a primarily carcinogenic substance, can aid the development of gastric cancer with a carcinogen.

Lymph node and organ metastases are rarely encountered in experimentally induced alterations. The pronounced malignancy of experimental tumors provides its own scale of problems as well. Since the carcinomas in question are, for the most part, highly differentiated, the definitive malignancy of the alterations can only be ascertained by the combination of several specific traits. Glandular proliferations with neoplastic similarities are in themselves no criteria of proof for malignancy, even if they descend beneath the serosa. Glands can thus be shifted up to the serosa by surgical manipulation and continue proliferating. This is particularly elucidated by experimental investigations concerning the development of cancer in the surgically treated stomach. It was possible to demonstrate that proliferating mucosal changes are a product of multiple factors. The proximity of different epithelial types alone, irrespective of the surgical method used, can have a proliferative effect on the gastric mucosa without the influence of a carcinogen. In accord with epidemiological data and clinical observations, the experimental findings also indicate a multifactorial etiology of carcinogenesis, whereby the various factors do not act singly, but rather in combination with each other. The experimental investigations thus exhibit the character of a relevant model for the better understanding of cancer in humans.

3 Precancerous Lesions of Gastric Cancer

Histology of Possible Precancerous Stages in the Stomach

E. Grundmann and W. Schlake

Precancerous changes have been divided into two groups: A *precancerous condition* is a generalized state associated with significantly increased risk of cancer; a *precancerous lesion* is a morphologically altered tissue in which cancer is more likely to occur than in its apparently normal counterpart. [Definition of a WHO-meeting (Can. 73.1)]. The present report includes only precancerous lesions. Regarding the broad spectrum of such lesions in the human stomach, nothing should be said here about the significance of atrophic gastritis as a possible precancerous condition, morphologically, nor shall the different types of polypoid lesions of the stomach, in general, be discussed. The problem of intestinal metaplasia being connected with a possibly increased risk of gastric carcinoma will be mentioned in view of the next paper (Correa, see p. 83).

Our interest should focus on the question, which histological changes in gastric mucosa – either in atrophic gastritis or in polypoid lesions or elsewhere – must be seen as indicators of precancerous conditions, i.e., as "Präkanzerose" (Hamperl [4]), in the strictest sense.

The practical point of our question relates to previously accumulated experience from other epithelial lesions, especially from squamous epithelium in the uterine cervix. For these tissues, classification into three different stages of dysplasia was internationally accepted. As a result, women showing these histological changes are now subjected to cytohistological monitoring at regular short intervals for effective control and prevention of actual carcinoma.

The term "dysplasia," adopted for squamous epithelium, is also gaining acceptance for glandular epithelia. The definition implies a high rate of reversibility of these changes, in analogy to squamous cell dysplasia. In the latter, it has been ascertained that some 50% of all dysplasias regress completely, some 30% remain stable for the whole life of the patient, and only 20% show progressive tendencies to malignancy during a certain period, varying between 2 months and 10 years. Only one-half of these (i.e., some 10% of the total) turn eventually into real carcinoma.

These rates will explain that a histological finding of dysplasia must be seen as nothing more than a risk factor which, in the stomach, will not be indicating resection, but only careful monitoring (Oehlert [8]).

Definition of Dysplasia

The main morphological features of precancerous nature are: cellular atypia, abnormal differentiation, and a disorganized mucosal architecture.

Cellular atypia is seen, principally, in every state of nontypical morphology. With regard to precancerous conditions, nuclear pleomorphism, including hyperchromasia, increased nucleocytoplasmic ratio, increasing cytoplasmic basophilia, and loss of cellular polarity may be the most important features.

Abnormal differentiation of gastric mucosa is manifested as follows: alteration or disappearance of secretory products from the gastric epithelium, and disappearance of differences between mucous cells, chief cells, and parietal cells. Intestinal metaplasia is a special type of abnormal differentiation which may turn into a possible precancerous structure with loss or reduction of goblet and Paneth cells in the metaplastic area.

Disorganized mucosal architecture is manifested by irregularity of crypt structures, back-to-back gland formation, and budding or branching of crypts, or, in some phases, by surface papillary growth.

In analogy to squamous epithelial dysplasia, gastric mucosal dysplasias are subdivided into four groups:

1) Inflammatory epithelial changes (this stage is, per definition, *not* a precancerous one).
2) Mild dysplasia.
3) Moderate dysplasia.
4) Severe dysplasia.

Histological Examples of the Different Dysplasias

1) Inflammatory epithelial changes (Fig. 1) are a regenerative reaction following more or less severe gastritis. Cellular atypias are few, abnormal differentiation does not exceed the picture of typical intestinal metaplasia, and mucosal architecture shows but very slight disturbance. These reactive changes are found in every chronic gastritis, but also in smaller or bigger polyps, or in the vicinity of gastric ulcers.
2) Mild dysplasia (Fig. 2) shows a shift in the nucleocytoplasmic ratio in favor of irregularly shaped, often hyperchromatic nuclei. Secretory vesicles are often visible. If there is intestinal metaplasia, the number of goblet and Paneth cells is somewhat reduced, and glandular architecture is generally irregular.
3) Moderate dysplasia (Fig. 3) shows an enhancement of the previous features. All the above changes are present, plus some areas where dark, spindle-shaped nuclei show a strong shift of nucleocytoplasmic ratio. Only isolated secretory vacuoles are found. In areas of intestinal metaplasia, reduction of goblet cells and Paneth cells is stronger, the disarray of mucosal architecture in gland tubules is more marked.
4) Severe dysplasia (Fig. 4) shows highly atypical nuclei with an even stronger shift of the nucleocytoplasmic ratio and severe nuclear pleomorphism: pitted nuclei, irregular granular or striated patterns, generalized hyperchromasia of nuclei, and no evidence of secretory vacuoles. If the condition was preceded by intestinal metaplasia, such areas show now complete loss of goblet cells and Paneth cells, and equally complete destruction of mucosal architecture. Normal glandular structures are seen in hazy outlines, they are replaced by less differentiated, actively proliferating cells.

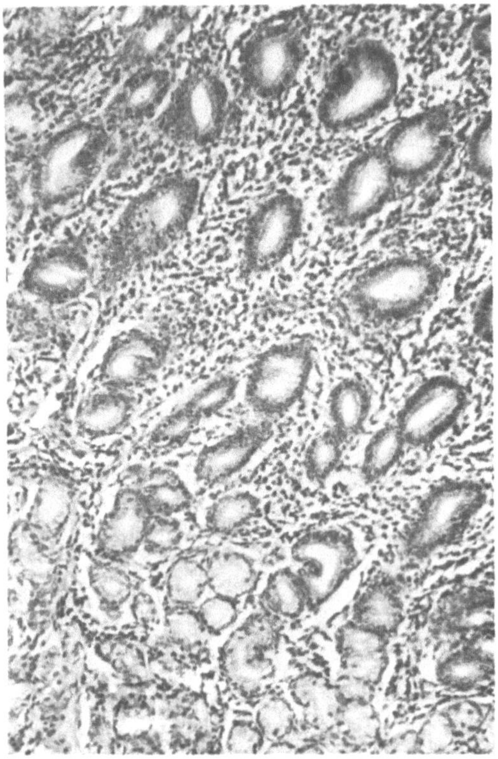

Fig. 1. Inflammatory epithelial changes in chronic gastritis, low-grade cellular atypia, slight disorders of mucosal architecture. (HE, × 150)

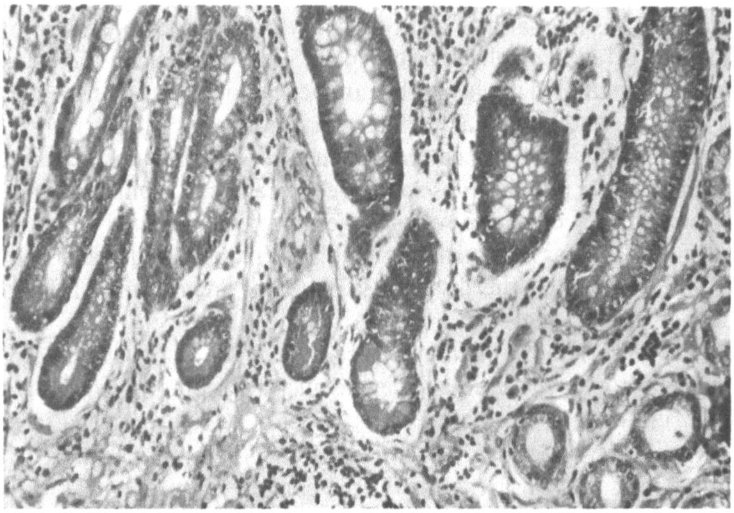

Fig. 2. Mild dysplasia in an area of intestinal metaplasia; shift of nucleocytoplasmic ratio, persisting secretory vesicles. (HE, × 150)

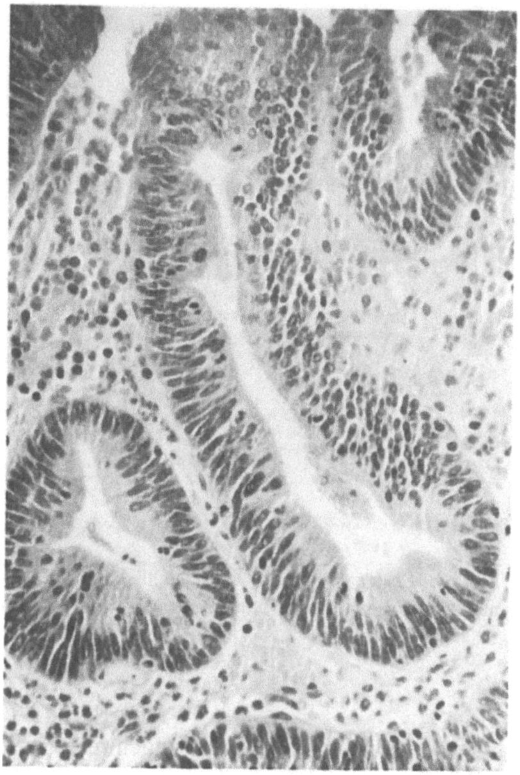

Fig. 3. Moderate dysplasia with highly hyperchromatic, often spindle-shaped nuclei, strong shift of nucleocytoplasmic ratio in favor of nuclei, heavy loss of secretory vacuoles, strongly disorganized mucosal architecture. (HE, × 150)

Compared with our previous definitions (Grundmann [2]) that had been adopted in some parts by Oehlert et al. [7, 8], the present definitions are more stricty delineated: certain changes that had been classified among mild dysplasias (see dysplasia I in Oehlert [8]) will now be evaluated as inflammatory reactive changes. Our present mild dysplasia corresponds, morpholoigically, to dysplasia II proposed by Oehlert [8] and, approximately, to Nagayo's "benign lesion with slight atypia" (Nagayo [6]). This author had described the many variations found in changes of the stage that we now call mild dysplasia.

Our moderate dysplasia corresponds to "severe dysplasia" as defined by Oehlert [8] and to the "borderline lesions" defined by Nagayo [6]. The most characteristic features are the dark-staining nuclei and their elongated shape and stratification which results, in some places, in palisade arrangements (Fig. 3).

The changes that we now call severe dysplasia had been defined as "probably carcinoma" by Nagayo [6]. Judging from our own observations, this condition may persist over a long time and even completely regress in some cases.

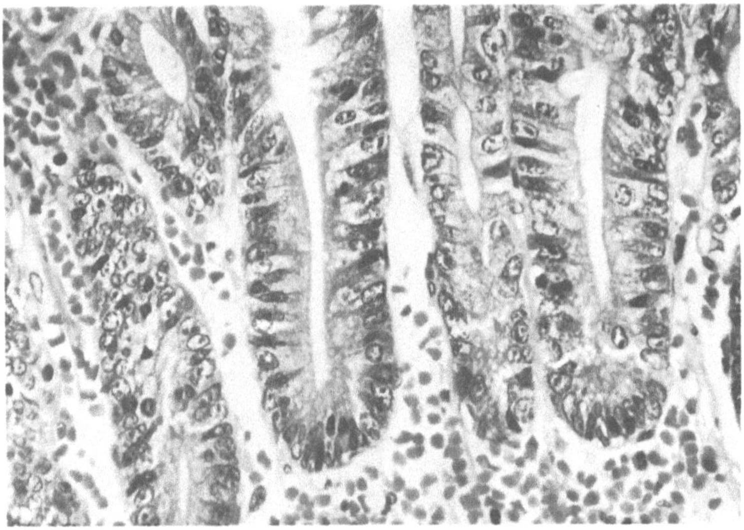

Fig. 4. Severe dysplasia with highly atypical nuclei, strong variations of nucleocytoplasmic ratio, marked nuclear pleomorphism and hyperchromasia. (HE, × 350)

In rats, after Billroth I stomach resection, enhanced by additional exposure to MNNG, certain histological changes were located in and near the anastomosed tissues, which were largely consistent with the degrees of dysplasia found in human stomachs (Fig. 5a, b). Under experimental conditions, these dysplastic changes are obligatory prestages of gastric carcinoma of the intestinal type [9].

Further proof for the precancerous nature of dysplasias is found in the occurrence of all described forms of dysplasia, in the vicinity of gastric carcinoma, particularly often near early gastric cancers.

An equally striking, though rare observation was that of some early gastric cancers that were limited to the upper layers of the mucosa. These are genuine intramucosal carcinomas (Versé [11]), i.e., early stages of early gastric cancer Beside and especially below these surface carcinomatous lesions, we regularly found evidence of severe dysplasia (Fig. 6), which suggested a direct analogy to squamous epithelial changes, where severe dysplasia may turn slowly or suddenly into carcinoma in situ.

However, the term "carcinoma-in-situ", per definition, a growth in a given tissue structure *instead* of normal cells, appears inappropriate in gastric mucosa and should not be adopted. As an example, the changes demonstrated in Fig. 6 must be seen as an actually carcinomatous growth penetrating the epithelial basement membrane of the glands and infiltrating the mucosal lamina propria.

So far, the dysplasias discussed here were all seen as possible precursors of intestinal type gastric carcinoma. However, advanced as well as early gastric carcinomas occur not only as intestinal type cancers, but also as diffuse type (classification by Laurén [5]). According to our own studies, this diffuse type

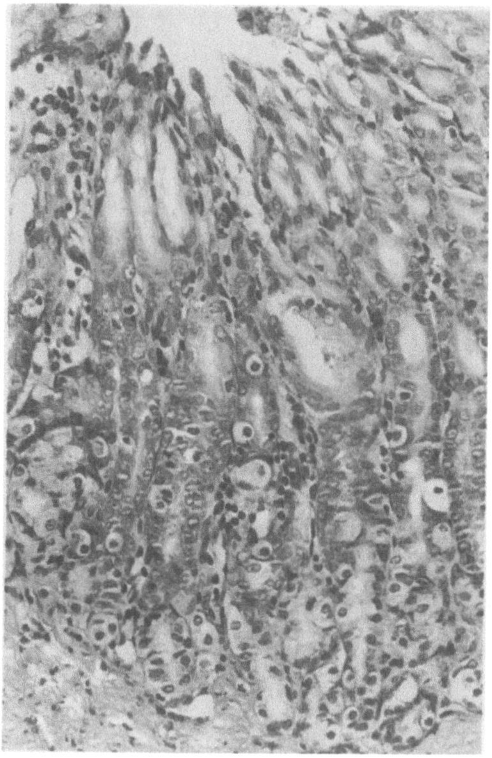

Fig. 5a. Mild dysplasia in rat stomach; area of gastric stump after Billroth I resection and MNNG administration. (HE, × 288)

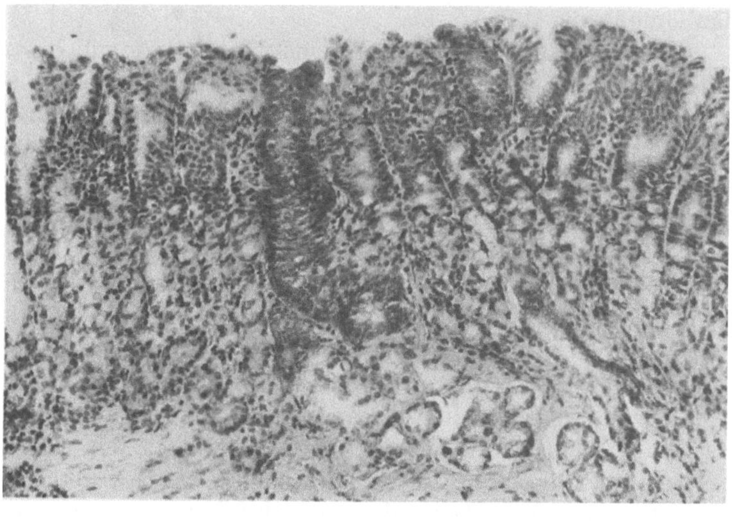

Fig. 5b. Moderate dysplasia in gland tubule of rat stomach, area near Billroth I resection after MNNG. (HE, autoradiogram, × 184)

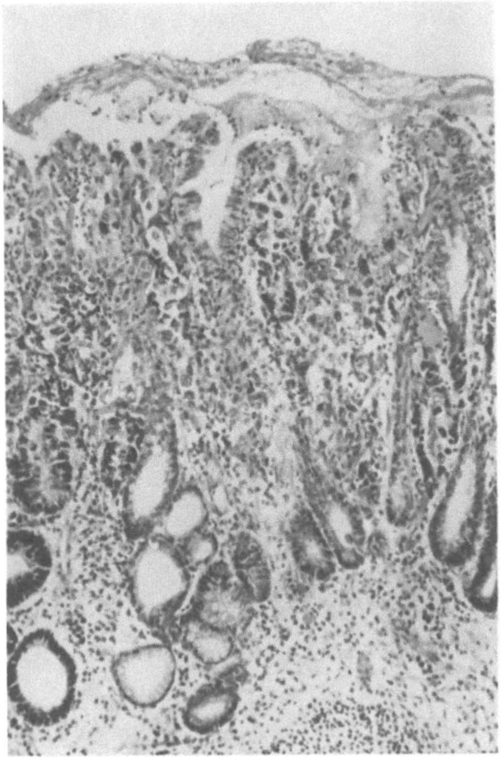

Fig. 6. Superficial mucosal (intramucosal) carcinoma of intestinal type; severe dysplasia below this lesion. (HE, × 150)

needs a subclassification into a signet ring cell type and an anaplastic type, including early gastric cancer (see Grundmann [3]). The coexistence of several histological types side by side in one early gastric cancer is a not an unfrequent finding; we prefer to call this picture a "mixed type early gastric cancer" (Schlake and Grundmann [10]).

A possible, minute form of signet ring cell carcinoma is seen in the "dripping" of single signet ring cells from the lower part of gland necks (Grundmann [1]). The earliest manifestation of anaplastic mucosal carcinoma was described as a "glandular neck dysplasia" in the antrum (Grundmann [2]). In both these very early subtypes of diffuse early gastric cancer, the most striking feature is that transformation of dysplastic into carcinomatous epithelium does always occur in the gland neck area.

Two additional cases may illustrate this observation: Fig. 7a shows a sector of gastric mucosa with superficial evidence of necrosis and fibrin. Immediately below this necrotic zone, dysplastic gland tubules are seen with mild dysplasia. Close to these, we observe strikingly clear vesicular cells. The architecture of gland tubules appears almost completely suppressed, some typical signet ring cells are present (Fig. 7b). These conditions must be interpreted as minute forms of signet ring cell carcinoma arising from mild dysplasia in the gland neck zone.

That anaplastic, early gastric cancer also develops from the gland neck area, may be illustrated by the second case: anaplastic early gastric cancer is limited to the area between gland necks and the mucosal surface. The mucosal carcinoma

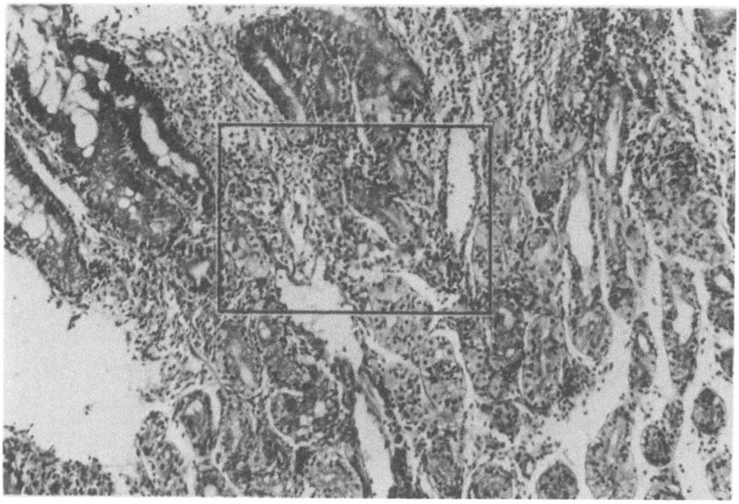

Fig. 7a. Gastric mucosa with mild dysplasia (*top: left*) and transition to minute form of early signet ring cell carcinoma (*center*). (HE, × 150)

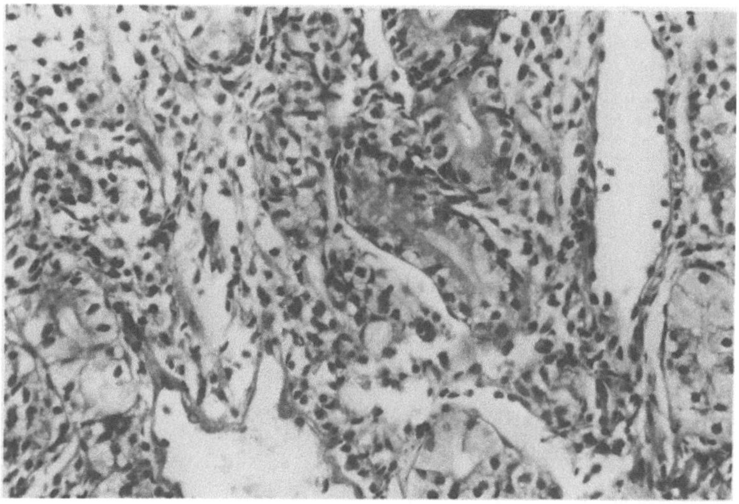

Fig. 7b. Insert of 7a: Minute form of signet ring cell early gastric cancer in the vicinity of mild intestinal metaplasia. Signet ring cell carcinoma arises from gland neck area. (HE, × 350)

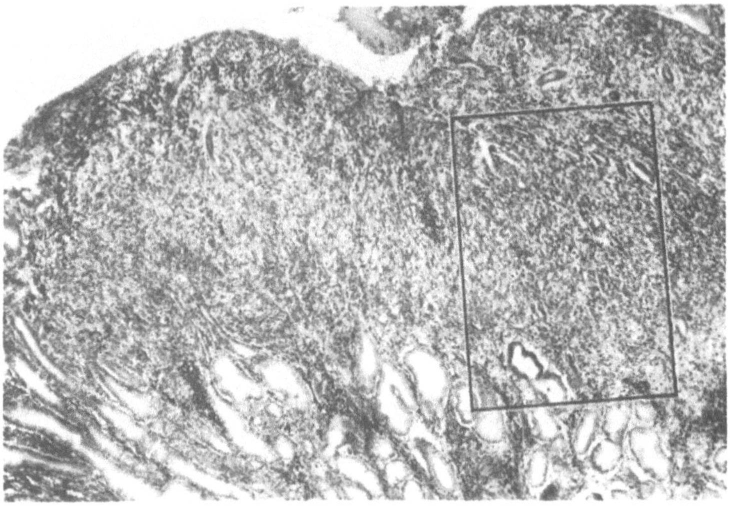

Fig. 8a. Anaplastic surface early gastric cancer developing from gland necks; superficial ulceration. (HE, × 150)

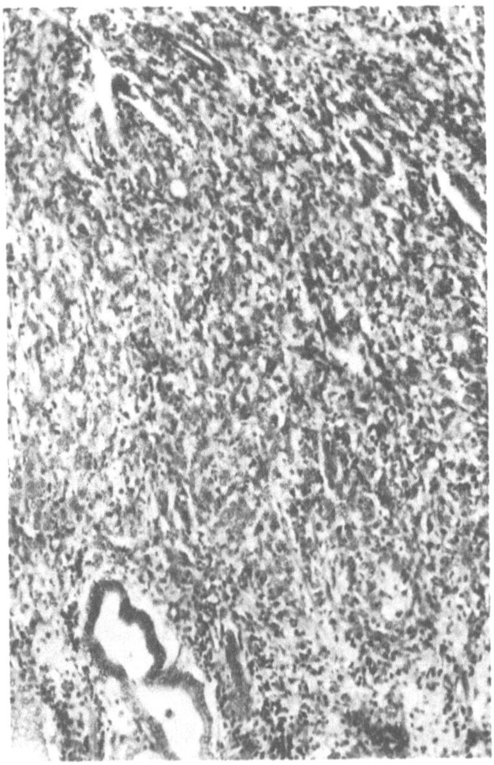

Fig. 8b. Insert of 8a: mild basal dysplasia of a gland tubule. (HE, × 350)

obviously did arise in the circumscribed area of gland necks to grow subsequently towards the lumen. This early gastric cancer also shows ulceration at its surface. In higher magnification (Fig. 8a, b), dysplastic gland tubules are again visible in the neighborhood of the anaplastic carcinoma (Fig. 8b, *bottom*).

Summary

In analogy to findings in other epithelial tissues, some possible precancerous lesions found in gastric mucosa are defined as dysplasia. They are divided into the three degrees of mild, moderate, and severe dysplasia, which are readily distinguished from nonprecancerous inflammatory, reactive changes of the epithelium.

Dysplasias are often found in the neighborhood of early gastric cancer as well as in superficial mucosal cancers of the stomach. They are situated either immediately bordering early gastric cancer lesions, or showing fluid transitions to the latter. These properties closely resemble those of squamous epithelial dysplasia. Early or minute forms of signet ring cell carcinoma and anaplastic carcinoma are found exclusively in the region of gland necks. Recent experiences suggest that particular attention should focus on these regions when one is looking for lesions which actually precede signet ring cell carcinoma and anaplastic carcinoma.

Analogous manifestations of dysplasia are found in the gastric stump of rats after Billroth I resection, with increasing frequency after additional administration of MNNG. According to our present knowledge, dysplasia of the human gastric mucosa should be interpreted as a possible precancerous lesion which presents no indication for stomach resection. It is only the genuine, early intramucosal carcinoma, limited to the interior layers of the mucosa, which must be seen as a fully developed carcinoma and should be subjected to adequate surgical intervention. Correct definition and visualization of dysplasia is an indispensable prerequisite for classifying those patients in appropriate risk groups.

References

1. Grundmann, E.: Histologie und Histogenese des Magenfrühkarzinoms. Therapiewoche *24*, 3824–3831 (1974)
2. Grundmann, E.: Histologic types and possible initial stages in early gastric carcinoma. Beitr. Pathol. *154*, 256–280 (1975)
3. Grundmann, E.: Early gastric cancer – today. Pathol. Res. Pract. *162*, 347–360 (1978)
4. Hamperl, H.: Präcancerose und Carcinoma in situ. In: Handbuch der Allgemeinen Pathologie. Vol. VI/5, p. 351–415. Berlin, Heidelberg, New York: Springer 1974
5. Lauren, P.: The two histological main types of gastric carcinoma: diffuse and so-called intestinal type carcinoma. An attempt at histo-clinical classification. Acta Pathol. Microbiol. Scand. *64*, 31–49 (1965)
6. Nagayo, T.: Histological diagnosis of biopsied gastric mucosae with special reference to that of borderline lesions. Gann Monogr. Cancer Res. *11*, 245–256 (1971)
7. Oehlert, W., Keller, P., Henke, M., Strauch, M.: Die Dysplasien der Magenschleimhaut und ihre klinische Relevanz. Dtsch. Med. Wochenschr. *100*, 1950–1956 (1975)

8. Oehlert, W.: Klinische Pathologie des Magen-Darm-Traktes. Stuttgart, New York: Schattauer 1978
9. Schlake, W.: Experimentelle Studien zur Histogenese des Karzinoms im Billroth-I-operierten Drüsenmagen der Ratte. Ph. D. Dissertation University of Münster 1978
10. Schlake, W., Grundmann, E.: Multifocal early gastric cancer of mixed type. Pathol. Res. Pract. *164* 331 – 341 (1979)
11. Versé, E.: Über die Entstehung, den Bau und das Wachstum der Polypen, Adenome und Karzinome des Magen-Darm-Kanals. Arb. Pathol. Inst. *1*, 1 – 40 (1908)

Dysplastic Changes in Intestinal Metaplasia of the Gastric Mucosa*

C. Cuello and P. Correa

The role of intestinal metaplasia as a precursor of the intestinal type of gastric cancer has received support from multiple fronts. Bonne and collaborators reported in 1938 that Chinese immigrants to Java had a high frequency of gastric cancer and high prevalence of "goblet-cell metaplasia" while both lesions were rare in the local natives [1]. Jarvi and Lauren in 1951 reported that the majority of gastric cancers originated in islands of intestinal epithelium [10]. Morson in 1955 documented the origin of small gastric carcinomas in areas of metaplasia [12]. Similar findings were reported in Japan by Nagayo [14]. Metaplasia has been induced with carcinogens in experimental animals [5, 11]. Studies of internal migration in Colombia have shown positive correlation between the prevalence of metaplasia in autopsies and the incidence of carcinoma [2]. Metaplasia is more frequent in Japan than in the United States [9]. Patients with metaplasia have about ten times greater risk of carcinoma than people with negative gastric biopsies [13].

A description of the dysplastic changes in stomachs with metaplasia is given here, based on our experience in the region of Nariño, Colombia, where gastric cancer frequency is extremely high [3].

Materials, Methods, and Results

Gastric biopsies (two from antrum and two from body) were performed in patients consulting for gastrointestinal symptoms in Nariño. The tissue was immediately fixed in 10% buffered formalin and brought to the Department of Pathology of the Universidad del Valle Mecial School in Cali for embedding, sectioning, and staining with hematoxylin eosin, PAS, and Alcian blue. Each biopsy was classified as: normal, superficial gastritis, or chronic atrophic gastritis with or without intestinal metaplasia, following previously published criteria [3]. The metaplastic and dysplastic changes were classified as follows:

Mature intestinal metaplasia: The glands are straight, short, tubular crypts of regular size and shape mostly occupied by alternating absorptive and goblet cells with large vacuoles of regular size (Figs. 1 and 2). Paneth and undifferentiated cells are seen at the bottom of the crypts. There is a well-developed brush border. The nuclei are small and round at the bottom of the crypts with some mitoses. The nucleoli are inconspicuous or absent. The lamina propria shows variable

* Work supported by contracts NO1-CP-53521 and NO1-CP-33286

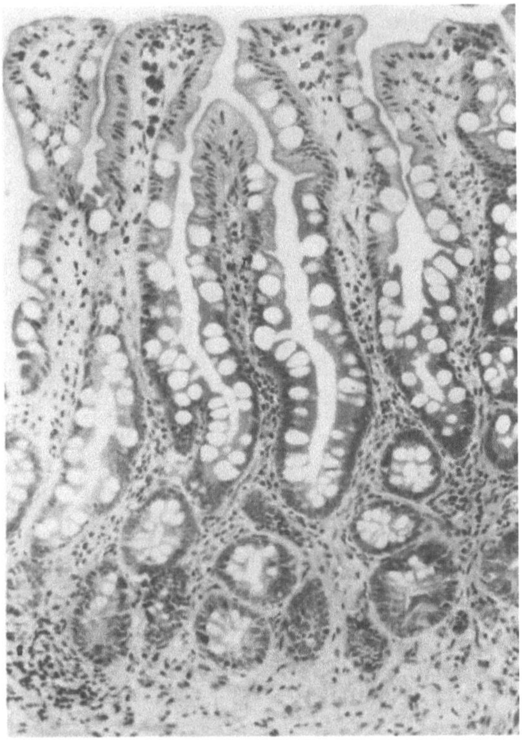

Fig. 1. Mature intestinal metaplasia. (HE, × 136)

amounts of lymphocytes and plasma cells. The affected mucosa is considerably thinner than the normal gastric mucosa.

Hyperplastic dysplasia, mild: The glands are of different size and shape with occasional cystic changes and branching (Figs. 3 and 4). An ill-defined brush border may be found. The epithelium shows a predominance of tall columnar cells with secretory microvesicles in the upper part of the cytoplasm. Goblet and Paneth cells are sparce and irregularly located. There is striking variability in the size of goblet cells. The nuclei are elongated, ovoid, hyperchromatic, and variable in size. A moderate number of mitoses is found. The nucleocytoplastic ratio is higher than in mature metaplasia. Pseudostratification is more prominent. A few nuclei surpass the basal half of the cell. The nucleoli are inconspicuous.

Hyperplastic dysplasia, severe: The architecture of the glands is the same as in the mild type, but the disarrangement ist more evident. The brush borders is ill-defined. The epithelial cells show a predominance of large cuboidal or low columnar cells. The nuclei are large, hyperchromatic or clear, oval, or round, located at the center of the cells. In some cases, pseudostratification is marked and some nuclei reach the surface of the cell. The nucleocytoplasmic ratio is markedly elevated. There is an increased number of mitoses and the nucleoli are enlarged (Fig. 5).

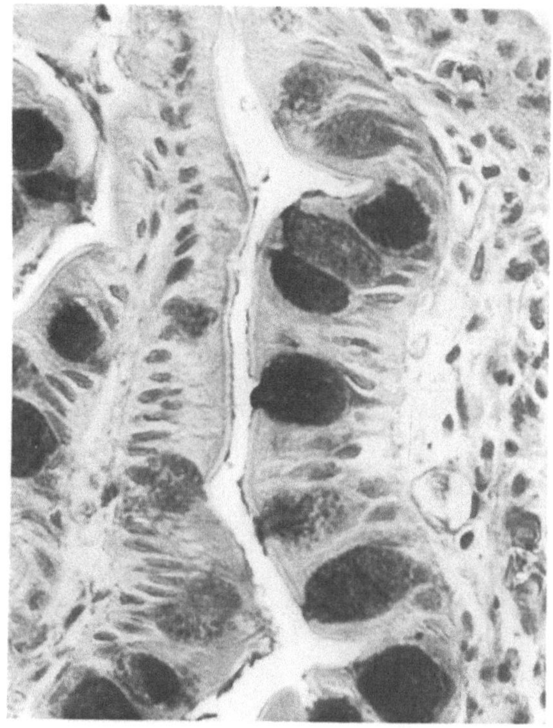

Fig. 2. Alcian blue stain of mature intestinal metaplasia demonstrating large goblets and well-defined brush border (HE, × 272)

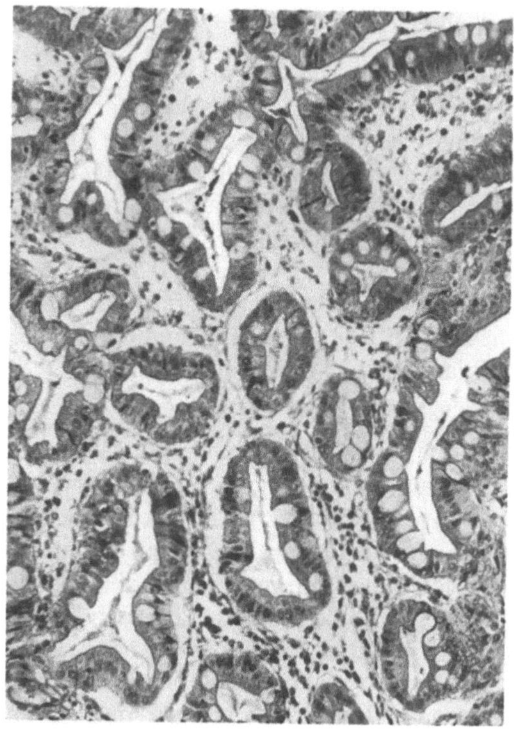

Fig. 3. Hyperplastic dysplasia, mild. (HE, × 168)

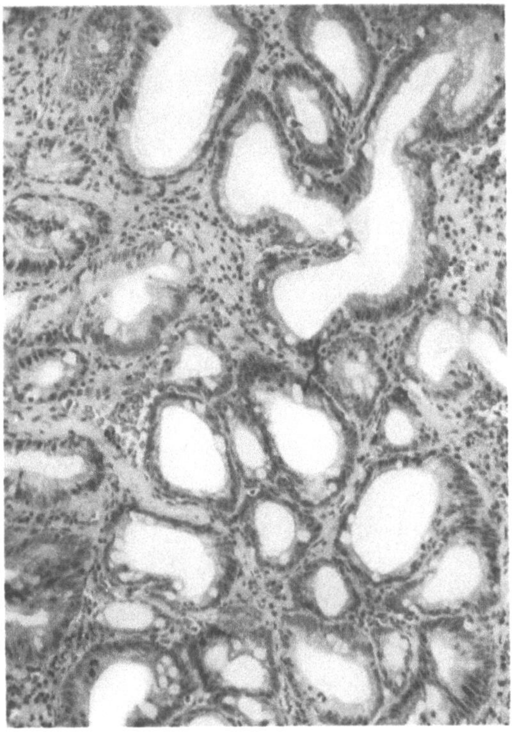

Fig. 4. Hyperplastic dysplasia, mild. (HE, × 168)

Adenomatous dysplasia, mild: This is characterized by a crowded proliferation of newly formed glands of regular tubular pattern, morphologically similar to the tubular adenoma of the large bowel (Fig. 6). The brush border is ill-defined. The epithelial cells are mostly of the tall columnar absorptive type with deeply eosinophilic cytoplasma. Scarce goblet and Paneth cells are irregularly distributed in the glands. Goblets of different size are present, with predominance of small droplets. The nuclei are elongated, hyperchromatic, and piled up, with prominent pseudostratification. Few nuclei reach the upper half of the cell. There is a moderate number of mitoses. The nucleocytoplasmic ratio is high and the nucleoli are inconspicuous.

Adenomatous dysplasia, severe: The same pattern of glandular architecture as in the mild type is seen, but dilatation of some tubules and simple branching are usually present (Figs. 7 and 8). The epithelial cells are similar to those of the mild type. Elongated, rod-shaped hyperchromatic nuclei of irregular size are seen. Pseudostratification is very striking with many nuclei reaching the cell surface. Mitoses are very frequent. The nucleocytoplasmic ratio is elevated. The nucleoli are inconspicuous. The lamina propria is less abundant because of the closely packed tubular proliferation.

Table 1 shows the diagnosis made in 123 biopsies, by age and sex. All males had some abnormality in their mucosa and only four females had normal mucosa. Simple atrophic gastritis was frequent in both sexes. Dysplastic

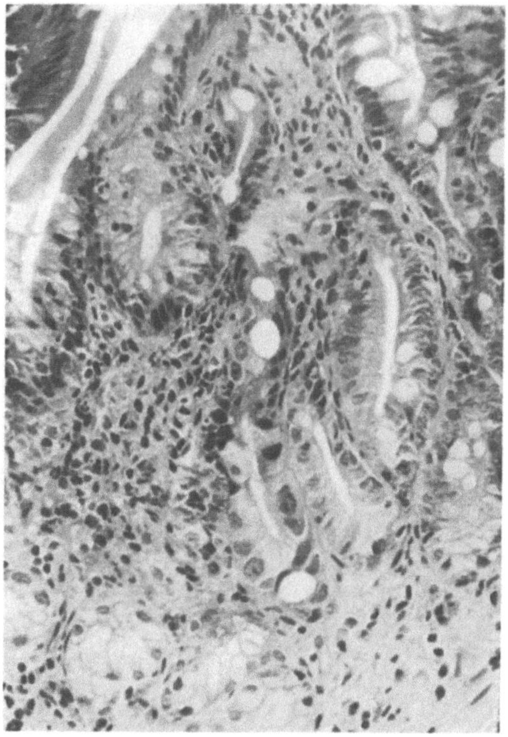

Fig. 5. Hyperplastic dysplasia, severe. (HE, × 208)

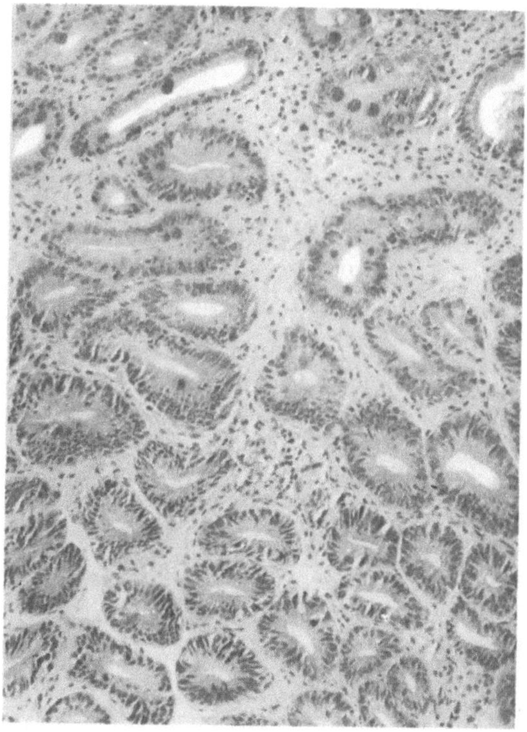

Fig. 6. Adenomatous dysplasia, mild. Alcian-blue stained irregular goblets (HE, × 136)

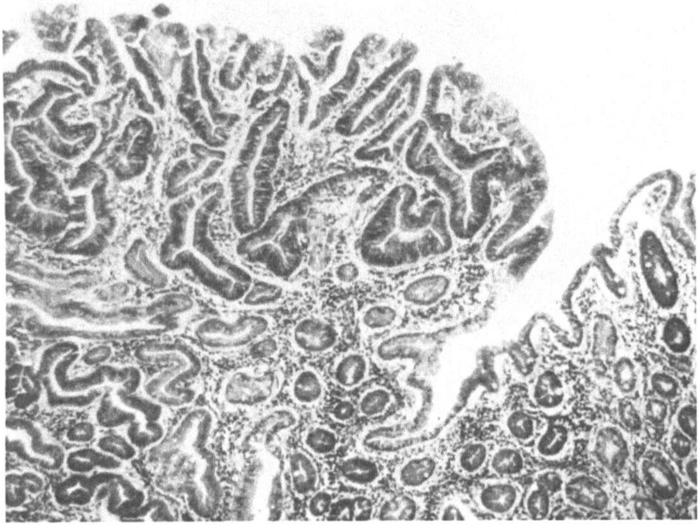

Fig. 7. Adenomatous dysplasia, severe. (HE, × 112)

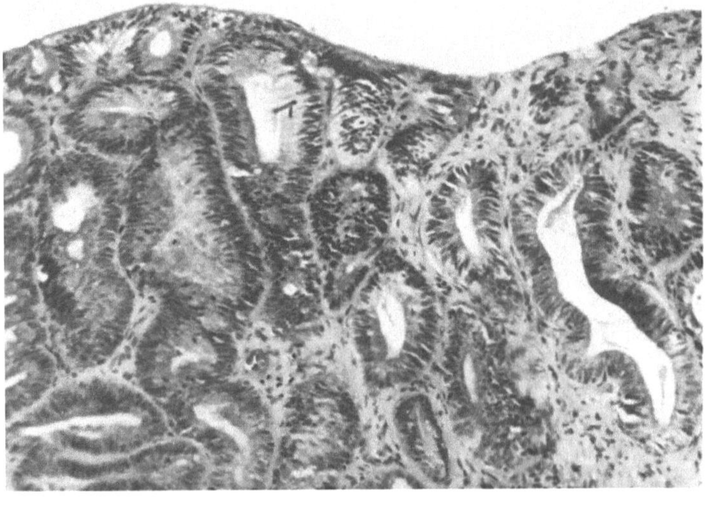

Fig. 8. Adenomatous dysplasia, severe. (HE, × 136)

Table 1. Prevalence of lesions by sex and age group

Age	*No. Cases*	*Normal*	*Superficial Gastritis*	*Chronic Atrophic Gastritis*		
				Simple	*MIM*	*DM*
		%	%	%	%	%
Males						
≤49	45	0	6.7	35.5	28.9	28.9
≥50	31	0	9.7	16.1	29.0	45.2
All ages	76	0	7.9	27.6	28.9	35.5
Females						
≤49	35	11.4	0	40.0	34.3	14.3
≥50	12	0	0	41.7	25.0	33.3
All ages	47	8.5	0	40.4	31.9	19.1

MIM = Mature Intestinal Metaplasia
DM = Dysplastic Metaplasia

metaplasia increased significantly with age, resulting in an apparent relative decrease with age for simple atrophic gastritis in males and mature metaplasia in females. The prevalence of dysplastic metaplasia is markedly higher in males than in females.

Discussion

The description and classification of lesions just offered differs somewhat from other classifications of gastric dysplasias published by Japanese and German investigators [7, 15, 16]. The differences, however, are more apparent than real. Some classifications are based on the study of the gastric mucosa surrounding overt neoplasms, especially small tumors. In such circumstances, there may be an over-representation of the more advanced atypias. Our material is from patients without gastric cancer, but belonging to a population where such a disease is very frequent. This provides a more broad variety of typical lesions, from mild to severe. We hope that the description of this spectrum of lesions will be useful to the practicing pathologist in his attempt to determine the degree of gastric dysplasias in a particular patient.

Our interpretation is that intestinal metaplasia appears first as multiple foci in a background of chronic atrophic gastritis. All the morphological evidence points to the fact that the dysplastic changes appear in glands that are already metaplastic. It seems, therefore, that there is a continuum of morphological changes from atrophic gastritis to metaplasia to dysplasia and finally to neoplasia. There is abundant epidemiologic and experimental evidence to support the view that these changes are of environmental origin. We should, therefore, abandon the concept that these lesions represent "heterotopias" originating in misplaced embryonic rests.

Obviously, not all cases progress to neoplasia. This may be because the persons die of other diseases (competing risks) before neoplasia has a chance to develop. It has been estimated, on the basis of cellular kinetic studies, that the preinvasive changes take about 24 years to develop [6]. The possibility that the dysplastic changes could be reversed either spontaneously or through such drugs as retinoid acid should be considered and explored. The experimental models now available provide an opportunity for such tests [11].

It should be noted that in some cases of gastric carcinoma none of the above described dysplastic changes are observed. Such carcinomas are usually of the "diffuse" type in which genetic predisposition seems to play a bigger role [2]. Diffuse carcinomas are expected to become relatively more frequent when a general decline in the incidence rate of gastric cancer has occurred, as observed in many Western societies at the present time.

References

1. Bonne, C., Hartz, Ph. H., Klerks, J. V., Posthuma, J. H. , Radsma, W., Tjokreonegoro, S.: Morphology of the stomach and gastric secretion in Malays and Chinese and the different incidence of gastric ulcer and cancer in these races. Am. J. Cancer *33*, 265–279 (1938)
2. Correa, P., Cuello, C., Duque, E.: Carcinoma and intestinal metaplasia of the stomach in Colombian migrants. J. Natl. Cancer Inst. *44*, 297–306 (1970)
3. Correa, P., Cuello, C., Duque, E., Burbano, L. C., García, F. T., Bolanos, O., Brown, C., Haenszel, W.: Gastric cancer in Colombia. III. Natural history of precursor lesions. J. Natl. Cancer Inst. *57*, 1027–1035 (1976)
4. Cuello, C., Correa, P., Haenszel, W., Gordillo, G., Brown, C., Archer, M., Tannenbaum, S.: Gastric cancer in Colombia. I. Cancer risk and suspect environmental agents. J. Natl. Cancer Inst. *57*, 1015–1020 (1976)
5. Feit, J., Svejda, M., Sochorová, M.: Experimental intestinal metaplasia of gastric mucosa of rats and its relationship to carcinoma. Neoplasma *14*, 285–290 (1967)
6. Fujita, S., Hattori, T.: Cell proliferation, differentiation, and migration in the gastric mucosa. In: Pathophysiology of carcinogenesis in digestive organs. Farber, E. et al. (eds.), pp. 21–36. Tokyo: University Press 1977
7. Grundmann, E.: Histologic types and possible initial stages in early gastric carcinoma. Beitr. Pathol. *154*, 256–280 (1975)
8. Haenszel, W., Correa, P., Cuello, C., Guzman, N., Burbano, L. C., Lores, H., Muñoz, J.: Gastric cancer in Colombia. II. Case-control epidemiology study of precursor lesions. J. Natl. Cancer Inst. *57*, 1021–1026 (1976)
9. Imai, T., Kubo, T., Watanahe, H.: Chronic gastritis in Japanese with reference to high incidence of gastric carcinoma. J. Natl. Cancer Inst. *47*, 179–196 (1971)
10. Jarvi, O., Lauren, P.: On the role of heterotopias of the intestinal epithelium in the pathogenesis of gastric cancer. Acta Pathol. Microbiol. Scand. *29*, 26–43 (1951)
11. Matsukura, N., Kawachi, T., Sasajima, K., Sugimura, T., Hirota, T.: Induction of intestinal metaplasia in the stomachs of rats by MNNG. J. Natl. Cancer Inst. *61*, 141–144 (1978)
12. Morson, B. C.: Carcinoma arising from areas of intestinal metaplasia in the gastric mucosa. Br. J. Cancer *9*, 377–385 (1955)
13. Muñoz, N., Matko, I.: Histologic types of gastric cancer and its relationship with intestinal metaplasia. Recent Results Cancer Res. *39*, 99–105 (1972)
14. Nagayo, T.: Histological diagnosis of biopsied gastric mucosa with reference to that of borderline lesions. In: Early Gastric Cancer, pp. 245–256. Baltimore, Tokyo: University Park Press 1972
15. Nagayo, T., Komagoe, T.: Histological studies of gastric mucosal cancer with special reference to relationship of histological pictures between the mucosal cancer and the cancer-bearing gastric mucosa. Gan *52*, 109–119 (1961)
16. Sugano, H., Nakamura, K., Tagaki, K.: An atypical epithelium of the stomach. In: Early Gastric Cancer, pp. 257–269. Baltimore, Tokyo: University Park Press 1972

Biological Significance of Dysplasias of the Epithelium and of Atrophic Gastritis

W. Oehlert

Systematic investigations on resected specimens carried out by Büchner [1] and Konjetzny [15, 16] during the 1920s and 1930s, have proved that particular cellular alterations occur very regularly in the vicinity of carcinomas of the stomach, and that these may be regarded as forming the earlier stages. This assumption of the earlier investigators was confirmed by findings obtained by light and electron microscopic examinations from different stages of the experimental carcinogenesis of the stomach in the rat and in the dog [13, 33]. These changes of the gastric mucosa are now commonly recognized as precancerous lesions. The definition of precancerous lesions covers alterations like chronic gastritis accompanied by mucosal atrophy and intestinal metaplasia. It also refers, however, to advanced processes of dedifferentiation of the gastric mucosa, as for example the borderline lesion [20], a proliferation of the glandular neck cells associated with atypical forms [9], the different varieties of dysplasia [11, 24, 20] and the carcinoma of the surface or intra-epithelial carcinoma [19, 28] or the carcinoma in situ, respectively [3]. From the scientific point of view, it might be interesting to find out whether these changes of the gastric mucosa within the resected specimens of the stomach are to be defined as facultative or obligatory precancerous lesions, but this is of no consequence to the treatment of the individual patient. The situation is quite different when the pathologist has to define similar alterations which have been detected in biopsy specimens. Should the investigator observe a change, which in his opinion is irreversible and will definitely lead to a fully developed carcinoma within a measurable period of time, he would be advised to give a detailed description to the clinician and suggest the removal of the affected stomach surgically. If, however, he believes that the particular form of "precancerous lesion" observed by him is still reversible, or if he is not able to decide on its further development, he may insist on additional investigation of this specimen. It could, however, be of assistance to the pathologist, if his decisions were supported by certain criteria which have been obtained from a sufficient number of long-term investigations which would allow him to make decisions on the further development of cellular changes. By making investigations which were regularly controlled over a period of 3 years, we were in a position to demonstrate that even severe dysplasias of the epithelium, which are histologically identical with intra-epithelial carcinomas or surface carcinomas, as defined by other authors [19, 28], and which resemble in every respect the borderline lesions described by Nagayo, are reversible in more than 50% of cases, and may remain unchanged for a period of many years in more than 30%. In contrast to this, Elster [9] holds the view that the borderline lesion is an irreversible process, which will definitely develop into a carcinoma.

Because of the uncertainty in judging alterations of the mucosa which precede the carcinoma of the stomach, Nagayo [22] suggested separating precancerous conditions from precancerous changes.

Precancerous lesions (Fig. 1) include adenomatous polyps, chronic gastritis accompanied by atrophy, intestinal metaplasia, and chronic gastric ulcer. If, in addition to these changes, an excessive cell proliferation, a cellular dedifferentiation accompanied by an enlargement of the proliferation area and an increase of the nuclear size, beside a disturbed nucleus-plasma ratio and a decrease of the mucus production occur, the precancerous change will develop into a precancerous condition. These precancerous changes should include our definition of dysplasia type III (Figs. 2 and 3), dysplasia type IV as defined by Ming, severe dysplasia described by Grundmann, Nagayo's borderline lesion as well as the neck cell proliferation accompanied by atypical nuclei defined by Elster. When taking the histological and cytological characteristics of these precancerous changes into consideration, one may assume that the precancerous condition will develop in a manner as shown in Fig. 4. As with the development of cancer in other tissues, we must assume that the almost entirely unknown and unobserved initial carcinogenic agent, which cannot yet be detected by the methods of investigation at our diposal, will eventually be revealed by the cocarcinogenic events, the most important being excessive cell proliferation. Because of the uncontrolled new formation of cells accompanied by a correspondingly shortened duration of life time of the epithelia of the surface, the closely related cellular dedifferentiation results in a loss of mucus secretion which in turn maintains the excessive new formation of cells following the alteration of the epithelium of the surface. This vicious circle ends up in the formation of the precancerous change with its varying definitions, such as dysplasia or borderline lesion. All the theoretical considerations and speculations so far available concerning the correctness of a particular definition take us no further from the point of view of clinical pathology, or observations made under the microscope, so long as we possess no more exact knowledge about the timing of the events of the changes. Even the application of transmission electron microscopy, screening electron microscopy, or the use of histochemical, cytochemical, and autoradiographic methods in the individual case will not allow us to decide whether these

Precancerous condition	+	Abnormal cellular proliferation Cellular dedifferentiation	=	Precancerous change
Adenomatous polyp Chron. atroph. gastritis Intestinal metaplasia Chronic ulcer		Enlargement of proliferation zone Increase of nuclear size Loss of mucus production		Dysplasia Type III (Oehlert) Dysplasia Typ IV (Ming) Borderline lesion (Nagayo) Neck cell proliferation (Elster)

Fig. 1. The formation of precancerous changes within precancerous conditions

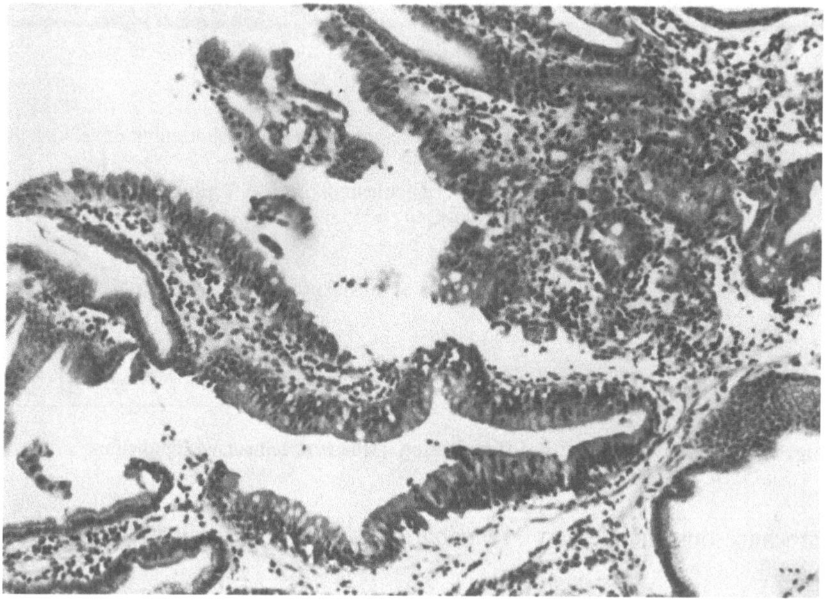

Fig. 2. Dysplasia type II, showing polypous changes within the area of anastomosis of a stomach after Billroth II resection for gastric ulcer, 12 years following operation. (HE, × 100)

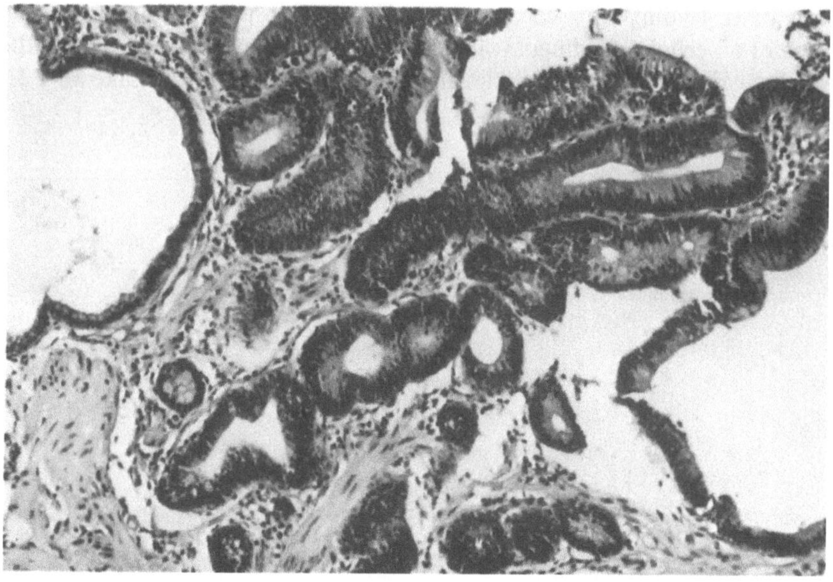

Fig. 3. Dysplasia type III with chronic atrophic gastritis (HE, × 100)

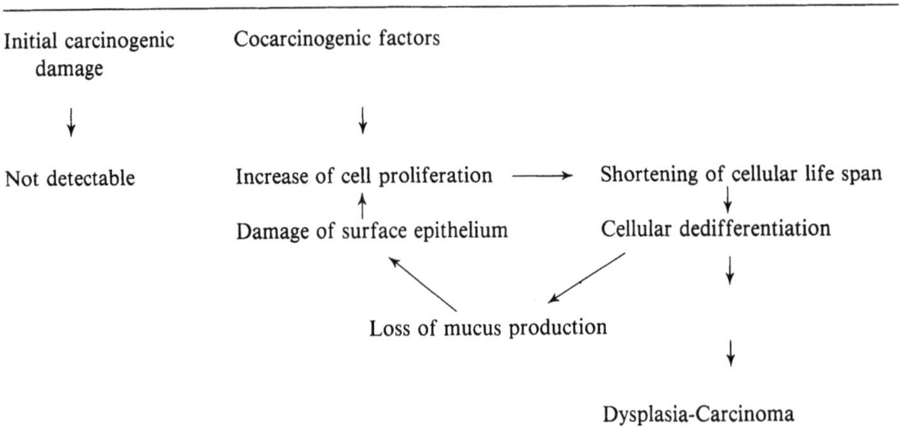

Fig. 4. Mechanism of cellular dedifferentiation in the stomach surface epithelium

precancerous changes are reversible or whether they will develop into a carcinoma.

If we *scrutinize* what little information we have on the timing of the events with regard to the development of the precancerous condition, the subsequent precancerous change resulting in the formation of the early carcinoma, and the diagnosis based on the clinical manifestation of the carcinoma, we may conclude, as stated by Siurala [31] and Fujita and Hattori [10], that the development of the microscopic carcinoma to an early carcinoma will take more than 10 years, i.e., from 16 to 24 years (Fig. 5). In this context, we would like to indicate that we are not in a position to fix the critical moment from which the irreversible growth originates leading to a carcinoma as Hutchinson assumed when he based his studies on cellular findings. It is assumed that the period of time from the onset of the early carcinoma until clinical manifestation will again take 16 – 27 years.

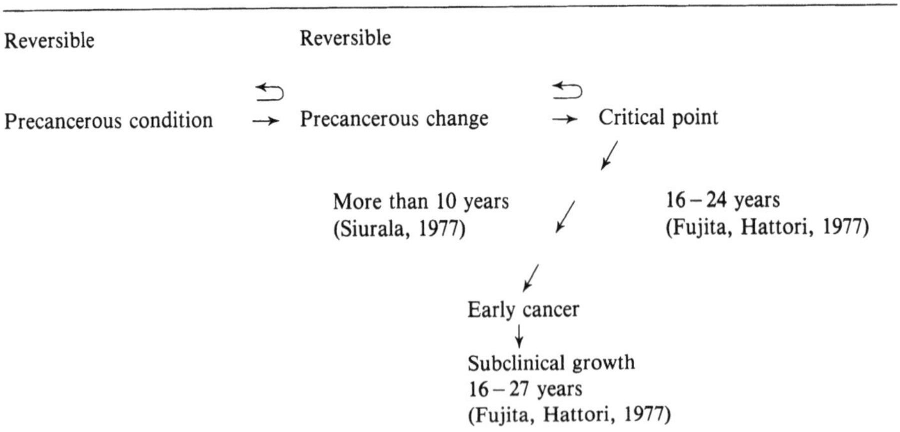

Fig. 5. Estimated time from the development of precancerous changes until the onset of early cancer

The aforementioned data show that we have to take long periods of time into consideration regarding the development of the carcinomatous growth within the mucosa of the stomach, but the exact determination of the critical moment which would justify a surgical intervention – except when a fully developed carcinoma is known to be present – is at present impossible (Fig. 5).

Since, consequently, the question regarding the further development of the precancerous change, which is decisive for the prognosis, cannot be answered from the definition of the cellular alteration *alone*, careful considerations should be made as to whether further parameters obtainable from biopsy material exist, which could offer more information on the biological or clinical significance of the precancerous change.

Biological Significance

A summary of the currently known mean life times of surface epithelia associated with precancerous conditions, precancerous changes, and carcinoma itself, show that on the one hand, there are considerable differences between normal and precancerous conditions (Fig. 6), but that on the other hand, there is no similar difference in regard to growth between the precancerous changes and the carcinoma (Table 1). This also applies to the determination of the ploidy pattern within normal epithelium, and epithelium showing inflammatory alterations or carcinomatous changes (Table 2). In comparing the diameters of nuclei in normal and precancerous conditions, a considerable increase in size can be seen. This is not found, however, when the diameters of cells from the precancerous and cancerous tissues are compared. There is a similar situation with regard to localization and enlargement of the indifferential zone of the gastric mucosa. Under normal conditions, this zone is localized within the area of the glandular necks (Fig. 7). An enlargement of the intermediate zone, which spreads also into the mucosal areas situated at a higher level, may be seen even in an uncomplicated inflammation. When a precancerous change occurs, the total width of the surface epithelium forms an intermediate zone similar to the conditions prevailing in a carcinoma. When comparing some parameters with regard to cell growth and cell differentiation, we may conclude that there are no measurable parameters based on biopsy material from which, in the individual case, clear information could be obtained on the biological significance of the precancerous change within the mucosa.

Clinical Significance

Since we presume that the rate at which a precancerous lesion develops into a carcinoma is not only determined by the autonomous factors within the lesion, but equally or more by the surrounding conditions to which the organisms react as a whole, it should be feasible to draw conclusions on the *clinical significance* of a precancerous change by considering the case history, the course of the disease, the characteristics of the pre-existing precancerous condition, and the histological alterations accompanying the precancerous change.

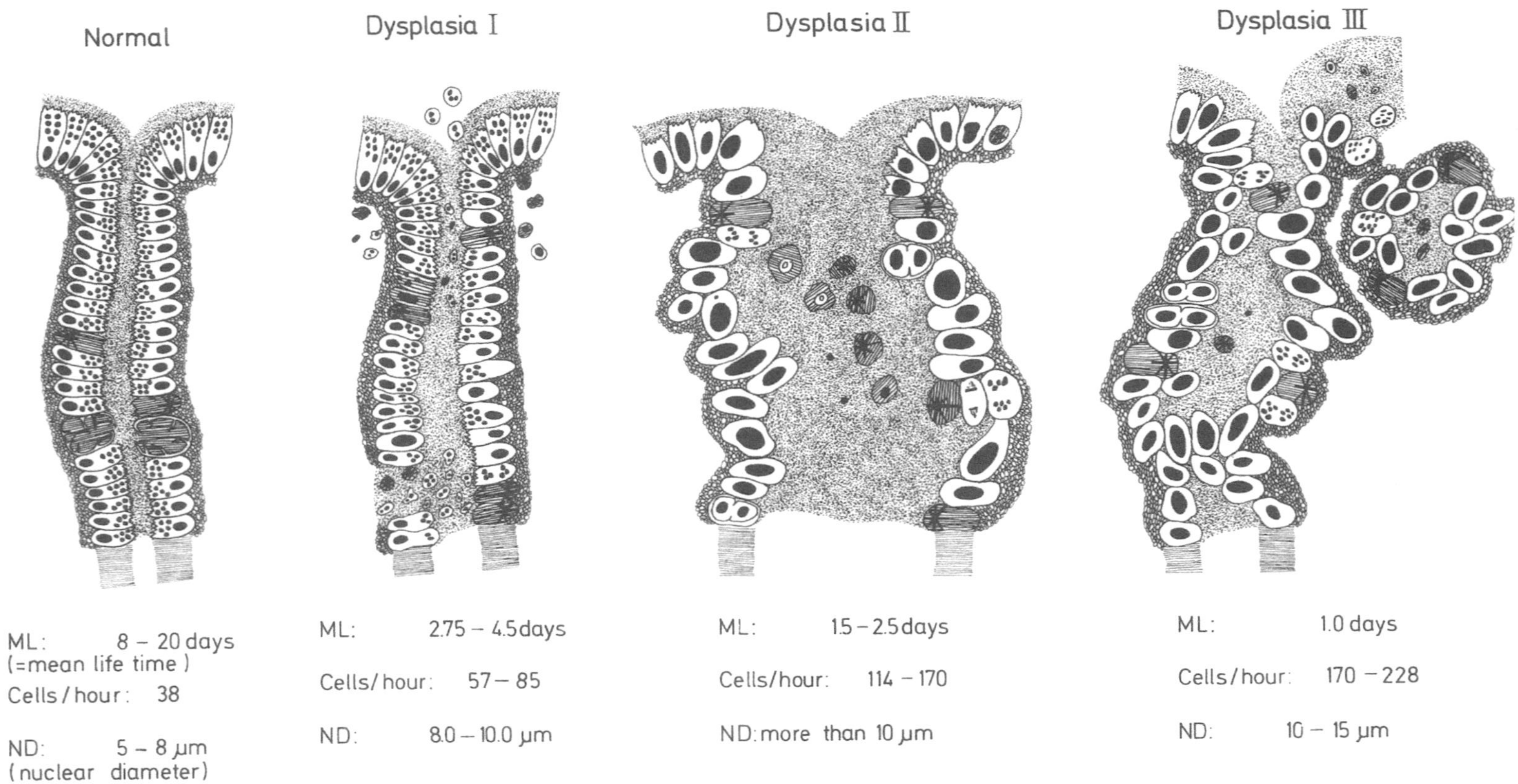

Fig. 6. Cell proliferation kinetics and nuclear diameter in the normal and dysplastic surface epithelium of the stomach

Table 1. Criteria of cellular proliferation; life span of surface epithelial cells (days)

Normal	Inflammation	Ulcus-wall	Atrophic gastritis	Intestinal metaplasia	Dysplasia Type III	Early cancer
8–20	2.7–4.5	1.00	1.25	1.5	1.0	1.0

Table 2. Criteria of cellular differentiation

a) *DNA-Content of surface epithelium*				
DNA	Normal	Ulcus-wall	Atroph. gastr.	Carcinoma
2n	90%	50%–75%	50%–75%	20%–50%
3–4n	10%	25%–50%	25%–50%	50%–80%
b) *Nuclear diameter: μm*				
Normal	Pernicious anemia	Dysplasia Type II	Dysplasia Type III	Carcinoma
5,8–7.9	7.9–10.5	more than 10	10–15	8–15

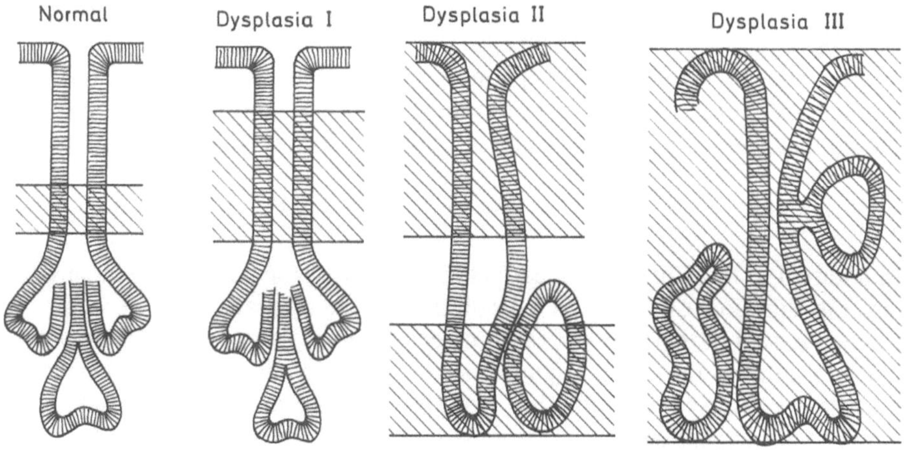

Fig. 7. Zone of cell proliferation with normal and dysplastic stomach epithelium

Genetic and Environmental Factors

All presently available results suggest that there are families with a high risk of developing a gastric carcinoma [31], and that members of such families are characterized by particular features. They may, for instance, belong to blood group A or be specially liable to develop a particular form of chronic gastritis. Investigations carried out by Correa et al. [2] have clearly proved that the development of gastric carcinoma following a precancerous condition and change is favored by a diet with a high nitrite content. Patients suffering from pernicious anemia are more frequently affected by carcinoma of the stomach than patients suffering from an uncomplicated chronic atrophic gastritis. The occurrence of precancerous changes in patients belonging to these risk groups should therefore be taken more seriously than the same event in patients who are not subject to similar factors.

General or Local State of Immunity

General or local states of immunity are of great importance when one considers the rapidity of the development and growth of cancer [31].

The breakdown of the local immunoresistance is determinant in regarding the transition of the precancerous change into a fully developed carcinoma and of the early carcinoma to the advanced carcinoma [26, 25]. Therefore, particular attention should be paid to all factors indicating a locally impaired state of immunity when determining the clinical significance of a precancerous change in the stomach. Among the clinical symptoms which indicate a reduced general or local state of immunity is an infection with candida albicans [18]. The biopsy material of some of our own investigations (Table 3) revealed that an infestation with candida albicans occurs far more often with carcinomatous ulcerations than with uncomplicated ulcers of the stomach. In as many as 31% of the ulcerations with carcinomatous changes which we observed, an infection with candida albicans was recognizable. These observations proved to be true even more frequently with exulcerated lymphomas of the stomach. An infection with candida albicans in the presence of eroding or ulcerative precancerous changes should therefore be considered as an indication of locally diminished immunity.

Time Factors

In addition to the aforementioned factors, the age of the patient and in particular, the duration of both the precancerous condition and the precancerous change, as well as their further development observed in control biopsies, are of importance when the clinical significance of precancerous changes of the gastric mucosa are being considered. Our own investigations revealed that in approximately 500 patients who were diagnosed as suffering from dysplasia type III, regression occurred in as many as 74%, whereas in 25.5%, the condition was still present after a year's observation (Table 4). After a period of more than 3 years, during which 46 patients who suffered from dysplasia type III continued to be regularly controlled, a regression could be observed in 15.3%, whereas in as

Table 3. Infestation of gastric ulcers with candida albicans in biopsies (1-year observation)

Total	104	100%	Investigated ulcers
Carcinomatous ulcer	60	57.6%	(133/60 = 45.11%)
Gastric ulcer without carcinoma	32	31.7%	(347/32 = 9.22%)
Lymphoma with ulceration	12	11.7%	(18/12 = 66.60%)

many as 76% of cases, a severe dysplasia continued to be present and to show no alteration. In 8.7% of cases, dysplasia type III had developed into an early carcinoma (Table 4). From these observations, we can conclude that in most cases severe dysplasias are reversible and that it would therefore be unjustified to suggest a surgical intervention solely on the grounds of cellular change. On the other hand, these findings show that dysplasias which have persisted for several years may develop into an early carcinoma and should then undergo surgical treatment when all other factors involved have been carefully considered and when a certain period of observation has passed.

Precancerous Conditions

As can be seen from Table 5, severe dysplasia develops in varying precancerous conditions, including particularly chronic gastritis, where the edge of a gastric ulcer or the anastomosis of a Billroth II operation may be considered to be specially liable to cellular dedifferentiation. Dysplastic change of the surface epithelium of mesenchymal benign tumors [23] and at the surface of adenomatous polyps of the gastric mucosa occurs relatively frequently. The removal of polyps of the gastric mucosa and of benign mesenchymal tumors within the submucosa, whether or not dysplastic changes have already developed, should

Table 4. Results of control-biopsies from patients with dysplasia II and III

Controlled after	Dysplasia	Number of patients	Recovered	Unchanged	Aggravated
2 months – 1 year	II	672 (100%)	437 (65.03%)	211 (31.40%)	24 (3.50%)
	III	498 (100%)	371 (74.50%)	127 (25.50%)	
1 – 2 years	II	268 (100%)	107 (39.93%)	150 (55.97%)	11 (4.10%)
	III	121 (100%)	61 (50.40%)	60 (49.60%)	
2 – 3 years	II	96 (100%)	32 (33.40%)	44 (45.80%)	20 (20.8%)
	III	152 (100%)	35 (23.00%)	117 (77.00%)	
More than 3 years	II	12 (100%)	–	12 (100.0%)	
	III	46 (100%)	7 (15.30%)	35 (76.00%)	4 (8.70%)

Table 5. Pathological changes in 2291 patients with the diagnosis: dysplasia Type II and Type III

Edge of gastric ulcer	432	18.85%
Scar of ulcer	210	9.26%
Edge of gastric erosion	272	11.86%
Chronic surface gastritis	166	7.24%
Chronic atrophic gastritis	521	22.74%
Anastomosis	385	16.80%
Polyps	12	0.50%
Mesenchymal tumors	7	0.30%
Early cancer	84	3.65%
Carcinoma	202	8.80%

be undertaken. There is nothing surprising about the relatively frequent occurrence of dysplastic change in the epithelium within the area of anastomosis of Billroth II resections for gastric ulcer. The frequency of development of precancerous conditions and precancerous changes within the area of anastomosis may be seen in Table 6, and in this connection, particular attention should be drawn to cystic changes when considering further development in the direction of malignancy [10]. Taking into consideration that 10 years after a Billroth II resection, there is an increased occurrence of gastric stump carcinomas [5, 30]; the presence of severe dysplasia near the anastomosis or in the remaining part of the stomach should be considered more seriously than a similar dysplasia with chronic atrophic gastritis.

Environmental Response to Precancerous Changes

Basing his investigations on histochemical findings, Heilmann [12] demonstrated that the mucus composition within the goblet cells of intestinal metaplasia in stomachs which had been removed because of a duodenal or gastric ulcer differs from that of the cancerous stomach. As can be seen in Table 7, there is an increased production of acid as opposed to neutral mucopolysaccarides. Heilmann [12] also described a recognizable cellular change of the intestinal metaplasia accompanying an increase of the goblet cells and a simultaneous reduction of the Paneth cells which he defined as "enterocolic metaplasia". This change equals intestinal metaplasia Type B which Siurala described in 1974 (Fig. 8 and 9). This progressing dedifferentiation, in comparison with differentiated intestinal metaplasia may be considered as a further step towards the development of a carcinoma. In determining the clinical significance, the occurrence of this enterocolic metaplasia and its characteristic, altered chemical composition of the mucus should be taken into consideration if, at the same time, a severe dysplasia is present. There is a similar situation after embryonic carcino-

Table 6. Pathological changes in anastomosis and gastric stump after B II resection (for gastric or duodenal ulcers)

Total number of cases	Normal gastric mucosa	Surface gastritis	Chronic atrophic gastritis	Intestinal metaplasia	Authors
114 (100%)	4 (3.5%)	58 (50.9%)	52 (45.6%)	–	Seifert 1976
50 (100%)	2 (4.0%)	10 (20.0%)	38 (76.0%)	11 (22.0%)	Domellöf 1976
108 (100%)	1 (0.92%)	–	–	24 (22.2%)	Serck-Hansen 1977
157 (100%)	11 (7.0%)	51 (32.5%)	95 (60.5%)	22 (12.7%)	Oehlert 1978
Total number of cases	**Cystic changes of gastric glands**	**Foveolar hyperplasia**	**Polypoid hyperplasia**	**Dysplasia II**	**Dysplasia III (severe)**
157 (100%)	120 (76.4%)	85 (54.2%)	32 (20.3%)	10 (6.4%)	3 (2.0%)

Table 7. Different mucus composition in the intestinal metaplasia of cancerous and noncancerous stomach

Diagnosis	Number of cases	Neutral	Acid	Mixed
Duodenal ulcer	48	6.2%	31.2%	62.5%
Gastric ulcer	36	16.0%	16.0%	66.9%
Carcinoma	67	5.9%	44.7%	49.2%

Production of acid mucus in the cancerous and noncancerous stomach (with and without intestinal metaplasia)

Diagnosis	Number of cases	Antrum	Intermedial zone	Corpus
Duodenal ulcer	102	14.7%	3.9%	2.9%
Gastric ulcer	44	13.6%	4.5%	–
Carcinoma	83	33.0%	19.1%	16.8%

from K. L. Heilmann: Gastritis – Intestinale Metaplasie – Karzinom, 1978 [12]

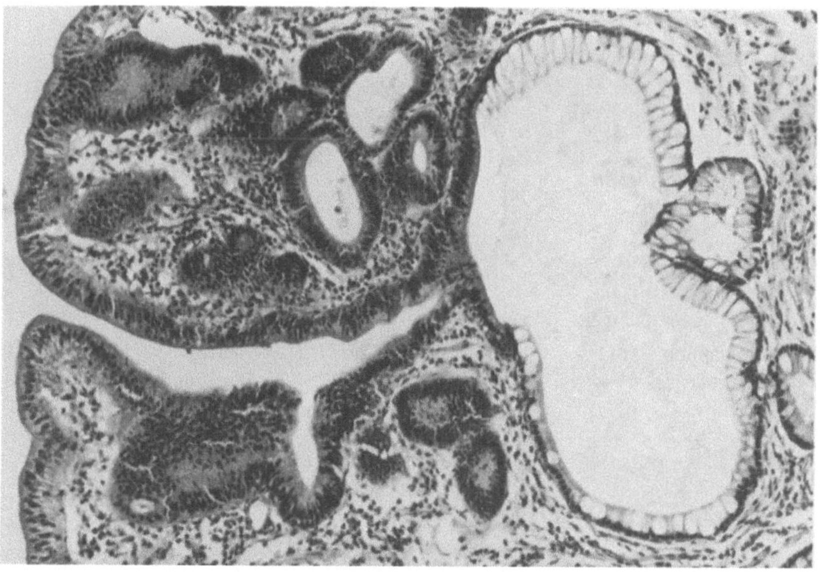

Fig. 8. Dysplasia type III with "enterocolic metaplasia" accompanied by the formation of a mucus cyst. (HE, × 100)

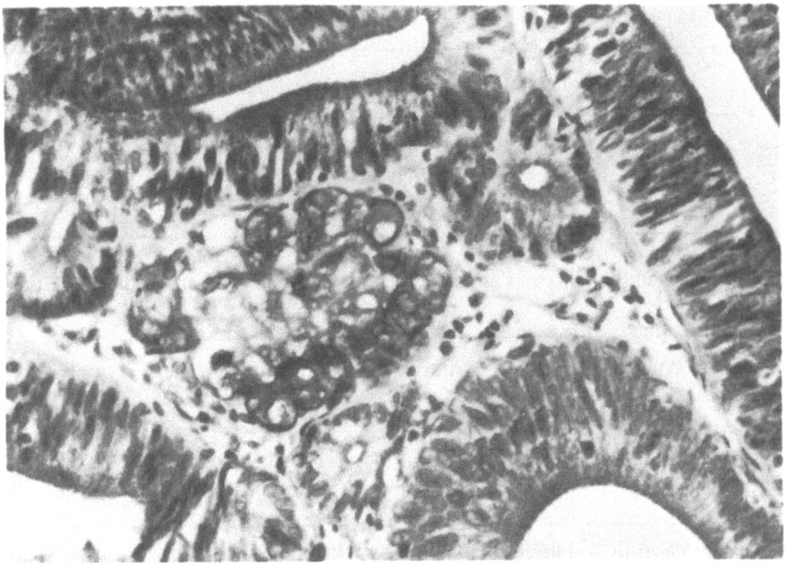

Fig. 9. Dysplasia of mucigenic cells within dysplasia III. (PAS, × 250)

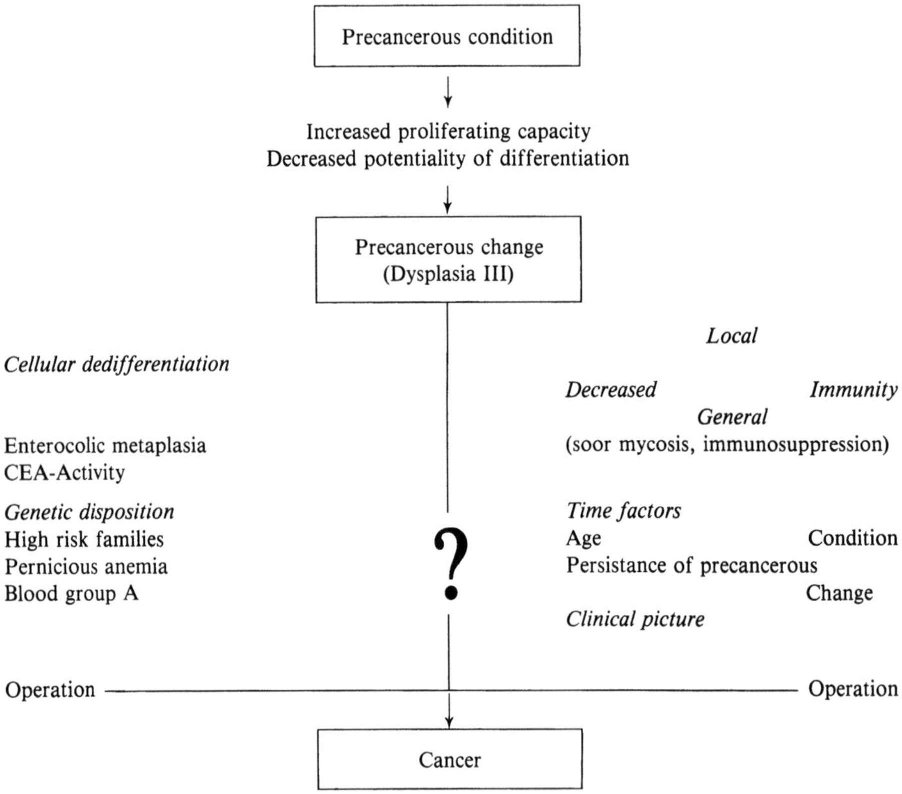

Fig. 10. Precancerous conditions, precancerous changes and factors which determine their clinical significance

genic antigen has been revealed in the tissue section under precancerous conditions. Siurala et al. [31] showed that not only the normal gastric mucosa, but also differentiated intestinal metaplasia, revealed no embryonic carcinogenic activity resembling the antigen, and that within dedifferentiated crypts of intestinal metaplasia similar activity may be found as occurs with the intestinal type of gastric carcinoma. Both the alteration of the mucus quality within enterocolic metaplasia and the manifestation of an embryonic carcinogenic activity resembling the antigen found in biopsy material should play a decisive role when the clinical significance of alterations present in individual cases is considered, if, at the same time, there is evidence of a severe dysplasia.

Conclusion

Although changes which, because of microscopic findings are known to be precancerous lesions, and which are defined in varying medical terms, may be considered as early stages of gastric carcinoma, their clinical significance – on which alone the further treatment will be based – should not be determined exclusively by the histological picture. A great number of additional factors, like genetic disposition, the altered general or local state of immunity, as well as time factors play decisive roles in the transition of precancerous changes towards tumor growth and with regard to the time involved (Fig. 10). Only if all these factors are taken into consideration it is possible to evaluate the changes found in the biopsy specimens and to suggest appropriate treatment in the individual case.

References

1. Büchner, F.: Die Histologie der peptischen Veränderungen und ihre Beziehungen zum Magenkarzinom. Veroeff. Kriegspathol. Konstitutionspathol. *18*, 1 – 125 (1927)
2. Correa, P., Cuello, C., Haenszel, W.: Epidemiology of premalignant gastric lesions, pp. 107 – 120. Tokyo: University Press 1977
3. Crespi, M., Bigotti, A., di Matteo, S.: Early gastric cancer. Grundmann, E., Grunze, H., Witte, S. (eds.), p. 60. In: early gastric cancer. Berlin, Heidelberg, New York: Springer 1974
4. Deschner, E. E., Lipkin, M.: Proliferation and differentiation of gastrointestinal cells in health and disease. In: Gastrointestinal tract cancer. Lipkin, M., Good, R. A., (eds.), pp. 3 – 24. New York, London: Plenum Medical Book 1978
5. Domellöf, L., Eriksson, S., Janunger, K. G.: Late occurrence of precancerous changes and carcinoma of the gastric stump after Billroth II resection. Acta Chir. Scand. *141*, 292 – 297 (1975)
6. Eastwood, G. L.: Progress in gastroenterology: Gastrointestinal epithelial renewal. Gastroenterology *72*, 962 (1977)
7. Elster, K., Kudlich, W.: Die diagnostische Effektivität der Gastrobiopsie. Endoscopy *4*, 162 (1972)
8. Elster, K.: False diagnosis in the diagnostics of early gastric cancer. In: Early gastric cancer. Grundmann, Grunze, Witte (eds.), p. 58. Berlin, Heidelberg, New York: Springer 1974
9. Elster, K.: Diskussion zum Thema: Magenfrühkarzinom. Therapiewoche *28*, 4996 (1978)
10. Fujita, S., Hattori, T.: Cell proliferation, differentiation and migration in the gastric mucosa: A study on the background of carcinogenesis. In: Pathophysiology of carcinogenesis in digestive organs. Farber, E. et al. (eds.), pp. 21 – 36. Tokyo: University Press 1977
11. Grundmann, E.: Histologic types and possible initial stages in early gastric carcinoma. Beitr. Pathol. *154*, 256 (1975)

12. Heilmann, K. L., Gastritis – Intestinale Metaplasie – Karzinom. Vergleichende quantitative und qualitative morphologische Untersuchungen. In: Gastroenterologie und Stoffwechsel. Bartelheimer, H., Kühn, H. A., Becker, V., Stelzner, F. (eds.), Vol. 13. Stuttgart: Thieme 1978
13. Kobori, O., Gedigk, P., Totovic, V.: Early changes of glandular stomach in Wistar Rats ingesting N-methyl-N'-nitro-N-nitrosoguanidine (MNNG): With special reference to light microscopic, electron microscopic, and enzyme histochemical study of the regenerating epithelium induced by MNNG. Z. Krebsforsch. *87*, 87 (1976)
14. Konjetzny, G. E.: Der Magenkrebs. Stuttgart: 1938
15. Konjetzny, G. E.: Der oberflächliche Schleimhautkrebs des Magens. Chirurg. *191*, 192 (1940)
16. Marks, J., Shuster, S.: The skin and gastrointestinal malignancy. In: Gastrointestinal Tract Cancer. Lipkin, M., Good, R. A. (eds.), pp. 509 – 534. New York, London: Plenum Medical Book 1978
17. Mason, M. K.: Surface carcinoma of the stomach. Gut *6*, 185 (1965)
18. Ming, S. C.: Dysplasias of the stomach. International Conference of Gastrointestinal Cancer 1977. Basel, München, Paris, London, New York, Sydney: Karger 1977
19. Nagayo, T.: Microscopical cancer of the stomach. A study on histogenesis of gastric carcinoma. Int. J. Cancer *16*, 52 (1975)
20. Nagayo, T.: Precursors of human gastric cancer: Their frequencies and histological characteristics, pp. 151 – 161. Tokyo: University Press 1977
21. Oehlert, W., Keller, P., Henke, M., Strauch, M.: Die Dysplasien der Magenschleimhaut. Das Problem ihrer klinischen Bedeutung. Dtsch. Med. Wochenschr. *100*, 1950 (1975)
22. Oehlert, W.: Klinische Pathologie des Magen-Darmtraktes. Stuttgart: Schattauer 1978
23. Orita, K., Kobayashi, M., Uchida, Y., Yumara, M., Yamamoto, I., Fukuda, H., Kaneda, S., Mammami, T., Kokuma, Y., Tanaka, S.: Reduction of concomitant cell-mediated immunity level in advanced cancer patients. Cancer immunology. GANN Monogr. Cancer Res. *16*, 141 (1974)
24. Piessens, W. F.: Evidence for human cancer immunity. A review. Cancer *26*, 1212 (1970)
25. Saito, T., Sasaki, O., Tamada, R., Iwamatsu, M., Matsukuchi, T., Inokuchi, K.: Follow-up studies of experimental stomach cancer in dogs. In: Pathophysiology of carcinogenesis in digestive organs. Farber, E. et al. (eds.), pp. 107 – 120. Tokyo: University Press 1977
26. Schade, R. O. K.: The borderline between benign and malignant lesions in the stomach. In: Early gastric cancer, Grundmann, E., Grunze, H., Witte, S. (eds.), p. 45. Berlin, Heidelberg, New York: Springer 1974
27. Seifert, E., Dittrich, H., Erd, W.: Gastrobioptische Untersuchungen am Resektionsmagen. Med. Welt *17*, 38 – 44 (1966)
28. Serck-Hansen, A., Schrumpf, E., Stadaas, J., Myren, J., Osnes, M.: Mucosal changes in the gastric stump 20 – 25 years after resection for ulcer. A follow-up study. International Conference of Gastrointestinal Cancer 1977, p. 273. Basel, München, Paris, London, New York, Sydney: Karger 1977
29. Siurala, M., Villako, K., Ihamäki, T., Kekki, M., Lehtola, J., Sipponen, P., Varis, K.: Atrophic gastritis. Its genetic and dynamic behavior and its relations to gastric carcinoma and pernicious anemia. In: Pathophysiology of carcinogenesis in digestive organs. Farber, E. et al. (eds.), pp. 135 – 150. Tokyo: University Press 1977
30. Spector, B. D., Good, R. A., Kersey, J. H.: Immunodeficiency diseases and malignancy. In: Gastrointestinal tract cancer. Lipkin, M., Good, R. A. (eds.), pp. 51 – 67. New York, London: Plenum Medical Book 1978
31. Sugimura, T., Kawachi, T.: Experimental stomach carcinogenesis. In: Gastrointestinal tract cancer. Lipkin, M., Good, R. A. (eds.), pp. 327 – 337. New York, London: Plenum Medical Book 1978
32. Twomey, J. J.: Immunological dysfunction with atrophic gastritis and gastric malignant. In: Gastrointestinal tract cancer. Lipkin, M., Good, R. A. (eds.), pp. 93 – 111. New York, London: Plenum Medical Book 1978

Significance and Location of Atrophic Gastritis and of Glandular Dysplasia in Benign and Malignant Gastric Disease

H. Meister, Ch. Holubarsch, O. Haferkamp, P. Schlag, and Ch. Herfarth

Introduction

Examination of human biopsy specimens from the stomach has shown that chronic atrophic gastritis (CAG) or intestinal metaplasia (IM) are often accompanied by proliferative changes of the superficial parts of gastric mucosa [2, 6]. These lesions are discussed as cancerous precursor stages, although no reliable data dealing with their biological behavior is available so far [3, 7]. The demonstration of such changes, particularly of severe dysplasia, often evokes questions concerning further diagnostic and therapeutic steps.

Without regard of the role of these conditions as possible premalignant changes, we were interested in knowing, how the distribution and frequency of CAG, IM, and different types of dysplasias associated with duodenal (UD) and gastric ulcers (UV) compare with the distribution and frequency of early (EC) and advanced carcinoma (CA) of the stomach. Therefore, we have examined gastrectomy specimens from patients operated on for benign ulcer disease or gastric cancer, whereby particular attention was paid to the extent of the inflammatory, metaplastic, and dysplastic mucosal lesions and the site of ulcer or cancer.

Material and Methods

Fifty stomachs resected for UD (n = 11), UV (n = 8), EC (n = 10), and CA (n = 21) have been investigated; the average age of each group was 63.5 years (58 – 73). Immediately after resection, the stomachs were opened along the greater curvature, pinned onto a cork board, and then placed into a 4% buffered formol fixative for a minimum of 48 h. The position of an ulcer or a tumor was noted on a diagram of the specimen. Following fixation, blocks of tissue (2.0 × 0.5 cm) were taken from the anterior wall, the lesser curvature, and the posterior wall. Additional tissue specimens were cut from the surroundings of large carcinomas; small tumors, early cancers, and ulcera were completely embedded, in addition to the routine specimens. Material was embedded in paraffin; sections 4 – 6 µm in thickness were cut stepwise and stained by hematoxylin and eosin. When signet-ring cell infiltration was suspected, PAS staining was also used. Histological classification of CAG, IM, and CA was performed in the conventional manner [1, 4, 5], EC was diagnosed according to Tasaka [8], dysplasias according to Grundmann [2] and Oehlert [6]. The histological findings were mapped out on diagrams.

Results

In all cases of ulcer disease or gastric cancer, CAG and IM were always present without any difference in distribution or frequency. In more than 50% of cases with UD, CAG and IM was demonstrable, in specimens with UV, EC, and CA, the frequency was mostly 100%. Mild and moderate dysplasia differed a bit in the stomachs with ulcer disease, but appeared in nearly the same amounts in EC and CA, as did CAG and IM. Only severe dysplasia, which was very rare in benign ulcer disease, was demonstrated in EC in 40% and in CA in 81% of the cases (Table 1). Within the different groups, CAG and IM exhibited an identical distribution pattern which was most comparable with that of mild and moderate dysplasia. In UD, for instance, these lesions occurred almost entirely in the pyloric region; in UV, they were additionally found in proximal areas. In EC and CA, their distribution pattern was comparable with their occurrence in UV. Severe dysplasia was found only sporadically at different sites in one stomach with UD and in one with UV. Severe dysplasia was most frequent in EC and CA and was most often located in those areas where cancerous lesions were demonstrable. Seventy percent of severe dysplasic lesions in EC and even 90% in CA were located within 2 cm of the malignant mucosal changes (Table 2).

Table 1. Frequency of chronic atrophic gastritis, intestinal metaplasia, and differing degrees of dysplasia in gastrectomy specimens from patients with duodenal or gastric ulcers or gastric cancer

Diagnosis	n	Gastritis[a] %	Dysplasia I %	Dysplasia II %	Dysplasia III %
Duodenal ulcer	11	54	54	27	9
Gastric ulcer	8	100	75	62	12
Early cancer	10	90	90	90	40
Advanced cancer	21	100	100	95	81

[a] Identical with values of chronic atrophic gastritis and metaplasia

Table 2. Histotopographical relationship between severe and cancerous mucosal lesions in gastrectomy specimens from patients with early and advanced gastric cancer

Cancer Border – Dysplasia III (distance in cm)	Early cancer	Advanced cancer
Less than 2 cm	70%	90%
More than 2 cm	30%	10%

Conclusion

In human stomach specimens resected for benign ulcer disease or gastric cancer, we found that only severe epithelial dysplasia exhibited a remarkable increase in frequency in the cases with early and advanced cancer, particularly in the immediate neighborhood of the malignant lesions. Chronic gastritis or mild and moderate dysplasia did not show such behavior. Their frequency and distribution could not be connected either with duodenal or gastric ulcer with certainty, or with early or advanced gastric cancer. In order to evaluate the importance of severe dysplasia as a possible premalignant change, all patients with severe dysplasia should be monitored continuously by gastroscopic check-ups.

References

1. Elster, K.: Histopathologie der Gastritis. Gastroenterologischer Fortbildungskurs. Praxis *4*, 17–28 (1973)
2. Grundmann, E.: Histologic types and possible initial stages in early gastric carcinoma. Beitr. Pathol. *154*, 256–280 (1975)
3. Hammar, E.: The localization of precancerous changes and carcinoma after previous gastric operation for benign condition. Acta Pathol. Microbiol. Scand. [A] *84*, 495–507 (1976)
4. Lauren, P.: The two histological main types of gastric carcinoma: Diffuse and so-called intestinal-type carcinoma. Acta. Pathol. Microbiol. Scand. *64*, 31–49 (1965)
5. Ming, S. G.: Gastric carcinoma: A Pathobiological classification. Cancer *39*, 2475–2485 (1977)
6. Oehlert, W., Keller, P., Henke, M., Strauch, M.: Die Dysplasien der Magenschleimhaut. Dtsch. Med. Wochenschr. *100*, 1950–1956 (1975)
7. Reynolds, K. W., Johnson, A. G., Fox, B.: Is intestinal metaplasia of the gastric mucosa a premalignant lesion? Clin. Oncol. *1*, 101–109 (1975)
8. Tasaka, S.: National collection of early gastric carcinoma. Jpn. Gastroenterol. Endosc. *4*, 4–14 (1962)

Endoscopic Therapy of Gastric Precancerosis

W. Rösch

Gastric precanceroses are by definition, lesions which will most probably degenerate or transform into gastric carcinoma over a period of time. According to our current knowledge, this applies only to two conditions: true gastric adenoma and the so-called borderline lesion, protruded type [1]. Both lesions are nowadays treated by endoscopic polypectomy, which, however, may be difficult from the technical point of view, since adenomas may exhibit a diameter of 3 to 5 cm and borderline lesions are usually broad-based and not very prominent. Therefore, surgical resection is advocated by many authors, especially in view of the possible malignant nature of the lesion, although preliminary follow-up data show that they grow very slowly (Elster, personal communication, 1978).

Adenomas and borderline lesions may harbor a clinically evident carcinoma, a fact which has to be kept in mind when endoscopic therapy is attempted. Serial sections are necessary to rule out early gastric carcinoma originating in these lesions. Furthermore, follow-up studies seem advisable in three month intervals to detect local recurrency. The mean age of three patients with adenoma and 15 patients with borderline lesions which were treated by endoscopic snareectomy was 72 years; follow-up studies disclosed two local recurrencies of 1 – 2 mm size. These were destroyed by Argon laser photo-coagulation, a method with selective penetrance of mucosa and submucosa [2]. Whereas adenomas are usually solitary lesions, borderline lesions are commonly multiple and may be associated with early gastric carcinoma at a different site. Endoscopic therapy is therefore only justified in patients with advanced age and when a carcinoma has definitely been ruled out. If histology reveals that infiltration of the tunica propria has occurred, but the carcinoma was excised in toto, the risk of regional lymph node metastases (in case of mucosal carcinoma, about 3.4%) has to be weighed against the risk of partial or total gastrectomy. Our experience of local endoscopic therapy of early gastric carcinoma, limited hitherto to four patients, is encouraging, although this can not be recommended as a standard therapy.

References

1. Nagayo, T.: Histological diagnosis of biopsied gastric mucosa with special reference to that of borderline lesions. Gan. *II*, 245 – 258 (1972)
2. Rösch, W., Frühmorgen, P.: Endoscopic therapy of premalignant and malignant gastric lesions. 4th World Congress of Digestive Endoscopy, Madrid 1978

Summary: Precancerous Lesions of Gastric Cancer

Dysplastic and metaplastic changes in the gastric mucosa must be observed discriminatingly with respect to their valency as precancerous lesions. Dysplasia, in its definition as a low- to high-grade epithelial alteration with a potential for transition to cancer, can today only be described phenomenologically. At present there are no certain criteria for determining the obligatory moment for the transition of a severe dysplasia to cancer in any one particular instance.

A great number of additional factors, like genetic disposition, the altered general or local state of immunity, as well as time factors play decisive roles in the transition of precancerous lesions to tumor growth.

Extreme difficulties are also encountered in attempting to quantify these changes in a uniform fashion, although cytophotometry is apt to offer valuable aid. The clinical consequences are regular endoscopic – bioptic controls for patients with low- and medium-grade dysplasias and strict bioptic supervision of high-grade dysplasias, as there is a high possibility that a cancer (early or advanced stage) is present in the vicinity of severe dysplasias. The bioptic demonstration of severe epithelial dysplasia without a lesion of the gastric mucosa is in itself insufficient to warrant surgical intervention.

The so-called mucosal cancer on the level of the tunica mucosa was particularly expounded as a special type of dysplastic or cancerous change of the epithelium. It is of special significance, because it has a different prognosis than the early cancer conventionally designated as mucosal type. This is supposedly based on the possibility of attaining remission. The question then arises as to how this lesion can be differentiated from the so-called borderline lesion or severe epithelial dysplasia. Risk factors for gastric cancer are not the inflammatory epithelial changes, but primarily the higher-grade epithelial dysplasias. The severe epithelial dysplasias are generally supposed to have a close relationship to the intestinal differentiated carcinomas, whereas carcinomas of the diffuse type can be found in largely normal gastric mucosa. The metaplasias, which can also be regarded as precancerous, must be subdivided into enteral and enterocolic metaplasias. The differentiated type of enteral metaplasia with proliferation of goblet cells and Paneth's cells can be often found in people with normal stomach, and in itself does not constitute a precancerous lesion. Enterocolic metaplasia occurs primarily in combination with ulcerated carcinomas. The differentiation of hyperplastic and adenomatous dysplasias comprises the same general aspects as the differentiation of intestinal metaplasia and dysplasia into various degrees of severity.

4 Risk Factors for Gastric Cancer

Duodenogastric Reflux and Epithelial Lesions

H. H. Lawson

Introduction

The present investigation was undertaken to establish whether or not duodenal contents affected gastric mucosa, as this could be of importance in the pathogenesis of gastritis, gastric ulceration, and gastric carcinoma.

Material and Methods

All experimental procedures were carried out on dogs and mice, and it is emphasized that each animal acted as its own control.

Standard histological techniques were used and whenever it was possible, the "Swiss roll" preparation was employed (Fig. 1), as described by Stein [22].

The term "chronic gastritis" is usually used to describe histological changes in the gastric mucosa, but the present author prefers the term "chronic gastric mucosal reaction"(C. G. M. R.), as the changes seen do not resemble typical chronic inflammation as described in standard texts of pathology.

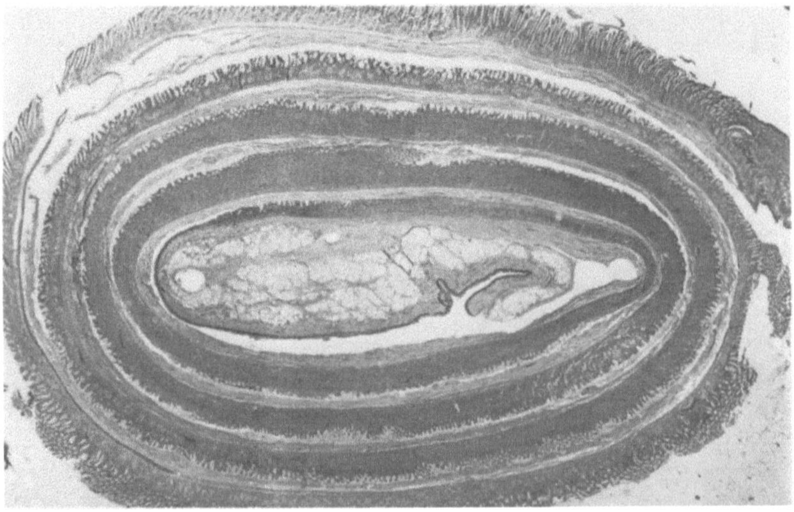

Fig. 1. Appearance of a typical "Swiss roll" preparation of mucosa

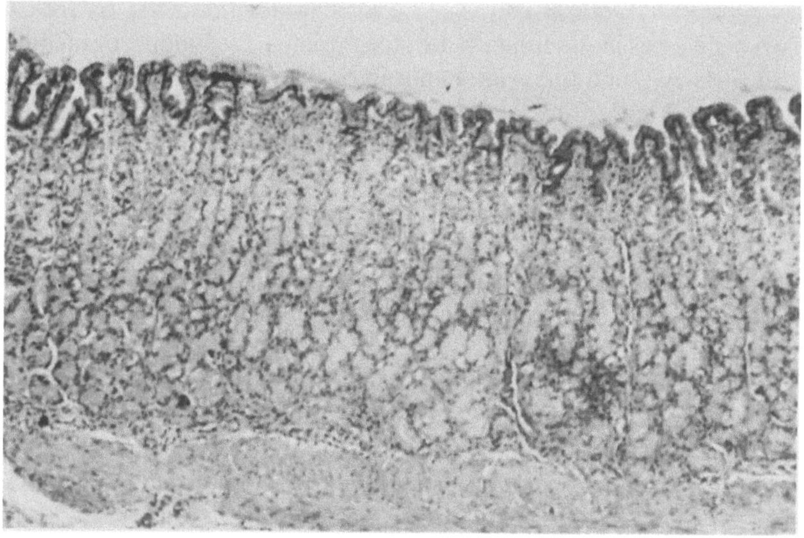

Fig. 2. Normal fundic gland area. Short gastric pits and well-defined areas of chief and parietal cells (× 65)

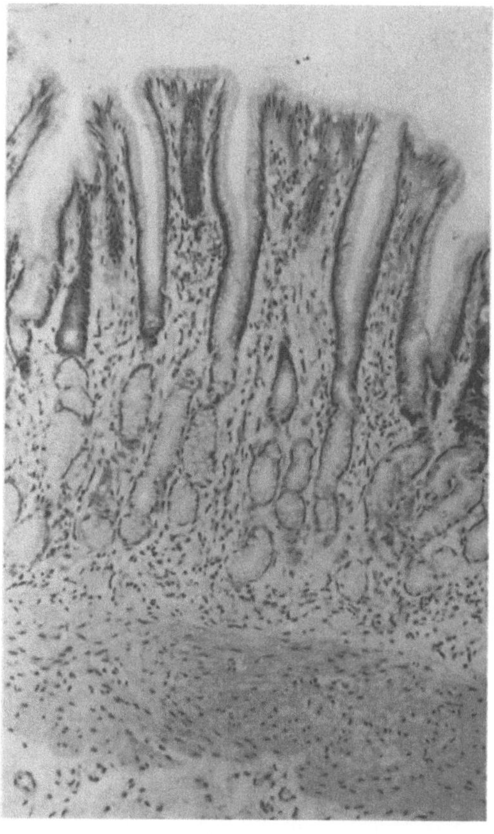

Fig. 3. Normal pyloric gland area. Deep gastric pits and well-defined areas of mucus secreting glands (× 65)

Results

Two main areas in the stomach are recognized – the fundus, or the fundic gland area (F.G.A.), and the pyloric antrum or the pyloric gland area (P.G.A.).

Figures 2 and 3 illustrate the appearance of the normal F.G.A. and P.G.A.

The gastric mucosa can be exposed to the effect of bile alone, or to the total effects of the duodenal contents by carrying out one or other type of pyloroplasty, partial gastrectomy, or by a procedure as illustrated in Fig. 4.

There are three varieties of the C.G.M.R. that may be seen in the early stages, though it is not possible to state which is the earliest. The surface epithelium looses its straight appearance and becomes mamillated or polypoid (Fig. 5).

The surface epithelium elongates and forms long fronds or papillae, and this is especially noticable in the F.G.A., where normally the pits are so shallow. This is so-called epithelial proliferation (Fig. 6), and the fact that there is abnormal epithelial proliferation may be confirmed by counting the number of mitotic figures seen in a single high powered field.

The third early change is pseudopyloric metaplasia, which can only be diagnosed with certainty in the F.G.A. Figure 7 illustrates the typical appearances of pseudopyloric metaplasia.

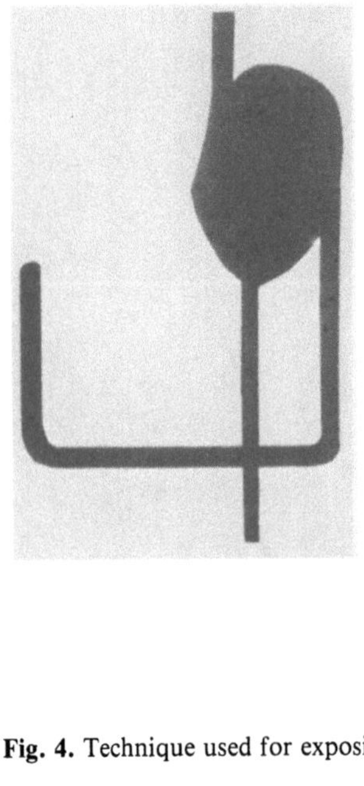

Fig. 4. Technique used for exposing the gastric mucosa to the effects of the total duodenal contents

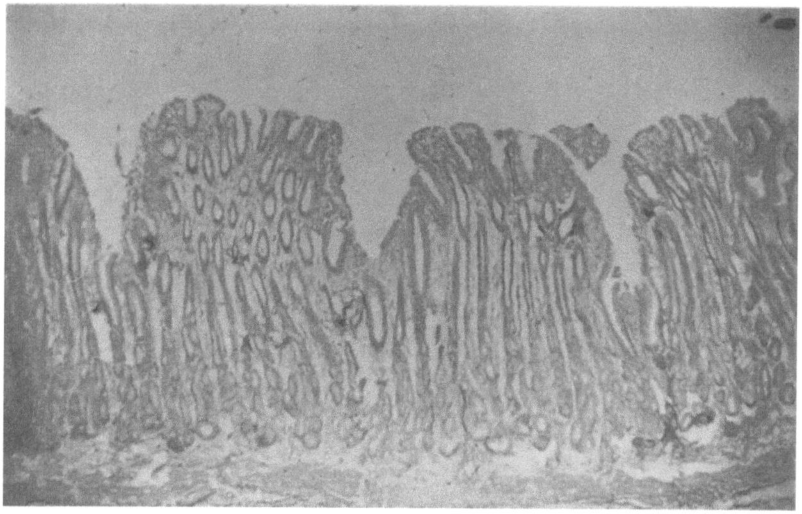

Fig. 5. Polypoid or mamillated gastric mucosa – an early manifestation of the chronic gastric mucosal reaction (× 65)

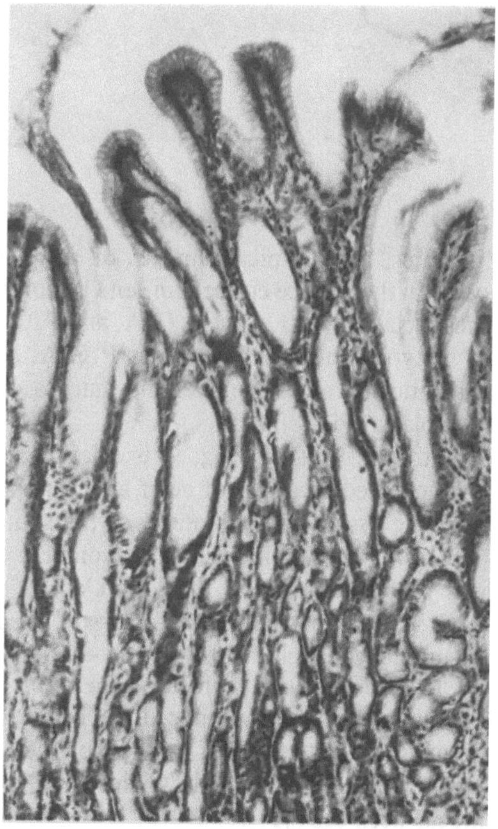

Fig. 6. Epithelial proliferation – a further early manifestation of the chronic gastric mucosal reaction (× 250)

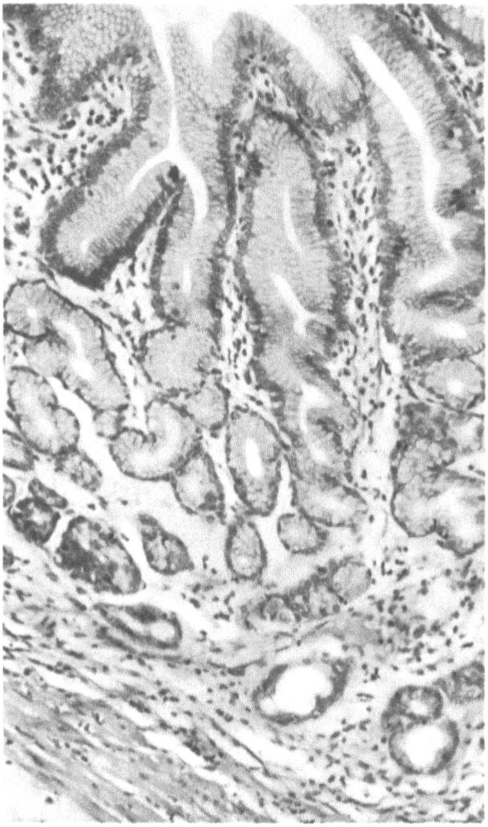

Fig. 7. Pseudopyloric metaplasia. The normal fundic gland area resembles pyloric gland mucosa (× 250)

Later, other typical changes of the C. G. M. R. develop. Goblet cells may occur in the surface epithelium, and be confined to that area, or they may replace the specialized cells of the F. G. A. and P. G. A. When this occurs, mucosa known to be typical normal F. G. A. or P. G. A. changes preoperatively in appearance dramatically, and resembles the mucosa of small bowel – so-called intestinal metaplasia (Fig. 8).

Atrophic gastritis (Fig. 9) is a late manifestation of the C. G. M. R., and is characterized by a loss of chief and parietal cells, which are replaced by mucus secreting tissue, with tortuosity of the glands, and cyst formation [7, 8, 13, 5].

Having shown that duodenal contents cause the C. G. M. R., an experiment was designed to see if the lesion could be reversed. It was shown that the C. G. M. R. in partial gastrectomy specimens reverted to histological normality, when bile was excluded by a Roux-en-Y procedure [12].

The mechanism by which regeneration occurred was then examined, using a rat model with X-ray induced C. G. M. R. and autoradiography with tritiated thymidine. Up to 10% of the new parietal cells were labeled, indicating that in regenerating mucosa, at least this number of cells was derived from original mucus neck cells [11].

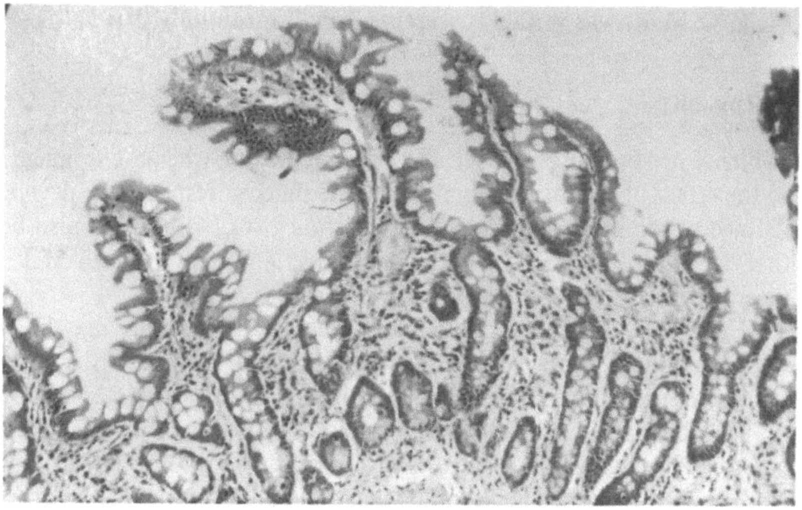

Fig. 8. Intestinal metaplasia of the normal fundic gland area (× 250)

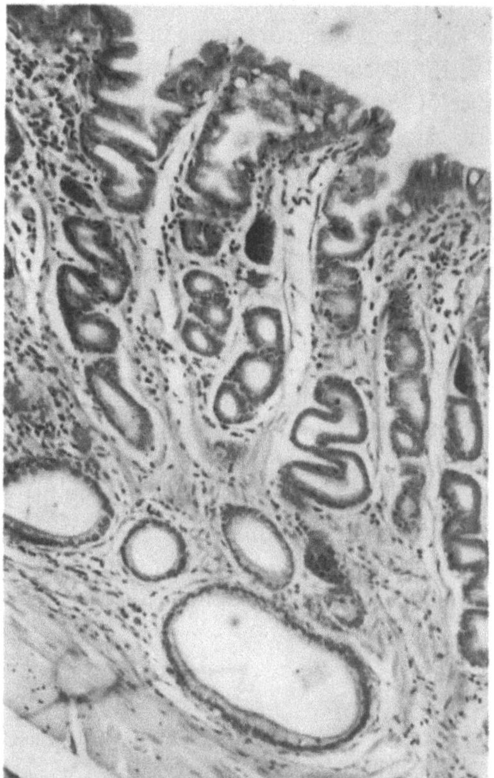

Fig. 9. Atrophic gastritis with loss of chief and parietal cells, tortuosity of glands, and the appearance of cysts on the lamina muscularis mucosa (× 250)

Using an explant model, it was then possible to show that mucosa affected by the C.G.M.R. was in fact susceptible to ulceration [9, 10].

Discussion

Evidence has been presented to show that in the dog when the stomach is exposed to the effect of the duodenal contents, the mucosa responds by developing well-defined histological changes described as the C.G.M.R. It has also been shown that again under experimental conditions, an area of C.G.M.R. becomes ulcerated when it is exposed to gastric contents.

These findings lend support to the view that bile reflux may be a factor of importance in the development of gastritis and chronic gastric ulceration as suggested by Schindler [20], Palmer [16], and du Plessis [1, 2, 3].

The fact that a Roux-en-Y conversion is effective in preventing bile from entering the stomach is well established, but the operation fell into disfavor because of the frequency of consequent stomal ulceration [6]. The present study offers an explanation for this phenomenon, and indicates why a vagotomy is essential. There is now considerable literature that indicates the successful use of a Roux-en-Y conversion in the treatment of postoperative alkaline reflux gastritis and esophagitis [18, 14, 23].

The relationship between the C.G.M.R. and the development of carcinoma of the stomach is not clear, but it is generally accepted that there is an increased risk of developing carcinoma in the gastric remnant following gastric surgery [21, 19, 15]. Because the histological changes seen in the C.G.M.R. following exposure of the mucosa to duodenal contents, are similar to those that occur in gastric carcinoma, a relationship between bile reflux and subsequent carcinoma is possible. Morson [16] has suggested that intestinal metaplasia may be the premalignant condition.

du Plessis [4] suggested that there may be two types of carcinoma, the one caused by bile reflux, the other by an external carcinogen.

Conclusion

Under experimental conditions, the duodenal contents cause the chronic gastric mucosal reaction (chronic gastritis) in the stomach of the dog. Such an area is susceptible to gastric ulceration. The chronic gastric mucosal reaction may be reversed by a procedure that protects the stomach from small bowel contents, and in regenerating mucosa, some of the chief and parietal cells are derived from mucus neck cells. A relationship between abnormal reflux of small bowel contents and the development of carcinoma of the stomach is suggested.

References

1. du Plessis, D. J.: Some aspects of the pathogenesis and surgical management of peptic ulcers. S. Afr. Med. J. *34,* 101 – 108 (1960)
2. du Plessis, D. J.: Gastric mucosal changes after operations on the stomach. S. Afr. Med. J. *36,* 471 – 478 (1962)

3. du Plessis, D. J.: The importance of the pyloric antrum in peptic ulceration. S. Afr. J. Surg. *1*, 3–11 (1963)
4. du Plessis, D. J.: The distribution of gastritis in carcinoma of the stomach. Br. J. Surg. *61*, 521–523 (1974)
5. du Plessis, D. J., Lawson, H. H.: Gastric mucosal alterations benign and malignant. In: Surgery Annual. Nyhus, L. (ed.), pp. 73–101. Appleton: Century Croft 1974
6. Lambley, D. G.: The case against gastrectomy with Y-anastomosis of peptic ulcer. Br. Med. J. *1*, 1588–1590 (1962)
7. Lawson, H. H.: The effect of duodenal contents on the gastric mucosa under experimental conditions. Preliminary communication. Lancet *1*, 469–473 (1964)
8. Lawson, H. H.: The effect of duodenal contents on the gastric mucosa under experimental conditions. S. Afr. J. Surg. *3*, 79–91 (1965)
9. Lawson, H. H.: Gastritis and gastric ulceration. Br. J. Surg. *53*, 493–496 (1966)
10. Lawson, H. H.: The lesser curvature of the stomach. Br. J. Surg. *55*, 625–627 (1968)
11. Lawson, H. H.: The origin of the specialised cells of the gastric mucosa. Br. J. Surg. *56*, 707 (1969)
12. Lawson, H. H.: The reversibility of post gastrectomy alkaline reflux gastritis by a Roux-en-Y loop. Br. J. Surg. *59*, 13–15 (1972)
13. Lawson, H. H.: The distribution and early morphology of the chronic gastric mucosal reaction. Br. J. Surg. *63*, 585–588 (1976)
14. Mackman, S., Lemmer, K. E., Morrissey, J. F.: Post operative reflux alkali gastritis and oesophagitis. Am. J. Surg. *121*, 694–697 (1971)
15. Morgenstern, L., Yamakawa, T., Seltzer, D.: Carcinoma of the gastric stump. Am. J. Surg. *125*, 29–38 (1973)
16. Morson, B. C.: The gastric mucosa and metaplasia. In: Surgery of the Stomach. 2nd ed. Boston: Little Brown 1973
17. Palmer, E. D.: Gastritis a re-evaluation. Medicine (Baltimore) *33*, 199–290 (1954)
18. Payne, W. S.: Surgical treatment of reflux oesophagitis and stricture associated with permanent incompetence of the cardia. Mayo Clin. Proc. *45*, 553–562 (1970)
19. Saegesser, F., James, D. L.: Cancer in the gastric stump after partial gastrectomy. (Billroth II Principle) for ulcer. Cancer *29*, 1150–1159 (1972)
20. Schindler, R.: Gastritis. London: Heineman 1947
21. Stalsberg, H., Taksdal, S. O.: Stomach cancer following gastric surgery for benign conditions. Lancet *11*, 1175–1177 (1971)
22. Stein, H. B.: A method for the histological examination of long strips of hollow viscera. S. Afr. J. Med. Sci., *2*, 117–120 (1937)
23. Van Heerden, J. A., Phillips, S. F., Adson, M. A., McIlrath D. C.: Postoperative reflux gastritis. Am. J. Surg. *129*, 82–93 (1975)

Nitrite and *N*-Nitrosocompounds in the Operated Stomach

P. Schlag, R. Böckler, H. Meyer, and D. Belohlavek

Nitrosamines are among the most potent chemical carcinogens known [6, 12] with which, at least in animal experiments, the induction of gastric cancer could be demonstrated [21, 25]. It has been suggested that nitrite and secondary amines present in food might react with each other in the environment of the human stomach to form these carcinogens [18, 20, 23]. Because in food stuffs secondary amines are in general present, intragastric nitrosamine formation occurs if there is a sufficient nitrite concentration in the gastric juice. The intragastric bacterial reduction of nitrate to nitrite is therefore very important [9, 15]. Bacterial overgrowth of the small bowel has been demonstrated after gastric surgery [1, 3, 5, 7, 8]. However, until now, little attention has been paid to the influence of the operative technique on the bacterial flora of the gastric juice [14, 22]. Concerning the cancer risk of the operated stomach [4], it was the aim of our investigation to evaluate experimentally the influence of different operative techniques on the composition of the bacterial gastric flora. In particular, we were interested in the production of bacterial nitrites in the stomach with respect to formation of carcinogenic nitrosamines.

Material and Methods

For our experiments, we used female SPF-Wistar rats, weighing 180 – 200 g. The following operative procedures were performed in groups of 15 animals (Fig. 1):

Group 1: Gastrotomy
The stomach was opened for a length of 1 cm along the great curvature and was closed as one layer with interrupted sutures. These animals were used as controls.

Group 2: Truncal Vagotomy
A typical truncal vagotomy was performed by medial laparotomy.

Group 3: Truncal Vagotomy and Pyloroplasty
In addition to a typical truncal vagotomy, a pyloroplasty for a length of 1 cm was performed.

Group 4: Antecolic Gastroenterostomy without Entero-enteroanastomosis
The small bowel, 2 cm distal to the ligament of Treitz, was anastomosed to the glandular stomach on the great curvature. Consequently, all duodenal contents, including bile and pancreatic juice were passed through the anastomotic region.

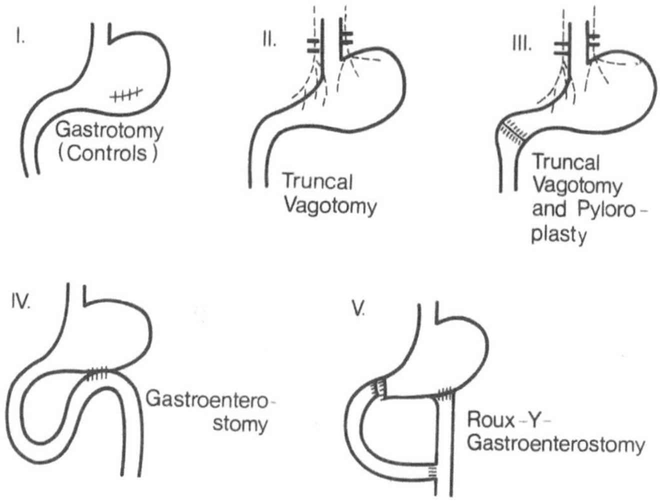

Fig. 1. Performed operative procedures in animal experiments

Group 5: Gastroenterostomy with a Roux-en-Y-Intestinal Loop
The pylorus was separated from the duodenum and the stumps were closed. Then, the small bowel was separated 2 cm distal to the ligament of Treitz. The distal part was then anastomosed to the glandular stomach on the great curvature and the proximal segment set to drain into the jejunum 3 cm below the gastroenterostomy (Roux-en-Y-method). Thus, a duodenogastric reflux was prevented.

All animals were kept in the same environment and fed identically throughout the period of the experiments. The rats were sacrificed in a carbon dioxide atmosphere 35–37 weeks postoperatively and immediately the abdomen was dissected. For bacteriological investigation, the gastric contents were removed with a wire loop from definited location within the stomach. In agreement with the literature [11], in the upper third of the stomach there was a lower amount of cultivatable microorganisms than in the distal third. The various groups were compared with regard to the variations exhibited in the lower third of the stomach.

Isolation and identification of anerobic germs was performed by the modified Hungate-roll-tube-technique [10] and of aerobic bacteria by the surface drop method [2].

Those plates on which more than ten, but fewer than 100 colonies grew, were chosen for quantitative evaluation. The total bacterial count was analyzed for the logarithmic analogue of microbes per 1 ml gastric content. For the nitrite assay, gastric juice was buffered to pH 9 with 5% Borax buffer in deionizied water and was measured quantitatively with the reagent of Gries-Illosway. *N*-nitrosocompounds were measured by the nitrite concentration produced by irritation with low wave ultraviolet in alkaline solution. This reaction described by Sander [17] forms a highly specific and sensitive test for *N*-nitrosocompounds.

Using a variance analysis with 95% confidence limits, the statistical significance of the difference between the groups was determined ($p < 0.05$).

Results

Animal Experiments

Various strains of bacteria could be found in the stomach (Table 1). Differences were found in the bacterial counts between the upper and lower parts of the stomach or duodenum (Fig. 2). The main total bacterial count was greater in the upper gastric segment; it was less in the duodenal contents and lowest in the lower part of the stomach. The amounts of nitrate reductase positive organisms were in the same proportions. The differences in bacterial count by the different operative techniques on the stomach was compared at location B.

Gastroenterostomy and vagotomy resulted in variations in the bacterial flora of the stomach. These changes apply partially to the total bacterial count, but especially to the ratio of nitrate reductase positive bacteria to total count (Fig. 3).

Table 1. Microorganism groups detected in the stomach of the rat

Aerobic bacteria	Anaerobic bacteria
Escherichia coli[a]	*Peptostreptococcus productus*[a]
Lactobacillus acidophilus[a]	*Eubacterium contortum*
Lactobacillus cellobiosus	*Bacteroides symbiosus*
Streptococcus faecalis	*Bifidobacterium* species
Streptococcus suis	*Clostridium* species

[a] Nitrate reductase positive bacteria

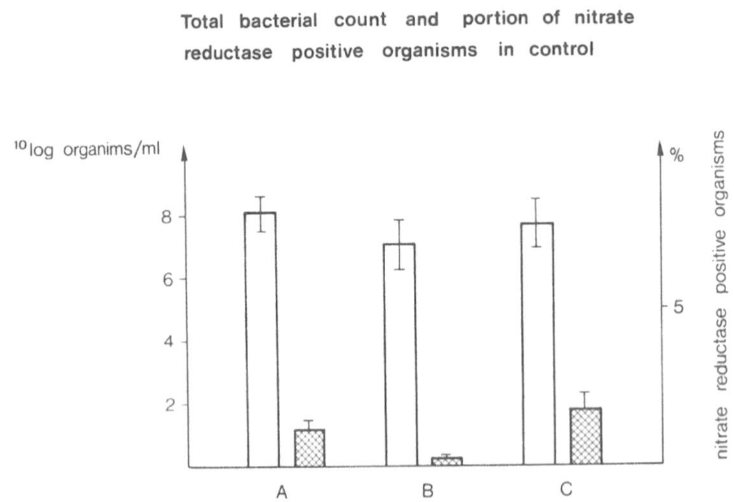

Fig. 2. Comparison of numbers of microorganisms in the stomach of the rat (*A* = upper 1/3, *B* = distal 1/3, *C* = duodenum)

After gastroenterostomy without entero-enteroanastomosis, the total bacterial count as well as the proportion of nitrate reductase positive organisms were significantly higher than in the gastrotomy group. Roux-en-Y-gastroenterostomy and vagotomy had no significant effect on the total bacterial count, but the ratio of nitrate reductase positive bacteria after Roux-en-Y-gastroenterostomy or vagotomy was significantly increased. Vagotomy with pyloroplasty promotes fewer of these changes than a vagotomy alone. The logarithm of the total count of nitrate reductase organisms of the gastroenterostomy without entero-entero-anastomosis was 6.5 ± 0.5 and was significantly higher than that in the gastrotomy group (3.6 ± 0.4). The nitrate reductase bacteria count was also significantly higher after Roux-en-Y-gastroenterostomy (5.5 ± 0.4) or vagotomy with (5.1 ± 0.5) and without pyloroplasty (5.9 ± 0.5) than in controls, but not as high as after gastroenterostomy without enteroanastomosis (Fig. 4). In correlation with the increase of nitrate decomposing bacteria after gastroenterostomy without entero-enteroanastomosis, the nitrite concentration in gastric juice was significantly higher than in controls. Nitrite concentration after Roux-Y-gastroenterostomy or truncal vagotomy with and without pyloroplasty was only two times higher and not yet more statistically significant than in controls (Fig. 5).

The presence of high nitrite concentration in gastric juice together with high bacterial count is followed by an increase of N-nitrosocompounds in the stomach, especially by gastroenterostomy without entero-enteroanastomosis (Fig. 6).

Clinical Findings

By standard conditions, gastric juice was aspirated by gastroscopy of normal individuals and individuals with operated stomach. Nitrite and N-nitroso-

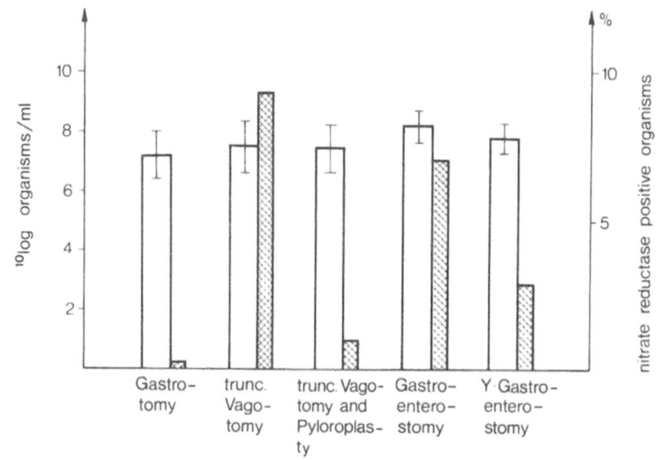

Fig. 3. Total bacterial counts and portion of nitrate reductase positive bacteria in the distal third of the stomach after various surgical procedures in animal experiments

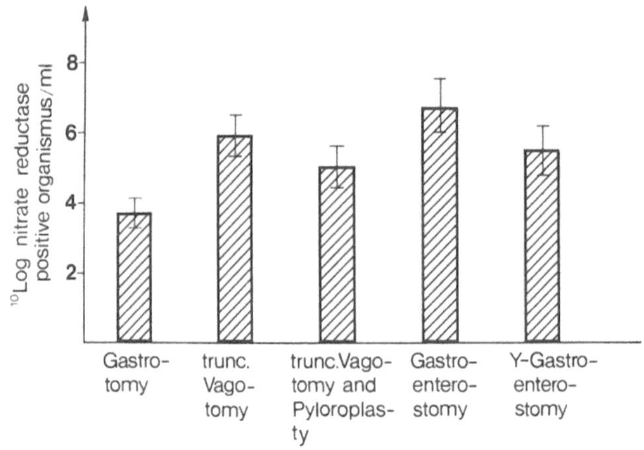

Fig. 4. Total counts of nitrate reductase positive bacteria after various surgical procedures in animal experiments

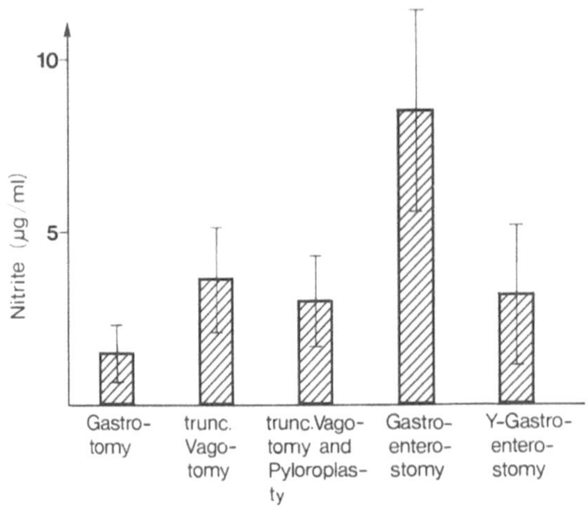

Fig. 5. Nitrite concentration in the gastric juice after various surgical procedures in animal experiments

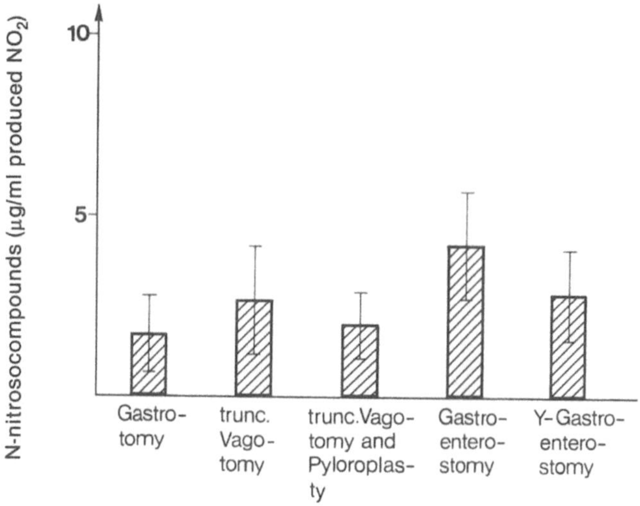

Fig. 6. *N*-nitrosocompounds in the gastric juice in correlation to the various operative procedures in animal experiments

compounds in the gastric juice were analyzed. A close relationship to our experimental findings exists (Figs. 7 and 8). The highest concentration of nitrite and N-nitrosocompounds was found in the Billroth II stomach, whereas these changes were less pronounced in the Billroth I stomach. We could not find differences in these parameters between controls and proximal gastric vagotomy.

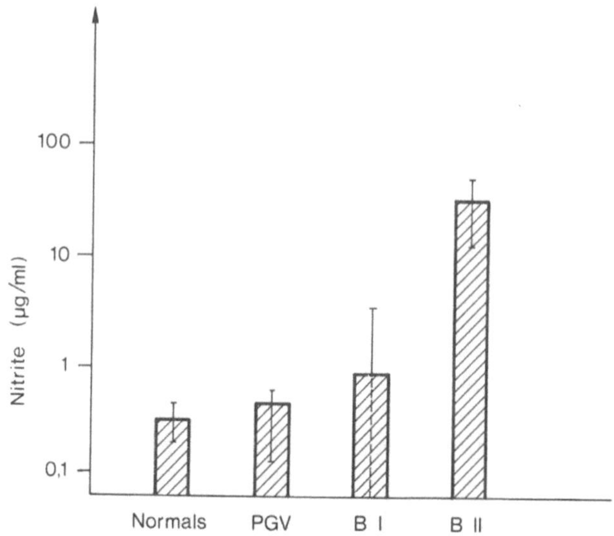

Fig. 7. Nitrite concentration in the gastric juice after various operative procedures in the human stomach

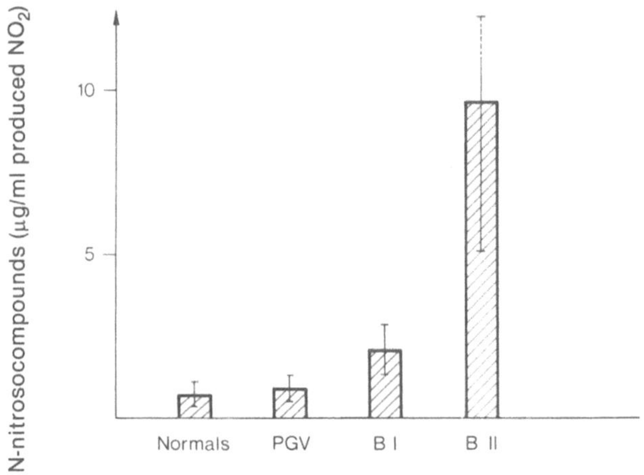

Fig. 8. *N*-nitrosocompounds in the gastric juice in correlation to various operative procedures in the human stomach

Discussion

Gastric surgery results in changes of bacterial flora not only in the bowel [1, 8, 24], but also in the stomach, as could be seen in our experiments. There are several suggested explanations for this. The bacteriostatic effect of gastric acid is unsettled [7, 15] and this could explain in part the changes in the bacterial flora after truncal vagotomy. However, achlorhydria does not necessarily result in bacterial overgrowth [3].

According to our experiments, after truncal vagotomy only the proportion of nitrate positive bacteria is increased, and we conclude that following vagotomy there is a qualitative change in the gastric flora.

Motility is another important factor for bacterial proliferation in the gut [5, 13]. After gastroenterostomy without entero-enteroanastomosis, the normal intestinal flow is disturbed and this effects an increase in the total bacterial count. Since, after gastroenterostomy without enteroanastomosis, the proportion of nitrate reductase positive organisms is increased, the higher total bacterial count results in a significant increase in nitrate decomposing bacteria. Roux-Y-gastroenterostomy without reflux promotes fewer of these changes. Truncal vagotomy leads not only to achlorhydria, but also gastric emptying is partially delayed. Therefore, vagotomy with pyloroplasty also promotes the shown changes less.

A high nitrite concentration in gastric juice is related to an increase in nitrate reductase positive organisms. The rate of N-nitrosation is determined by the concentration of nitrosable amine and the square of the nitrite concentration [19, 20]: Thus, the higher nitrite concentration found in gastric juice may be sufficient to allow intragastric formation of nitrosamines [9, 16, 23].

The presence of a high nitrite concentration together with a high total bacterial count in gastric juice is especially after gastroenterostomy without entero-enteroanastomosis, conductive in *N*-nitrosation. This leads to an intragastric increase of *N*-nitrosocompounds. In the Billroth II resected stomach, the effect of a gastroenterostomy is added to an achlorhydria by partial gastric resection. Therefore, these changes are more frequent than in the Billroth I resected stomach. Proximal gastric vagotomy probably does not lead to a disturbance of gastric emptying and gastric pH is not significantly influenced, thus, no differences in this group in comparison to normal individuals were found. Intragastric formation of *N*-nitrosocompounds [23, 18] may be a serious and dangerous factor in the development of cancer in the operated stomach. Of course, it cannot be concluded that all detectable *N*-nitrosocompounds are carcinogen and that present carcinogenic nitrosamines are always shown in relevant concentration [15, 16]. However, an increased intragastric development of *N*-nitrosocompounds should be considered as a cocarcinogenic factor. Intragastric *N*-nitrosation may induce malignant transformation, especially in the susceptible mucosa of the operated stomach [4, 25]. Because nitrite and *N*-nitrosocompounds in the gastric juice are dependent on operative technique, this should be taken into consideration for gastric surgery.

Conclusion

In animal experiments gastroenterostomy without enteroanastomosis or truncal vagotomy resulted in an increase of nitrate reductase positive organisms in the stomach. An increase in nitrate reductase positive bacteria is related to a higher nitrite concentration in gastric juice. The presence of high nitrite concentration together, with high bacterial count is followed by an increase of *N*-nitrosocompounds in the stomach.

Variations in nitrite concentration and N-nitrosocompounds in human gastric juice after various operative procedures on the stomach showed a close relationship to our animal experiments.

Because intragastric *N*-nitrosation, which may induce malignant transformation, is largely dependent on operative technique, this should be taken into consideration for gastric surgery.

References

1. Berndt, H.: Dysbiose nach Magenoperation und ihre Behandlung. Z. Inn. Med. *24,* 377 (1969)
2. Braun, O. H., Dehnert, J., Haenel, H., Müller-Beuthow, W., Reuter, G., Reploh, H.: Methoden der bakteriologischen Stuhluntersuchung. Zentralbl. Bakteriol. [Orig.] *200,* 405 (1966)

3. Cregan, J., Dunlop, E. E., Hayward, N. J.: Bacterial content of human small intestine in disease of stomach. Br. Med. J. *1953 2,* 1248
4. Dahm, K., Rehner, M. (eds.): Das Karzinom im operierten Magen. Stuttgart: Thieme 1975
5. Dixon, J. M. S.: Fate of bacteria in small intestine. J. Pathol. Bacteriol. *79,* 131 (1960)
6. Druckrey, H., Steinhoff, D., Beuthner, H., Klärner, P.: Prüfung von Nitrit auf chronisch toxische Wirkung an Ratten. Arzneim. Forsch. *13,* 320 (1963)
7. Goldstein, F., Wirts, C. W., Josephs, L.: Bacterial flora in the small intestine. Gastroenterology *42,* 755 (1962)
8. Greenlee, H. B., Vivit, R., Paez, J., Dietz, A.: Bacterial flora of the jejunum following peptic ulcer surgery. Arch. Surg. *102,* 250 (1971)
9. Hawksworth, G. M., Hill, M. J.: Bacterial and N-nitrosation of secondary amines. Br. J. Cancer *25,* 520 (1971)
10. Holdeman, L. V., Moore, W. E. C.: Anaerobe laboratory manual. Anaerobe Laboratory, Virginia Polytechnic Institute and State University, Blacksburg Va 1972
11. Kunstyr, I.: Some quantitative and qualitative aspects of the stomach microflora of the conventional rat and hamster. Zentralbl. Veterinaermed. [A] *21,* 553 (1974)
12. Magee, P. N., Schoental, R.: Carcinogenesis by nitrosocompounds. Br. Med. Bull. *20,* 102 (1964)
13. Merkle, P., Meyer, H., Ecknauer, R.: Mucosafunktion und Keimbesiedlung bei mechanischem Dünndarmileus der Ratte. In: Ileus. Eckert, P., Richter, H. (eds.). Stuttgart: Thieme 1978
14. Outryve, van M., Huybrechts, W., Blaauw, A. M., de Weerdt, G. A., Beke, R., Barbier, F.: Jejunal bile salts and microflora in patients with partial gastrectomy. Am. J. Gastroenterol. *69,* 550 (1978)
15. Ruddell, W. S. J., Bone, E. S., Hill, M. J., Walters, C. L.: Gastric juice nitrite. Lancet *1976 13,* 1037
16. Ruddell, W. S. J., Bone, E. S., Hill, M. J., Walters, C. L.: Pathogenesis of gastric cancer in pernicious anaemia. Lancet *1978 11,* 521
17. Sander, J.: Eine Methode zum Nachweis von Nitrosaminen. Z. Physiol. Chem. *348,* 852 (1967)
18. Sander, J., Schweinsberg, F., Menz, H. P.: Untersuchungen über die Entstehung carcinogener Nitrosamine im Magen. Z. Physiol. Chem. *349,* 1961 (1968)
19. Sander, J.: Nitrosaminsynthese durch Bakterien. Z. Physiol. Chem. *349,* 429 (1968)
20. Sander, J., Schweinsberg, F.: Wechselbeziehungen zwischen Nitrat, Nitrit und kanzerogenen N-Nitrosoverbindungen. Zentralbl. Bakteriol. Hyg. *156,* 299 (1972)
21. Sagimura, T., Katachi, T.: Das experimentelle Magencarcinom. Leber, Magen, Darm *6,* 80 (1976)
22. Schlag, P., Wonka, W., Meyer, H., Feyerabend, G., Merkle, P.: Bakterielle Besiedlung und Nitritbildung im Magen nach Gastroenterostomie. Langenbecks Arch. Chir. *344,* 109 (1977)
23. Sen, N. P., Smith, D. C., Schwinghamer, L.: Formation of N-nitrosamines from secondary amines and nitrite in human and animal gastric juice. Cosmet. Toxicol. *7,* 301 (1969)
24. Smith, W.: Observation on the flora of the alimentary and factors affecting it composition. J. Pathol. Bacteriol. *89,* 95 (1965)
25. Taylor, H. W., Lijinsky, T.: Tumor induction in rats by feeding hepamethylene-inine and nitrite in water. Cancer Res. *35,* 812 (1975)

Risk of Carcinoma in the Gastric Remnant After Gastric Resection for Benign Conditions

G. Clémençon

General Frequency of Carcinoma in the Operated Stomach

Up to 1950, carcinoma of the gastric remnant after resection for a benign lesion seemed to be a rare disease. Morgenstern et al. [25] estimated the number of patients with cancer of the gastric stump mentioned in the world literature up to the year 1972 to be about 1100. Kühlmayer and Rokitansky [22] collected among 50000 autopsies at the Institute of Pathology of the University of Vienna, 363 cases with gastric resections type Billroth I, Billroth II, or gastroenterostomies and found 40 cancers in this material. This corresponds to an incidence of 11% compared to 5.3% gastric cancers in nonoperated stomachs among the 49637 other autopsies. Hilbe et al. [17] found in their necropsy material 5.4% cancers among nonoperated stomachs, but a frequency double as high in resected stomachs. Stalsberg and Taksdal [39] report that among 630 cases of gastric cancer, the frequency of previous gastric surgery for benign conditions, 25 years or more before death, was six times the frequency among matched controls. Even if one objects that necropsy material is biased by preselection in some way, one cannot deny the higher incidence of gastric stump cancer. There are few prospective studies based on endoscopically examined patients. From 1968 to 1974, Pesendorfer et al. [29] found 16% gastric stump cancers among their patients with resected stomachs. Schmid et al. [35] evaluated 24000 gastroscopies and found 609 patients with gastrojejunostomy, after an interval of at least 5 years after gastric resection, 39 of them had gastric stump cancer (6.4%). Furthermore, they detected five cancer cases among patients with gastroduodenostomy (6.2%). Thus, in contrast to other authors [2, 12, 15, 25], the incidence is not different between Billroth I and II in their material. However, the frequency of cancer varies considerably in the four involved infirmaries of this group, from 11.5% to 4.6%.

Frequency of Carcinoma in the Operated Stomach in Our Own Material

There may be preselection among hospitalized patients and in autopsy material, depending on regional pecularities. We have tried to avoid this selection problem by evaluating a collective represented by ambulatory patients of five scientifically active gastroenterologists during the years 1968 – 1974. In this period, 6341 upper panendoscopies were performed. Among these were 346 gastrojejunostomies (Billroth II), 58 gastroduodenostomies (Billroth I), and 130 other gastric operations. Twenty-three gastric stump cancers were found (6.65%) among the 346 patients with Billroth II resection for a benign lesion; none in the other groups. In comparison, there were 279 gastric cancers (0.95%) among 29361 patients who had never been submitted to gastric surgery. There was no significant age difference at operation between patients with gastrojejunostomy and gastric stump cancer (39.19 years) and those with gastrojejunostomy without carcinoma (40.52 years). The mean interval from gastric resection to the manifestation of carcinoma was 23.8 years, which was comparable to the data of other authors (Table 1).

Importance of the Postoperative Interval

The mean age of the 23 patients with resected stomachs and carcinoma was 62.62 years, that of the 279 patients with gastric cancer in the nonoperated stomach 64.45 years; again there was no significant difference. Thus, it seems that age is of importance for both patient groups and one would expect that carcinoma incidence will augment with increasing interval. Our figures show this assumption to be correct. Up to 9 years after resection, none of 187 patients with gastric resection after Billroth II had cancer of the gastric remnant, but 6 (8.72%) of 69 patients 10 – 19 years after resection, and 15 of 70 patients 20 and more years later (21.4%). Thus, with an interval of 10 and more years, the overall incidence of gastric stump cancer is 15.1% (Table 2).

Table 1. Mean interval between gastric resection for a benign lesion and diagnosis of gastric stump cancer

Gerstenberg et al.	(1965)	23 years
Kobajashi et al.	(1970)	23 years
Stalsberg et al.	(1971)	26.4 years
Morgenstern et al.	(1973)	24 years
Schmid et al.	(1976)	23 years
Clémençon et al.	(1976)	23.8 years

Table 2. Carcinoma in the gastric remnant after Billroth II resection; importance of the postoperative interval

Interval (years)	Billroth II resected patients		Incidence of cancer of the gastric stump[a]	
	n	With carcinoma		
<9	187	0	0%	
10 – 19	69	6	8.7%	15.1%
≧20	70	15	21.4%	

Clémençon G. et al.: Dtsch. med. Wschr. *101*, 1015 – 1020 (1976)

[a] Two of the 23 cases of cancer in the gastric remnant are not considered in this table, since in one case, the diagnosis of the initial lesion leading to gastric resection and in the other, histology were not known

The figures of Schmid et al. [35] are similar: the incidence of gastric stump cancer was 2.3% for an interval of 5 – 14.9 years, 9.5% 15 – 29.9 years, and 15.7% 30 and more years after resection. In conclusion, the resected stomach shows a higher risk for developing carcinoma than the nonoperated stomach. The longer the interval after gastric resection, the higher the incidence of carcinoma. Or, in our patient collective: the patient with a resected stomach and a postoperative interval of more than 10 years had one chance in eight to suffer from cancer of the gastric remnant.

Statistical Problems and Expected Risk

However, things have changed these past 10 years. Surgery has chosen a new tactical proceeding. Instead of mutilating resections, methods preserving the continuity of the gastric organ are applied nowadays, such as highly selective vagotomy. Resections are limited to malignant diseases. Thus, in conjunction with the decline of the number of resected stomachs, a decrease of gastric stump cancer incidence will ensue. But regional differences may remain. I have tried to evaluate the situation for the next 10 years at my place of residence in Switzerland in the canton of Solothurn. Questionnaires were sent to five surgical departments asking for statistical material concerning gastric resections during the period from 1948 to 1968. The information was incomplete and in the statistics of earlier years, no difference was made between gastric resection with gastrojejunostomy (Billroth II) or with gastroduodenostomy (Billroth I). By interpolation, the following results: the frequency of gastric resection has declined impressively in the last 10 years. During the period from 1962 to 1968, the frequency of resection was at its highest. In the two main hospitals, highly selective vagotomy is performed routinely. In all surgical departments together, about 1860 patients were submitted to gastric resection corresponding to 0.8% of our residential population of 222 200. Assuming the incidence of gastric stump cancer to average 10%, we would have to expect 180 cases of gastric stump carcinoma within the next 10 years, a figure probably too high. In our aforementioned study, we did not examine asymptomatic patients [2]. With this in mind, we should estimate that only about 10% of patients with a resected stomach would have to consult their gastroenterologist for upper abdominal distress. This would reduce the aforementioned figure to 186. Of these patients, 93 had gastric resection in the period from 1948 to 1957, therefore producing 18 new cases of gastric stump cancer in accordance with a carcinoma risk of 20% 20 and more years after resection. The other 93 patients, operated on in the period 1958 – 1968 would then yield in the next 10 years in accordance with their postoperative interval of 10 – 29 years and a risk of about 15%, 14 new cases of stump cancers. Thus, in the canton of Solothurn we would have to expect among patients submitted to gastric resection during the period from 1948 to 1968, 32 new cases of carcinoma in the gastric remnant. I hardly need to point out how problematic this kind of calculation is. However, should we really intend to provide thoroughly organized prophylatic measures, we would have to submit yearly about 1800 patients to gastroscopy in our residential canton. Great social, financial, and organizational problems would thus emerge.

Table 3. Gastric stump cancer among patients of two gastroenterologists in the Swiss canton of Solothurn

Examiner	Period	Upper endoscopies (n)	Billroth II	Billroth I	Gastric stump cancers (Billroth II)	%
Miller	1 January 71 – 31 December 74	2030	95	27	7	7.37
	1 January 75 – 31 December 77	2040	57	31	3	5.2
Clémençon	1 January 71 – 31 December 74	1837	66	5	5	7.58
	1 January 75 – 31 December 77	1462	102	17	2	1.96

In contrast to the author group of Vienna detecting an incidence of 16% gastric stump cancers during the period 1968–1974 Pesendorfer et al. [29] and Pötzi et al. [30] found only 11 carcinomas (4.5%) from 1974 to 1976 among 244 patients submitted to stomach resection for a benign condition. They explain the lower incidence by the fact that during these 2 years, more asymptomatic patients had been submitted to gastroscopy than before. However, in this investigation, the postoperative interval was not taken into consideration.

Domellöf et al. [10] found in a prospective study among 459 Billroth II patients, a gastric stump cancer incidence of only 2.3%. They included asymptomatic patients and, furthermore, the great majority of these patients had a postoperative interval of not more than 20 years. Of their patients, 140 had died by the time of investigation, only 60 of them being submitted to necropsy. In this latter group, three carcinomas were detected. Of the patients, 105 refused examination. Analyzing our patient collective in the period from 1 January 1975 to 31 December 77, we also noticed a declining incidence.

Again, most of the patients in Table 3 have a postoperative interval of not more than 15 years. All these figures stress the importance attached to the postoperative interval when evaluating the frequency of cancer in the gastric remnant.

Importance of Atrophic Gastritis

None of the 23 cancers detected by our group were early cancers [5]. Early cancer in gastric remnants are detected more frequently these last years [16, 27,31], and from January to June 1978, I detected two cases. Histological changes are frequent near the anastomosis in resected stomachs and many authors point out the importance of chronic atrophic gastristis [13, 25, 36, 38, 40]. We examined

Table 4. Histology of Billroth II – resected stomachs 10–27 years after resection

Normal gastric mucosa	0
Superficial gastritis	11 (29.5%)
Chronic-atrophic gastritis	16 (43.0%)
Chronic-atrophic gastritis with intestinal metaplasia	8 (21.5%)
Stump cancers	2
	37

37 patients (Table 4) who had stomach resection for duodenal ulcer 10–27 years ago and none of them showed a normal histology of the gastric mucosa near the stoma [5].

It is surprising that in our patient collective, chronic atrophic gastritis with intestinal metaplasia and severe epithelial dysplasia was not more frequent, since most gastric cancers in the resected stomach are localized near the anastomosis [20, 21, 25]. Hammar [16] found among 65 patients with a resected stomach and a mean postoperative interval of 20 years, who had to be submitted to gastric surgery again, in the resected specimens, nine cases of precancerosis, 22 cases of early cancer, and 34 carcinomas with invasive growth.

In accordance with what has been explained hitherto, the incidence of carcinoma in the gastric remnant is undoubtedly higher than it is in the nonoperated stomach. This incidence can be compared to the frequency of gastric cancer in pernicious anemia [33, 37].

Importance of Duodenogastric Reflux

In addition to this statement, it would be of importance to know if there are some other risk factors promoting carcinoma in the gastric remnant. Palmer [28], Thompson [40], Du Plessis [11], Lawson [23] and others have attached importance to duodenogastric reflux as a possible etiological factor for chronic atrophic gastritis. Regurgitated bile, especially bile acids and salts, exert a noxious effect on gastric mucosa [8, 14, 19]. The gastric mucosal barrier is destroyed, since the detergent effect of bile acids leads to dissolution of the gastric mucus, thus promoting back-diffusion of H^+. In addition to bile acids and salts, other substances might exert this unwanted effect. We were able to detect and identify lysolecithin in gastric secretions [1, 4]. In the stomachs of patients with gastric ulcer, atrophic gastritis, and erosions, hemolytic substances including lysolecithin were more often discovered than in normal stomachs [3]. Furthermore, hemolytic substances were also found in resected stomachs (unpublished). Lysolecithin is a metabolite of lipid metabolism and is produced by the action of phospholipase A on lecithin which is excreted in the bile. This substance has a pronounced cytotoxic effect and promotes hemolysis in very low in very low concentrations. Johnson et al. [18] found lysolecithin in gastric ulcer stomachs and discussed its possible role in the pathogenesis of peptic ulcer disease. Davenport [9] demonstrated H^+ back-diffusion in the canine stomach after instillation of lysolecithin. Bile reflux is expected to occur quite often in resected stomachs, the frequency ranging from 60% to 90% in the literature. We observed bile reflux in 63.7% of Billroth II patients (Table 5).

However, one may notice that reflux is not a constant phenomenon. During the last 3 years, we performed gastroscopy a second time in 18 of 141 Billroth II patients. Seven proved again to have reflux (38.9%). This means that if no reflux can be observed on one examination, it may be detected on another occasion. We feel, that bile reflux is dependant on the operation technique. Occasionally, one is surprised to observe a pseudopyloric function of the anastomosis. Schindler [34] found among 41 patients with a resected stomach, only four with normal histology and all of them showed a rhythmic pseudopyloric function of the stoma. May it be a consequence of bile reflux or because of other reasons, chronic atrophic gastritis is frequent in the resected stomach; achlorhydria or hypochlorhydria will follow finally. Although it seems inadmissible to make comparisons in analogy to experimental work with nitrosoguanidines in animals, these experiments may uncover a possible way in pathogenesis of gastric carcinoma. Nitrosamines are produced in the stomach, mainly in a neutral milieu, and may deploy a deleterious effect only if the normal mucosal barrier is destroyed [6].

Multifactorial Pathogenesis of Carcinoma in the Gastric Stump

Thus, many factors are involved in the genesis of gastric stump cancer. If resection were the main promoting factor to cancer development, then the average age of about 60 years in patients with carcinoma in the gastric remnant and those with a cancer in the nonoperated stomach could hardly be explained. As Schmid et al. [35] point out, there is a negative correlation of the age at operation and the age at cancer manifestation. This statement has validity for our patients, too. The younger the patient at operation, the longer the interval to cancer development and vice versa. Undoubtedly, atrophic gastritis with or without intestinal metaplasia is one of the factors promoting carcinoma [32]. But it cannot be considered a precancerosis if not accompanied by severe epithelial dysplasia. Even then, regression of the process seems possible as Oehlert et al.

Table 5. Bile reflux in the resected stomach (among the last 1000 upper endoscopies)

Resection with:	n	Patients with reflux	%
Gastrojejunostomy	77	49	63.7
Gastroduodenostomy	15	11	73.3

[26] could show. There is no characteristic symptomatology allowing suspicion of gastric stump carcinoma at the beginning. Unrelated and vague dyspeptic troubles may motivate the patient to seek medical help. The awareness of a higher cancer frequency in the resected stomach is one of the reasons why early cancer has been detected more often lately.

Conclusion

1) Carcinoma of the stomach remnant 10 or more years after gastric resection for a benign condition represents a serious risk.
2) The mean interval between gastric resection and manifestation of gastric stump cancer is about 24 years. There is a negative correlation between the age at operation and the age at cancer manifestation.
3) The following should have an annual gastroscopic control:
   Patients with gastric resection at an age up to 40 years and a postoperative interval of 20 years.
   Patients with gastric resection at an age of more than 40 years after a postoperative interval of 10 years.
4) Patients with a resected stomach and proven chronic biliary reflux should have an yearly gastroscopic control after a postoperative interval of 10 years.
5) Patients with severe epithelial dysplasia in the gastric remnant should have regular short-termed endoscopic controls.
6) Any patients with a resected stomach and upper abdominal distress should have gastroscopy.

References

1. Bürgi, W., Kaufmann, H., Clémençon, G.: Isolierung, Identifizierung und quantitative Bestimmung von Lysolecithin im menschlichen Magensaft. Schweiz. Med. Wochenschr. *105,* 1814–1819 (1975)
2. Clémençon, G., Baumgartner, R., Leuthold, E., Miller, G., Neiger, A.: Das Karzinom des operierten Magens. Dtsch. Med. Wochenschr. *101*, 1015–1020 (1976)
3. Clémençon, G., Bürgi, W.: Hämolysierende Substanzen im Magensekret, Häufigkeit des Lysolecithin-Nachweises. Schweiz. Med. Wochenschr. *107,* 952–956 (1977)
4. Clémencon, G., Bürgi, W., Kaufmann, H.: Lysolecithin im nächtlichen Magensekret (Abstrakt). 1st Congress of the society for Gastroenterology in Bavaria 24–25 October 1973
5. Clémençon, G., Gloor, F.: Ist die chronisch atrophische Gastritis eine Präkanzerose? (in press)
6. Correa, P., Haenszel, W., Cuello, C., Tannenbaum, St., Archer, M.: A model for gastric cancer epidemiology. Lancet *1975 II,* 58–59
7. Dahm, K., Werner, B.: Das Karzinom im operierten Magen. Dtsch. Med. Wochenschr. *100,* 1073–1078 (1975)
8. Davenport, H. W.: Destruction of the gastric mucosal barrier by detergents and urea. Gastroenterology *54*, 175–181 (1968)
9. Davenport, H. W.: Effect of lysolecithin, digitonin and phospholipase A upon the dog's gastric mucosal barrier. Gastroenterology *59*, 505–509 (1970)
10. Domellöf, L., Eriksson, S., Janungen, K. G.: Carcinoma and possible precancerous changes of the gastric stump after Billroth II resection. Gastroenterology *73*, 462–468 (1977)
11. Du Plessis, D. J.: Gastric mucosal changes after operations on the stomach. S. Afr. Med. J. *36*, 471–478 (1962)

12. Gerstenberg, E., Albrecht, A., Krentz, K., Voth, H.: Das Magenstumpfkarzinom: Eine Spätkomplikation des operierten Magens? Dtsch. Med. Wochenschr. *90*, 2185–2190 (1965)
13. Gjeruldsen, S. T., Myren, J., Fretheim, B.: Alterations of gastric mucosa following a graded partial gastrectomy for duodenal ulcer. Scand. J. Gastroenterol. *3*, 465–470 (1968)
14. Grant, R., Grossmann, M. J., Wang, K. J., Jvy, A. C.: The cytolytic action of some gastrointestinal secretions and enzymes on epithelial cells of the gastric and duodenal mucosa. J. Cell. Comp. Physiol. *37*, 137–161 (1951)
15. Griesser, G., Schmidt, H.: Statistische Erhebungen über die Häufigkeit des Karzinoms nach Magenoperation wegen eines Geschwürleidens. Med. Welt *15*, 1836–1840 (1964)
16. Hammar, E.: The localization of precancerous changes and carcinoma after previous gastric surgery for benign condition. Acta Pathol. Microbiol. Scand. (A) *84*, 495–504 (1976)
17. Hilbe, G., Salzer, G. M., Hussl, H., Kutschera, H.: Die Carcinomgefährdung des Resektionsmagens. Langenbecks Arch. Klin. Chir. *323*, 142 (1968)
18. Johnson, A. G., McDermott, J. S.: Lysolecithin: A factor in the pathogenesis of gastric ulceration? Gut *15*, 710 (1974)
19. Jvey, K. J., Den Besten, L., Clifton, J. A.: Effect of bile salts on ionic movement across the human gastric mucosa. Gastroenterology *59*, 683–690 (1970)
20. Kobayashi, S., Prolla, J. C., Kirsner, J. B.: Late gastric carcinoma developing after surgery for benign conditions. Am. J. Dig. Dis. *15*, 905–912 (1970)
21. Krause, U.: Late prognosis after partial gastrectomy for ulcer. Acta. Chir. Scand. *114*, 341–354 (1957)
22. Kühlmayer, R., Rokitansky, O.: Das Magenstumpfcarcinom als Spätproblem der Ulcuschirurgie. Langenbecks Arch. klin. Chir. *278*, 361–375 (1954)
23. Lawson, H. H.: Effect of duodenal contents on the gastric mucosa under experimental conditions. Lancet *1964 I*, 469–472
24. Miller, G.: personal communication 1978
25. Morgenstern, L., Yamakawa, T., Seltzer, D.: Carcinoma of the gastric stump. Amer. J. Surg. *125*, 29–38 (1973)
26. Oehlert, W., Keller, P., Henke, M., Strauch, M.: Die Dysplasien der Magenschleimhaut. Dtsch. Med. Wochenschr. *100*, 1950–1956 (1975)
27. Osnes, M., Løtveil, T., Myren, J., Serek-Hansen, A.: Early gastric carcinoma in patients with a Billroth II partial gastrectomy. Endoscopy *9*, 45–49 (1977)
28. Palmer, E. D.: Gastritis. A revaluation. Medicine (Baltimore) *33*, 199–290 (1954)
29. Pesendorfer, F. X., Afschar, S., Henschel, E., Weiss, W.: Das Magenstumpfcarcinom aus endoskopischer Sicht. Fortschr. Gastroenterol. Endoskopie 117–121 (1974)
30. Pötzi, R., Pesendorfer, F. X., Denk, H., Wewalka, F.: Makroskopische und histologische Befunde am operierten Magen. Z. Gastroenterol. *15*, 627–629 (1977)
31. Rehner, M., Soehendra, N., Eichfuss, H. P., Dahm, K., Eckert, P., Mitschke, H.: Frühkarzinome im (Billroth-II-)Resektionsmagen. Dtsch. Med. Wochenschr. *99*, 533–534 (1974)
32. Reynolds, K. W., Johnson, A. G., Fox, B.: Is intestinal metaplasia of the gastric mucosa a premalignant lesion? Clin. Oncol. *1*, 101–109 (1975)
33. Schell, R. F., Dockerty, M. B., Comfort, M. W.: Carcinoma of the stomach associated with pernicious anemia. Surg. Gynecol. Obstet. *98*, 710–720 (1954)
34. Schindler, R.: Gastritis. New York: Grune & Stratton 1947
35. Schmid, E., Vollmer, R., Adlemg, J., Blaich, E., Goebell, H., Heinkel, K., Kimmig, J. M., Probst, M.: Zur endoskopischen Diagnose des Karzinoms im operierten Magen. Z. Gastroenterol. *14*, 521–530 (1976)
36. Seifert, E., Dittrich, H., Erd, W.: Gastrobioptische Untersuchung am Resektionsmagen. Med. Welt *17*, 38–44 (1966)
37. Shearmann, D. J. C., Finlayson, N. D. C., Wilson, R., Samson, R. R.: Carcinoma of the stomach and early pernicious anaemia. Lancet *1966 II*, 403–405
38. Simon, L., Figus, A. J., Bajtai, A.: Chronic gastritis following resection of the stomach. Am. J. Gastroenterol. *60*, 477–487 (1973)
39. Stalsberg, H., Taksdal, S.: Stomach cancer following gastric surgery for benign conditions. Lancet *1971 II*, 1175–1177
40. Thompson, H.: Gastritis in partial gastrectomy specimens. Gastroenterology *36*, 861–876 (1959)

Remarks on Frequency and Pathogenesis of Primary Gastric Stump Cancer

W. Peitsch

Since gastric resection of the Billroth-II type has been standard procedure in surgical treatment of gastric and duodenal ulcer disease in the last 40 years, an increase of primary gastric stump carcinomas can be observed.

More than 3 000 cases of primary gastric stump cancers have been published, but today it is not generally accepted that the risk of developing a cancer in the gastric remnant after different surgical procedures (Billroth I, Billroth II, vagotomy, or gastrojejunostomy) [2, 5, 7, 9, 13, 14, 15, 17] and the basic illness (gastric or duodenal ulcer, chronic atrophic gastritis) [7, 12] is higher compared to the risk of stomach cancer among the normal population.

Most of the analyses report clinical cases of gastric stump carcinomas [3, 13] or therapy and prognosis and correlate the frequency of primary gastric stump cancer with the number of operated gastric carcinomas or ulcer resections during the same period [2, 13, 15].

Possible Statistical Procedures and Their Limitations

1) Prospective controlled analyses must cover 5 – 30 years, because the interval from operation to the development of a cancer is more than 20 years [12, 13].

2) Postmortem studies have little importance, because there is a high incidence of carcinomas in university clinics; at death no information concerning the basic illness at the time of operation can be given. Postmortem studies give no data indicative of the absolute frequency of gastric stump carcinomas; they merely allow correlation of the frequency of gastric stump carcinomas with the frequency of primary gastric carcinomas in nonoperated persons from the same autopsy pool.

3) The importance of data obtained by random-sample routine endoscopy is controversial [2, 17], because only patients with gastric pain are examined. The endoscopist has no data concerning the basic illness at the time of operation or the operative procedure (e.g., Billroth II with or without enteroanastomosis).

Requirements for Prospective and Retrospective Studies

Prospective and retrospective studies have to include a great number of patients, e.g., 500 – 1000. They must cover more than 20 years, and all patients in the study have to be operated on using the same technique. Data concerning the basic illness at the time of primary operation, localization of the ulcer, and the benign histology of ulcer or gastritis must be present. However, 20 or 30 years ago ulcers were classified according to their localization in stomach or duodenum and not in relation to the amounts of gastric acid.

Finally there must be a comparision to a group of patients from the same area and with the same basic illness treated nonsurgically, because nonoperated gastric and duodenal ulcer patients and patients without gastric illness have different cancer risks [19, 20, 21].

Actual Rate of Gastric Stump Cancer

Prospective studies with a long observation time do not exist, all "prospective analyses" [6, 14, 18] are one or two endoscopic examinations of a group of resected stomachs conducted within a short period after an interval of 20–25 years (Table 1). Therefore the frequency of gastric stump carcinomas is too low (0.85% – 3.7%) [14, 18]. These prospective studies only give the cancer frequency after gastric resection at *one* observation point, e.g., after 20 years, not the cancer risk of the whole group. Only the relationship between stump cancer frequency in postmortem examinations of all resected stomach patients and the gastric cancer mortality among the normal population shows the cancer risk after resection for peptic ulcer, since all patients of this group can develop a primary gastric stump cancer.

The frequency of gastric stump carcinomas (1.3% – 8.9%) differs in relation to the observation time and the number of patients [12, 15]. Analytical data for a great number of patients indicate a cancer frequency among patients with Billroth-II resected stomachs of 7.7% – 14.4% [7, 10, 12].

Table 1. Actual rate of gastric stump carcinomas (so-called prospective analysis)

Author	Year	Follow-up time years	Number of patients *n*	Incidence of cancer %
Domellöf et al. (Billroth I)	1977	10–22	108	3.7
Domellöf et al. (Billroth II)	1977	18–26	228	3.7
Schrumpf et al. (Billroth II)	1977	20–25	108	3.7
Peitsch, Becker (Billroth II)	1978	5–40	104	1.8
Rösch, Prütting (Billroth II)	1978	>15	117	0.85

Influence of the Basic Illness on Cancer Frequency

Gastric resection after gastric ulcer shows a different cancer frequency to resection after duodenal ulcer (Tables 2, 3). After gastric ulcer resection, long-term studies show a cancer incidence of 13.2% – 16% [7, 12]. But also in patients with conservatively treated gastric ulcer, gastric cancer develops in 10.7% within 28 – 50 years [7]. In a group of patients with chronic atrophic gastritis it developed in 10% within 10 – 15 years [1, 19, 21]. This is important to know, since nearly all statistics correlate only the gastric stump carcinoma risk after gastric ulcer resection with the risk of the normal population.

After duodenal ulcer resection the stump cancer incidence is lower. Only 7.1% – 9.1% of patients who died more than 5 years after gastric resection had a stump cancer at death. But in this group no control group with medically treated duodenal ulcer disease and an observation time of 30 years or longer exists to correlate the cancer risk of the operated and nonoperated patients.

Table 2. Frequency of gastric cancer after partial gastrectomy (Billroth II) for gastric ulcer (retrospective analysis)

Author	Number of patients *n*	Incidence of cancer %	Follow-up time years
Griesser, Schmidt (1964)	419	16.0	28 – 50
Helsingen, Hillestad (1956)	25	40.0	10 – 35
Peitsch, Becker (1977)	91	13.2	5 – 40
Conservative treatment			
Griesser, Schmidt (1964)	253	10.7	28 – 50

Table 3. Frequency of gastric cancer after partial gastrectomy (Billroth II) for duodenal ulcer (retrospective analysis)

Author	Number of patients *n*	Incidence of cancer %	Follow up time years
Griesser, Schmidt (1964)	99	9.1	28 – 43
Helsingen, Hillestad (1956)	12	8.3	10 – 35
Peitsch, Becker (1977)	211	7.1	5 – 40
Conservative ulcer treatment		?	

Interval Between Gastric Resection and Development of Cancer

Approximate time intervals between gastric resection and diagnosis of gastric stump cancer are shown in Table 4. The interval ranges from 5 to 37 years, most cases appearing 26–37 years after the primary gastric resection. Only 1.9% – 4.7% of all patients dying 5 to 15 years after the partial gastrectomy had a cancer of the gastric remnant. Perhaps in this period a gastric resection has a protective effect against cancer, in correlation with the cancer incidence after medically treated gastric ulcer or chronic atrophic gastritis.

However, 26–30 years after gastric resection 22% of these patients died of gastric cancer. These findings illustrate the high risk of stump cancer in the resected stomach after a cancer-free interval of more than 15 to 20 years. The cancer-free interval decreases with increasing age of the patients at the time of primary resection for peptic ulcer, and the interval seems to be shorter after gastric ulcer resection, in correlation with duodenal ulcer resection.

Frequency of Gastric Cancer in Postmortem Studies

The postmortem studies of Kühlmayer and Rokitansky [11] and Hilbe et al. [9] show a cancer frequency in the resected stomach of 8.9% – 10.7%; in their

Table 4. Frequency and interval of gastric stump cancer after gastric resection for benign diseases

Death after gastric resection (years)	Number of patients	Number of gastric stump cancers	Percentage of gastric stump cancers
5–11	43	2	4.7
11–15	53	1	1.9
16–20	76	6	7.9
21–25	52	4	7.7
26–30	50	11	22.0
31–37	28	3	10.7

Table 5. Frequency of gastric cancer an autopsy statistics (Billroth-II resection)

Author	Number of		Frequency
	Patients	Carcinomas	%
Kühlmayer, Rokitansky (1954)	290	31	10.7
Hilbe et al. (1968)	350	31	8.9
Control groups without gastric resection			
Kühlmayer, Rokitansky (1954)	50000	2650	5.3
Hilbe et al. (1968)	9857	533	5.4

patients the cancer mortality is twice as high as the cancer mortality of the normal population (Table 5).

However, in postmortem studies we should expect a higher cancer incidence than in retrospective studies, because not all stump carcinomas are diagnosed clinically. Postmortem studies of today could be expected to reveal a higher cancer frequency than those of 20 years ago, because more and more patients with peptic ulcers survive 20 years and more after their partial gastrectomy.

Billroth-I Resection, Gastrojejunostomy

Very few details are known about the cancer risk of a stomach resected using the Billroth-I procedure; only Griesser and Schmidt tackle this in their retrospective study of 104 patients who had undergone gastric ulcer resection [7] – a cancer frequency of 8.3% was found. Data for Billroth-I duodenal ulcer resection do not exist.

The low frequency of clinical observations of carcinoma in the gastric remnant after Billroth-I resection does not say anything about the cancer risk of a Billroth-I resected stomach, because in mid-Europe only a small number of patients are resected using this method.

Data for the cancer risk of a stomach with peptic ulcer, treated by gastrojejunostomy, are also difficult to interpret. Prospective analyses do not exist and retrospective long-term observation studies are rare, because partial gastrectomy in ulcer therapy displaced gastrojejunostomy more than 40 years ago, specially in duodenal ulcer disease and pyloric stenosis.

Only one retrospective study [12] exists, and 124 dead gastric ulcer patients treated by gastrojejunostomy were involved. This analysis shows an increased cancer frequency of nearly 20%.

Animal Experimental Studies

In animal experimental models several groups [4, 16] have tried to show the frequency of gastric cancer after different operative procedures (Table 6); this

Table 6. Frequency of gastric cancer in animal experiments

Author	Number of animals n	Incidence of cancer %
	Billroth-I resection	
Dahm and Werner (1973)	37	40.5
	Billroth-II resection	
Dahm and Werner (1973)	29	34.5
	GE without enteroanastomosis	
Schlag et al. (1977)	30	0
	GE with Roux-en-Y-anastomosis	
Schlag et al. (1977)	15	0

depends upon the analogy of the pathogenesis of gastric cancer in resected stomachs of animals with the pathogenesis of gastric stump cancer in human beings.

The extensive studies of Dahm and Werner [4] with Wistar rats show a cancer frequency of the gastric stump of 34.5% after Billroth-II resection without Braun's enteroanastomosis, but one of 40.5% after Billroth-I resection. Nonoperated rats in the control group in no case developed a gastric cancer by the same cancerigenic exposition. To show the influence of the intestinal reflux in development of cancer in the rat stomach, Schlag et al. [16] performed gastrojejunostomies with and without Roux-en-Y anastomosis with the same carcinogenic exposition as Dahm and Werner, but could not produce gastric carcinomas.

Discrepancies Between Clinical and Experimental Studies

1) The animal experimental model is not identical with the human stomach at the time of operation, because in patients we find a pathologic gastric mucosa with gastritis or peptic ulcer over many years, but in the animals a healthy stomach with an unnaturally high carcinogen exposition exists.

2) Different groups explain the same histologic findings in different ways; one group describes a carcinoma while another describes a benign lesion.

3) In the animal model no lymphogenic metastases are to be seen; this is not the case in humans. In the rat the stump carcinoma immediately invades the jejunal mucosa, but in humans the jejunal mucosa is a barrier to the cancer for a long period [15].

4) Experimental studies show a higher incidence of carcinomas after B-I than B-II resection. Retrospective studies with a long observation time yield converse results.

5) Conservatively treated gastric ulcers have a carcinoma rate of 10%; corresponding animal experimental models do not exist.

6) Gastrojejunostomy in ulcer treatment shows a frequency of carcinoma of between 13% and 22%, whereas in experimental studies no carcinomas occur.

Pathogenetic Factors in the Development of Carcinomas in the Operated Stomach

Retrospective studies over a long observation time, animal experimental models with different operative procedures in ulcer treatment, and pathophysiologic reflections show that the risk of cancer development increases with the coincidence of hypochlorhydria, bile reflux into the stomach, pancreatic reflux, and development of a high nitrite concentration in the stomach (see p. 120ff.). All operative procedures that cause these factors must have a high stomach cancer risk.

Incidence of Cancer in Treatment of Peptic Ulcer

After Billroth-II resection of the stomach without side-to-side enteroanastomosis in *gastric* ulcer treatment, stump carcinoma occurs as often or more often than after medical treatment. The cancer risk increases with the interval after operation.

Perhaps a Billroth-II resection with antecolic gastrojejunostomy and side-to-side jejunojejunostomy without bile reflux have lower stump cancer incidences. But today these findings are only pathophysiologic reflections; no prospective studies exist.

After treatment of *gastric* ulcer by gastrojejunostomy alone with obligate bile reflux, only *one* retrospective clinical study shows a higher cancer incidence, but these results could not be reproduced in experimental models.

Clinical and experimental studies do not allow definitive conclusions concerning cancer risk after Billroth-I resection, but there seems to be a higher cancer frequency after this operation than is expected and published.

No retrospective and prospective long-term observation studies after ulcer treatment by vagotomy exist.

The same problems affect the results for stomach cancer risk after *duodenal* ulcer treatment. Exact data showing a cancer risk of 7% – 9% only exist after Billroth-II resection without Braun's enteroanastomosis. All other operative techniques and the medically treated duodenal ulcer do not allow definitive judgements on gastric cancer risk.

References

1. Cheli, R., Santi, L., Ciancymerla, G., Canciani, G.: A clinical and statistical follow-up study of atrophic gastritis. Dig. Dis. *18*, 1061 – 1066 (1973)
2. Clémençon, G., Baumgartner, R., Leuthold, E., Miller, G., Neiger, A.: Das Karzinom des operierten Magens. Dtsch. Med. Wochenschr. *101*, 1015 – 1020 (1976)
3. Dahm, K., Werner, B.: Experimentelles Anastomosenkarzinom. Ein Beitrag zur Pathogenese des Magenstumpfkarzinoms. Langenbecks Arch. Chir. *333*, 211 – 236 (1973)
4. Dahm, K., Eichen, R., Werner, B., Kozuschek, W.: Gastroenterale Anastomose und Carcinom im operierten Magen. Chirurg *47*, 494 – 495 (1976)
5. Domellöf, L., Eriksson, S., Janunger, K. G.: Late precancerous changes and carcinoma of the gastric stump after Billroth I resection. Am. J. Surg. *132*, 26 – 31 (1976)
6. Domellöf, L., Eriksson, S., Janunger, K. G.: Carcinoma and possible precancerous changes of the gastric stump after Billroth II resection. Gastroenterology *73*, 462 – 468 (1977)
7. Griesser, G., Schmidt, H.: Statistische Erhebungen über die Häufigkeit des Karzinoms nach Magenoperation wegen eines Geschwürleidens. Med. Welt *35*, 1836 – 1840 (1964)
8. Helsingen, N., Hillestad, L.: Cancer development in the gastric stump after partial gastrectomy for ulcer. Ann. Surg. *143*, 173 – 179 (1956)
9. Hilbe, G., Salzer, G. M., Hussl, H., Kutschera, H.: Die Carcinomgefährdung des Resektionsmagens. Langenbecks Arch. Klin. Chir. *323*, 142 – 153 (1968)
10. Krause, U.: Late prognosis after partial gastrectomy for ulcer. Acta Chir. Scand. *114*, 341 – 354 (1957)
11. Kühlmayer, R., Rokitansky, O.: Das Magenstumpfkarzinom als Spätproblem der Ulcuschirurgie. Langenbecks Arch. Klin. Chir. *278*, 361 – 375 (1954)
12. Peitsch, W., Becker, H. D.: Frequency and Prognosis of primary gastric stump carcinomas. Front. Gastrointest. Res. (in press)

13. Radomsky, J., Ungeheuer, E., Lüders, K.: Das Magenstumpfkarzinom. Dtsch. Ärzteblatt *75*, 1007 – 1010 (1978)
14. Rösch, W., Prütting, E.: Das Karzinom im operierten Magen (Stumpfkarzinom) – Analyse eines endoskopischen Untersuchungsguts. Kliniksarzt *7*, 386 – 390 (1978)
15. Schlag, P., Merkle, P., Meister, H.: Zur lokalen Tumorausbreitung des Karzinoms und des Karzinomrezidivs im operierten Magen. Med. Welt *28*, 810 – 812 (1977)
16. Schlag, P., Meister, H., Feyerabend, G., Merkle, P.: Der Einfluß des duodenogastrischen Refluxes auf das Epithel an der gastroenteralen Anastomose. Langenbecks Arch. Chir. *344*, 207 – 217 (1977)
17. Schmid, E., Vollmer, R., Adlung, J., Blaich, E., Goebell, H., Heinkel, K., Kimmig, J. M., Probst, M.: Zur endoskopischen Diagnostik des Karzinoms im operierten Magen. Gastroenterologie *14*, 521 – 530 (1976)
18. Serck-Hanssen, A., Schrumpf, E., Stadaas, J., Aune, S., Myren, J., Osnes, M.: Mucosal changes in the gastric stump 20 – 25 years after resection for ulcer: A follow-up study. Digestion *16*, 273 (1977)
19. Siurala, M., Salmi, H. J.: Long-term follow-up of subjects with superficial gastritis or a normal gastric mucosa. Scand. J. Gastroenterol. *6*, 559 – 563 (1971)
20. Siurala, M., Varis, K., Wiljasalo, M.: Studies of patients with atrophic gastritis: A 10 – 15 year follow-up. Scand. J. Gastroenterol. *1*, 40 – 48 (1966)
21. Walker, I. R., Strickland, R. G., Ungar, B., Mackay, I. R.: Simple atrophic gastritis and gastric carcinoma. Gut *12*, 906 – 911 (1971)

Prospective Studies in Patients with Resected Stomach and Stump Carcinoma

W. Rösch

The problem whether the resected stomach predisposes to the development of gastric carcinoma can only be solved by prospective studies. These are difficult to perform since patient fluctuation and multimorbidity interfers with a precise evaluation of the patient's risk to develop or die from gastric carcinoma. The age distribution of gastric carcinoma in the nonresected and the resected population are identical, the risk of develop gastric carcinoma is considered in a given population to be between 0.5% and 2%, most probably around 1.2%.

The few studies which were hitherto performed in asymptomatic patients to get an idea about the incidence of carcinoma of the gastric stump are listed in Table 1.

Schrumpf et al. [4] examined 108 of 421 patients with partial resection who were offered a gastroscopy. Although the gross aspect of the anastomosis was unsuspicious, histology revealed infiltrating carcinoma in four patients, severe dysplasia was seen in three.

Domellöf et al. [2] performed an endoscopic follow-up in 214 of 459 patients 20 years after Billroth II resection. Three patients with stump carcinoma were found among 140 deceased patients at the follow-up. Six carcinomas, among which two were early carcinomas, were diagnosed in the follow-up group. One patient had multifocal precancerous alterations of the stoma, two had tubular adenoma, and 20 (9.3%) had regenerative polyps. No difference was found in the ratio of original duodenal-gastric ulcer in patients with carcinoma or polyps when compared to other patients. The same authors reexamined also 74 patients 10–22 years after Billroth I resection and found four cases of carcinoma of the gastric stump. Another eight patients had regenerative polyps and one a tubular adenoma.

Table 1. Prospective studies in patients with partially resected stomach

Authors	Operation	Follow-up	*n*	Stump carcinoma	Early cancer
Domellöf et al. (1976)	Billroth I	10–22 years	74	4 (5.4%)	2
Domellöf et al. (1977)	Billroth II	20 years	214	6 (2.8%)	2
Schrumpf et al. (1977)	Billroth II	20–25 years	108	4 (3.7%)	3
Rösch et al. (1978)	Billroth II	15 years	117	1 (0.85%)	1

Our own experience covers 117 patients who were asked for routine endoscopy because the Billroth II resection was performed more than 15 years ago. Only one early gastric carcinoma was detected.

Analysis of the histological type according to Lauren's classification shows that of the 15 carcinomas listed in Table 1, seven were of the diffuse type, seven of the intestinal type, and one unclassifiable. A correlation to chronic atrophic gastritis, intestinal metaplasia, cystic dilatation of the gastric glands, or biliary reflux could not be established. Repeated gastroscopic examinations are recommended from 15 years after surgery. Schrumpf et al. [4] asks 20 biopsy specimens be taken from the distal part of the gastric stump within 2 cm of the anastomosis at equal intervals around the stoma, to achieve early detection of stump carcinoma.

References

1. Domellöf, L., Eriksson, S., Janunger, K. G.: Late precancerous changes and carcinoma of the gastric stump after Billroth I resection. Am. J. Surg. *132*, 26 – 31 (1976)
2. Domellöf, L., Eriksson, S., Janunger, K. G.: Carcinoma and possible precancerous changes of the gastric stump after Billroth II resection. Gastroenterology *73*, 462 – 468 (1977)
3. Rösch, W., Prütting, E.: Das Karzinom im operierten Magen. Analyse eines endoskopischen Untersuchungsguts. Klinikart *7*, 386 – 390 (1978)
4. Schrumpf, E., Serck-Hanssen, A., Stadaas, J., Aune, S., Myren, J., Osnes, M.: Mucosal changes in the gastric stump 20 – 25 years after partial gastrectomy. Lancet *1977 II*, 467 – 469

Gastric Polyps and Gastric Cancer

P. Hermanek

For many years, the relationship between gastric polyps and gastric carcinoma have been discussed. In this regard, the hamartomatous and the mesenchymal polyps can be neglected, only the so-called epithelial polyps should be taken into consideration. It is important to differentiate between nonneoplastic (tumor-like) and neoplastic epithelial polyps [3]. The so-called hyperplasiogenous polyp, according to Elster [2], can be regarded as a nonneoplastic lesion.

The neoplastic epithelial polyps, the adenomas, are far less frequent than the nonneoplastic polyps; the frequency is less than 5% of all gastric polyps. In our opinion, the adenomas are precursors of carcinoma, therefore, the development of infiltrating carcinoma in an adenoma must be taken into account. In our patients, 5 of 109 early gastric carcinomas (5%) have arisen in adenomas.

Carcinomas in nonneoplastic (hyperplastic, regenerative, hyperplasiogenous) polyps are extremely rare. The importance of these polyps is, that independent carcinomas frequently occur in the stomach with polyps. In our experience, 11 of 109 patients with early gastric carcinoma (10%) had coexisting hyperplastic polyps. For the radiologists and endoscopists, these polyps were sometimes more impressive than the carcinomas. Therefore, after the diagnosis of a hyperplastic polyp, one has to look for coexisting early gastric carcinomas with great care.

Another problem deals with the follow-up examinations after surgical or endoscopical polypectomy. The results of our team are presented in Table 1. It

Table 1. Follow up: nonneoplastic gastric polyps
Surgical and Medical Clinic Erlangen, Oct. 31, 1978

	n	Gastric carcinoma discovered after polypectomy
After surgical therapy[a]		
Follow-up time ≥ 5 years	27	4 (15%)
< 5 years	22	2 (9%)
Total	49	6 (12%)
After endoscopic polypectomy[b]		
Average follow-up time 4.5 years	21	1 (2%)

[a] Bötticher et al. 1975
[b] Unpublished data

must be stressed that the surgical patients were treated at a time when gastroscopy was not yet performed regularly before operation. It seems possible that some of the carcinomas recognized later on were existent, but were not diagnosed at the time of polypectomy.

Although to date, the number of patients mentioned in Table 1 is small, we think that caution is mandatory. Therefore all patients with polyps, hyperplastic polyps included, should be considered as patients with higher risk for stomach cancer and should be reexamined regularly.

References

1. Bötticher, R., Bünte, H., Hermanek, P., Rösch, W.: Magenpolypen. Prognose und Therapie. Dtsch. Med. Wochenschr. *100*, 167 – 170 (1975)
2. Elster, K.: Histologic classification of gastric polyps. In: Pathology of the gastrointestinal tract. Morson, B. C. (ed.), Berlin, Heidelberg, New York: Springer 1976
3. Oota, K.: Histological typing of gastric and oesophageal tumours. WHO, Geneva 1977

Summary: Risk Factors in Gastric Cancer

Even in the unoperated stomach, the duodenogastric reflux is in a position to provoke proliferative changes of the gastric mucosa. It thereby remains unclear, whether the proliferation of epithelium is in the first instance caused by inflammatory or metaplastic changes, or whether direct influences on the part of the duodenal contents affect the gastric mucosa in a proliferatory fashion. The observation, that a modification of environmental parameters within the stomach may lead to the endogenous development of carcinogenic substances, seems to be of interest. Achlorhydria in particular may have a pacemaker function in this respect. The fact that other risk factors for gastric cancer exist apart from the duodenogastric reflux is elaborated by the immunological gastritis in pernicious anemia, Morbus Menetrier, and by the hyperplastic gastric polyp. It is therefore extremely probable that aside from the duodenogastric reflux and exogenous noxae, genetic factors play their part in this process. The significance of the operated stomach as a risk factor for gastric cancer is indisputable.

The variously described models of experimental cancer induction in the operated stomachs of animals indicate that proliferative changes in the gastric mucosa may be the result of numerous factors. The proximity of different epithelia alone, without regard to the surgical method employed or to exogenous or endogenous influences of carcinogens, can have a proliferative effect on the gastric mucosa.

Although the figures for the frequency of cancer of the gastric stump vary considerably, there can be no doubt about the danger of a cancer developing in the operated stomach. A review of various collective statistics cannot to date decide the question of whether the B-I-resected stomach is prone to the same cancer risk as the stomach resected according to Billroth II. It also remains uncertain, whether the type of the original ulcer correlates significantly with the frequency of cancer development in the surgically treated stomach. These uncertainty-factors provide strong indications for constant endoscopic controls of patients with operated stomachs beginning with the 15th postoperative year.

The supervision of such patients is of particular importance, because cancer of the gastric stump exhibits no independent symptomology, and because patients with gastric resections generally tend to interpret ensuing complaints as a direct consequence of their previous operation.

5 Diagnostic Procedures for Classification of Gastric Cancer

Significance of Diagnostic Procedures for Preoperative Staging

W. Rösch

Introduction

The prognostic aspect of gastric carcinoma has not essentially changed, although endoscopy has contributed to a rise of early gastric carcinomas from 3% to about 15% among the resectable cases. The rate of primarily inoperable patients amounts to 10%, in an additional 30%, laparotomy reveals inoperability [32]. Since exploratory laparotomy carries a risk of 2.6% [8], preoperative staging using a variety of noninvasive techniques is advisable.

The precise judgement of local tumor extension and depth infiltration is difficult and asks for a combination of techniques, although there is, in general, a close correlation between horizontal spread and vertical infiltration in carcinomas of the protruding type [25]. Nevertheless, the results of preoperative staging, especially of local tumor growth, are always preliminary and may prove completely wrong during laparotomy.

Judgement of Local Tumor Extension

Radiology is still in many centers the first diagnostic procedure to get an idea about the size of the carcinoma. It is especially valuable in advanced carcinoma of the diffuse type, whereby a linitis plastica pattern often indicates inoperability.

Endoscopy is nowadays mandatory for preoperative histological confirmation, especially in regard to the differentiation between intestinal and diffuse type of carcinoma according to Lauren or Ming. In case of scirrhous growth, discontinuous tumor infiltration underneath a normally appearing mucosa may render the endoscopic judgement of tumor extension impossible.

In many gastroenterological centers, early gastric carcinoma amounts nowadays for 15% – 22% of all gastric carcinomas diagnosed [28]. Although even in Japan, the reliability of endoscopic correct interpretation of early gastric carcinoma varies between 52.8% and 86.4% [16], tumor size is a fairly good indicator of prognosis. Gonvers et al. [10] have shown that a diameter of less than 2 cm means operability without limitation. In early gastric cancer of the polypoid type, endoscopic snare-ectomy may even confirm the presence of surface carcinoma when the malignant growth was excised in toto. In type IIb, IIc, and III, however, the endoscopic aspect is not conclusive, although the endoscopist will often make the presumptive diagnosis of an early gastric carcinoma. Following endoscopic polypectomy of a small gastric carcinoma, marking with Indian ink seems advisable as is the case in small flat lesions in the proximal stomach to point the tumor localization to the surgeon for consecutive laparotomy, unless total gastrectomy is planned [38]. Another alternative is intraoperative gastroscopy to indicate the ideal line of resection in case of a small tumor which can not be palpated or localized properly [34].

Identification of esophageal involvement during endoscopy is occasionally decisive for transabdominal or transthoracic approach. According to Kobayashi and Watanabe [15], esophageal involvement can be ruled out reliably when the cardia is patulous symmetrically, whereas narrowing of the gastro-esophageal junction indicates tumor infiltration.

An additional problem is the common occurrence of multiple malignant growths as seen in at least 7.5% of early gastric cancer patients [27]. On subtle histological examination, multicentric carcinomatous foci, most commonly in the immediate vicinity of the tumor, are found in up to 20% [14]. Nevertheless, this observation does not, even in Japan, call for gastrectomy *en principe.* The experience of Scandinavian authors that some carcinomas of the gastric stump may be detected by taking circular biopsies from the anastomotic ring has still to be confirmed [33].

The presumptive diagnosis of early gastric carcinoma, which in our experience is possible in about 92% of cases, asks for two consequences: (1) since in early gastric carcinoma the 5-year survival rate is between 90% and 98%, this patient should be treated by the best surgeon available with the lowest mortality figures, and (2) the resected specimen should be carefully evaluated by the pathologist in embedding the entire lesion for serial sectioning and, if possible, subtle search for additional microscopic foci in the tumor-distant mucosa.

Preoperative Evaluation for Metastases

All patients with gastric carcinoma in whom curative surgery is scheduled should have preoperative evaluation for liver and peritoneal metastases. This approach includes rectal and gynecological examination, scintigraphy, ultrasonography, and peritoneoscopy, in some cases computerized tomography and angiography may be of an additional help (Table 1). The fate of patients with extensive liver metastases is rather poor: Berndt and Gütz [3] report a death rate of 20% within 3 weeks after laparotomy and of 30% during hospitalization, Zittel and Beck [39] cite a death rate of 58% within 4 weeks after laparotomy, whereas after laparoscopy, the death rate was 7.5%. The value of endoscopic transmural lymphography [31] has to be debated because the rate of false positives and false negatives is rather high. The position of computerized tomography in preoperative staging is not yet settled, however, preliminary experience shows that it may be used for demonstration of extensive lymph node involvement. Since the diagnostic accuracy of liver scanning in the detection of space-occupying lesions is unsatisfactory (Table 2), we submit all our patients prior to surgery to peritoneoscopy. This examination allows an evaluation of the transmural tumor extension and the demonstration of hepatic as well as serosal

Table 1. Diagnostic accuracy in liver metastases

Authors	Peritoneo-scopy	Scinti-graphy	Ultrasono-graphy	Angio-graphy	CT
Sauer et al., 1973	80%	79%	–	–	–
Bekier, 1974	–	74%	–	–	–
Lerona et al., 1974	–	92%	–	92%	–
Lutz et al., 1975	–	48%	59%	–	–
Vido et al., 1975	95%	89%	–	–	–
Horica et al., 1975	71%	62%	–	–	–
McArdle, 1976	–	–	76%	–	–
Bryan et al., 1977	–	96%	94%	–	88%
Pokieser et al., 1977	–	81%	80%	84%	–
Vicary and Shirley, 1978	–	–	87%	–	–
Own Results, 1978	87%	–	–	–	–

Table 2. Diagnostic accuracy of liver scan in %

Authors	n	Space-occupying lesion		No space-occupying lesion	
		Correct positive	False negative	Correct negative	False positive
Nagler et al., 1963	548	95	5	65	35
Lin et al., 1970	221	94	6	63	37
Covington, 1970	387	61	39	79	21
Drum, 1972	344	90	10	63	37
Bekier, 1974	197	74	26	98	2
Sauer et al., 1974	136	79	21	84	16
Horica et al., 1975	106	64	36	95	5
Angehrn et al., 1976	90	73	27	91	9

metastases which should be proven by biopsy [13]. Current experience in 83 patients with definite metastases showed that peritoneoscopy revealed metastatic growth in 62 (75%) and suspected metastases, as proven by biopsy, in an additional 10 (12%) patients. Thus, only 13% were missed. We feel that exploratory laparoscopy should replace exploratory laparotomy because of the lower risk [19].

Since not all metastases are reaching the liver surface and can be detected by peritoneoscopy, our patients are, in addition, submitted to ultrasonography. If space-occupying lesions are suspected in the ultrasonogram, percutaneous fine-needle aspiration biopsy is performed under ultrasonographic guidance. The results of this time-saving procedure which, too, carries a very low risk, are listed in Table 3.

Conclusion

By careful radiological and endoscopic examination of the stomach, a fairly precise outlining of the tumor growth can be obtained. Preoperative staging

Table 3. Results of percutaneous fine-needle aspiration biopsy

Lundquist (1970)	85% positive
Johansen and Myren (1971)	58% positive
Lutz et al. (1973)	77% positive
Thommesen (1973)	57% positive
Brase et al. (1973)	79% positive

should include peritoneoscopy to rule out peritoneal and hepatic metastases as proven by biopsy and scintigraphy or ultrasonography combined with percutaneous fine-needle aspiration biopsy unless palliative surgery is indicated. The considerable risk of exploratory laparotomy in patients with far advanced gastric carcinoma can in many cases be avoided by subtle preoperative staging.

References

1. Angehrn, F. G., Schmid, P., Prescia, R., Horica, C. A., Koelz, H. R., Herz, R., Cueni, B., Schmid, M., Akovbiantz, A., Heinzel, F., Landolt, M., Haemmerli, U. P., Blum, A. L.: Lebermetastasen: Diagnostischer Wert von Bluttests, Szintigraphie und Laparoskopie. Dtsch. Med. Wochenschr. *101*, 1047–1055 (1976)
2. Bekier, A.: Leistungsfähigkeit der Leberszintigraphie bei der Suche nach herdförmigen raumfordernden Parenchymerkrankungen. Schweiz. Med. Wochenschr. *104*, 729–732 (1974)
3. Berndt, H., Gütz, H. J.: Laparoskopie bei Magenkrebs. Z. Gastroenterol. *3*, 317–322 (1965)
4. Brase, A., Paul, F., Bockslaff, H., Atay, A.: Früherkennung von Lebermetastasen durch kombinierten Einsatz von Szintigraphie und Feinnadelbiopsie. Munch. Med. Wochenschr. *115*, 99–102 (1973)
5. Bryan, P. J., Dinn, W. M., Grossman, Z. D., Wistow, B. W., McAfle, J. G., Kieffer, S. A.: Correlation of computed tomography, gray scale ultrasonography and radionuclide imaging of the liver in detecting space-occupying processes. Radiology *124*, 387–393 (1977)
6. Covington, E. E.: The accuracy of liver photoscan. Am. J. Roentgenol. *109*, 742–744 (1970)
7. Drum, D. E., Christacopoulos, J. S.: Hepatic scintigraphy in clinical decision making. J. Nucl. Med. *13*, 908–912 (1972)
8. Fock, G., Koskipuro, H.: Mortality of exploratory laparotomy. Ann. Chir. Gynaecol. Fenn. *56*, 266–269 (1967)
9. Galvan, G., Pohl, G. B.: Klärung von Speicherdefekten im Leberszintigramm durch gezielte perkutane Feinnadelpunktion. Med. Klin. *69*, 2071–2074 (1974)
10. Gonvers, J. J., Realini, S., Arnold, J., Birchler, R., Capitaine, Y., Fasel, J., Fontoilliet, Ch., Loup, P., Séchaud, R., Hofstetter, J. R.: Valeur prognostique du status endoscopique dans le cancer gastrique. Schweiz. Rundschau Med. (Praxis) *66*, 1585–1590 (1977)
11. Horica, C. A., Pescia, R., Akovbiantz, A., Haemmerli, U. P., Jäger, M., Landolt, M., Schmid, M., Weitzel, M., Blum, A. L.: Diagnose von Lebermetastasen und primärem Hepatom mit Scintigraphie, Laparoskopie und Laparotomie. Schweiz. Med. Wochenschr. *105*, 1708–1711 (1975)
12. Johansen, S., Myren, J.: Fine-needle aspiration biopsy smears in the diagnosis of liver disease. Scand. J. Gastroenterol. *6*, 583–588 (1971)
13. Jori, G. P., Peschle, C.: Combined peritoneoscopy and liver biopsy in the diagnosis of hepatic neoplasm. Gastroenterology *63*, 1016–1019 (1972)
14. Karpas, C. M., Payson, B. A., Rechtschaffen, J.: Intestinal metaplasia and multicentric carcinoma of the stomach. N. Y. State J. Med. *71*, 1190–1195 (1971)
15. Kobayashi, S., Watanabe, H.: Endoscopic identification of esophageal involvement by carcinoma of the stomach. Am. J. Gastroenterol. *65*, 416–418 (1976)

16. Kobayashi, S., Sugiura, H., Kasugai, T.: Reliability of endoscopic observation in diagnosis of early carcinoma of the stomach. Endoscopy *4*, 61 – 66 (1972)
17. Lerona, P. T., Go, R. T., Cornell, S. H.: Limitations of angiography and scanning in diagnosis of liver masses. Radiology *112*, 139 – 145 (1974)
18. Lin, S. R., Mansfield, C. M., Kramer, S.: Liver scanning in patients with suspected or proven cancer. Am. J. Roentgenol. *108*, 98 – 101 (1970)
19. Lindner, H., Kirchhof, M.: Explorative Laparoskopie oder Laparotomie? Münch. Med. Wochenschr. *119*, 143 – 146 (1977)
20. Lundquist, A.: Fine-needle aspiration biopsy for cytodiagnosis of malignant tumor in the liver. Acta Med. Scand. *188*, 465 – 470 (1970)
21. Lutz, H., Weidenhiller, S., Rettenmaier, G.: Ultraschallgezielte Feinnadelbiopsie der Leber. Schweiz. Med. Wochenschr. *103*, 1030 – 1033 (1973)
22. Lutz, H., Katterle, D., Petzoldt, R.: Ultraschalldiagnostik von Lebermetastasen. Leber Magen Darm *5*, 223 – 227 (1975)
23. McArdle, C. R.: Ultrasonic diagnosis of liver metastases. J. Clin. Ultrasound *4*, 265 – 268 (1976)
24. Nagler, W., Bender, M. A., Blau, M.: Radioisotope scanning of the liver. Gastroenterology *44*, 36 – 42 (1963)
25. Okabe, H.: Growth of early gastric cancer. Gann Monograph on Cancer Research No. 11. pp. 67 – 79. Baltimore, London, Tokyo: University Park Press 1972
26. Pokieser, H., Czembirek, H., Mayrhofer, H., Urbanek, A., Kahn, P., Weiss, W., Base, W.: Einsatz und Leistungsbreite von Szintigraphie, Sonographie und Angiographie bei umschriebenen Leberprozessen. Roentgenblaetter *30*, 53 – 63 (1977)
27. Rösch, W.: Primär multiple Karzinome des Verdauungstrakts. Dtsch. Med. Wochenschr. *98*, 1872 – 1874 (1973)
28. Rösch, W.: Diagnose und Prognose des Magenfrühkarzinoms. In: Ergebnisse der Gastroenterologie 1977. Ritter, U., Classen, M. (eds.), pp. 128 – 136. München: Demeter 1977
29. Sauer, R., Müller, J.: Der Wert der Kolloid- und Leberszintigraphie sowie der Laparoskopie und Leberserologie bei der Diagnose von Lebergeschwülsten. Schweiz. Med. Wochenschr. *104*, 1085 – 1091 (1974)
30. Sauer, R., Fahrländer, H., Fridrich, R.: Comparison of the accuracy of liver scans and peritoneoscopy in benign and malignant primary and metastatic tumours of the liver. Scand. J. Gastroenterol. *8*, 389 – 394 (1973)
31. Schacht, U., Jünemann, A., Becker, H. J., Huth, F., Moschinski, D., Palomba, P. P.: Erste Ergebnisse der Lymphographie des menschlichen Magens. Dtsch. Med. Wochenschr. *99*, 616 – 618 (1976)
32. Schwemmle, K.: Chirurgische Behandlung des Magenkarzinoms. Munch. Med. Wochenschr. *117*, 281 – 286 (1975)
33. Schrumpf, E., Serck-Hanssen, A., Stadaas, J., Aune, S., Myren, J., Osnes, M.: Mucosal changes of the gastric stump 20 – 25 years after partial gastrectomy. Lancet *1977 II*, 467 – 469
34. Spilker, G., Geile, D., Ultsch, B., Erdt, A.: Intraoperative Gastroskopie. In: Fortschritte in der Endoskopie. W. Rösch (ed.), pp. 139 – 144. Erlangen: Perimed 1976
35. Thommesen, P.: Der Wert der Kombination von Leberszintigraphie und Feinnadelaspirationsbiopsie bei Lebermetastasen. Fortschr. Röntgenstr. *118*, 194 – 197 (1973)
36. Vicary, F. R., Shirley, I.: Ultrasound and hepatic metastases. Br. J. Radiol. *51*, 596 – 598 (1978)
37. Vido, I., Hundeshagen, H., Becker, H., Schmidt, F. W.: Vergleich laparoskopischer und szintigraphischer Befunde bei chronischer Hepatitis, Leberzirrhose und Lebertumoren. Dtsch. Med. Wochenschr. *100*, 129 – 132 (1975)
38. Waldmann, D., Oehlert, W.: Die intramurale Tuschemarkierung – eine praktikable Methode zur präoperativen endoskopischen Intestinalwandmarkierung. Endoscopy *10*, 141 (1978)
39. Zittel, R. X., Beck, K.: Die Bedeutung der Laparoskopie in der Chirurgie. Dtsch. Med. Wochenschr. *88*, 1999 – 2004 (1963)

Biological Markers for Staging of Gastric Cancer?

B. Heymer and A. Quentmeier

In the strict sense of the term, biological markers of tumors are substances – such as enzymes, hormones, or antigens – which are produced by the respective tumor and released into the body fluids where they may be detected. However, in a broader sense, the term includes characteristic reactions of the organism against the tumor, such as the formation of antibodies or cellular immune factors to tumor antigens. There are several examples of the successful application of such biological markers for the diagnosis or postoperative follow-up of human malignancies: the determination of AFP in liver carcinoma [13], of β-HCG in chorionic carcinoma [15], of CEA in colon carcinoma [14], and of EBV-antibodies in Burkitt lymphoma [9].

In the present report, the question is raised whether such markers are also available for gastric cancer (GC) and – if so – whether they can assist in staging. The attempt to answer this question will be divided into three sections: first, a description of general biological markers without specificity for GC; second, a discussion of markers with restricted specificity for GC; and third, a presentation of preliminary results obtained with the application of one of these markers.

General Biological Markers Without Specificity for Gastric Cancer

Many parameters have been studied in patients with GC for their potential to monitor tumor stage, effect of treatment, or prognosis. A small selection of these general biological markers is given in Table 1. None of them possesses any specificity for GC, but all of them appear to be correlated with tumor stage. The phytohemagglutinin-mediated (PHA) lymphocyte stimulation and the dinitrochlorobenzene-induced (DNCB) skin reaction represent a measure of cellular immunity. Both have been found to be significantly decreased in many patients with GC. In general, it holds true that the PHA- and DNCB-response is the weaker, the more advanced the neoplastic process [19, 2, 3, 10, 7]. Beta$_2$-microglobulin (Table 1) is a small molecular weight polypeptide which normally occurs in all body fluids in minute amounts. Approximately 75% of patients with GC show significantly increased (>2.4 μg/ml) β_2-microglobulin serum concentrations [5]. In addition, there appears to be some correlation with tumor stage. However, the serum levels of this marker are considerably influenced by renal function, that means they do not exclusively reflect tumor spread [5]. Similary (Table 1), tissue polypeptide antigen (TPA), a single chain polypeptide, present

Table 1. General biological markers in gastric cancer

Marker assay	Specificity for GC	Findings in pat. with GC	Correlation with GC stage	Ref.
PHA Lymphoc. stim.	∅	Decreased in 80–90% of pat.	(+)	[19]
DNCB Skin reaction	∅	Decreased in >60% of pat.	(+)	[2, 3, 10, 7]
β_2-microglobulin RIA, serum	∅	Increased in 75% of pat.	(+)	[15]
TPA HIA, serum	∅	Increased in 73 ± 10% of pat.	+	[1]

PHA = phytohemagglutinin
DNCB = dinitrochlorobenzene
RIA = radioimmunoassay
TPA = tissue polypeptide antigen
HIA = hemagglutination inhibition assay
GC = gastric cancer

in a large variety of human neoplasms, is found in highest titers in the sera of patients with metastazing malignancies [1]. While 73 ± 10% of such patients have pathologic serum-TPA-concentrations (>0.09 units/ml), only 2 ± 1% of healthy subjects show TPA values in this range [18]. Nevertheless, the clinical application of the general biological markers listed in Table 1 is limited by the fact that they are not specific for GC and that they may be influenced by factors unrelated to tumor stage.

Markers with Restricted Specificity for Gastric Cancer

In contrast, the second group of markers (Table 2) does possess a certain degree of specificity for GC. The migration inhibition factor (MIF), released upon exposure of lymphocytes to appropriate antigens, represents one of the mediators of cellular immunity. If autologous tumor antigen extracted from GC is employed in the migration inhibition test (MIT), a profound decrease in MIF-production by lymphocytes of patients with GC is evident, which closely parallels the tumor stage (Table 2): the more advanced the GC, the less frequently MIF is detectable. Although the significance of these findings is substantiated by the observation that they are in agreement with the results of the PHA-lymphocyte-stimulation and the DNCB-skin-testing (Table 1; [19, 2, 3, 10, 7]), the application of the MIT with autologous tumor antigen is restricted by the fact that such tests can only be performed postoperatively. When homologous rather than autologous antigen is employed, the assay system is much less specific, giving false positive results in 9% of patients with non-neoplastic disease of the stomach and in 3% of healthy subjects [25].

Table 2. "Specific" biological markers in gastric cancer (GC)

Marker assay	Specificity for GC	Findings in pat. with GC	Correlation with GC stage	Ref.
MIF MIT, autolog. Tu-Ag	+	Stage I + II: 44% pos. Stage III: 37% pos. Stage IV: 13% pos.	+	[7, 23]
FSA RIA, gastric juice	(+)	Detectable in 96% of pat.	∅	[14, 22, 12]
CEA RIA, serum	(+)	Increased in 54% of pat.	(+)	[16, 24, 20, 8, 4, 14, 5, 21]

MIF = migration inhibition factor
MIT = migration inhibition test
FSA = fetal sulfoglycoprotein antigen
RIA = radioimmunoassay
CEA = carcinoembryonic antigen
GC = gastric cancer

FSA and CEA in Gastric Cancer

Two further biological markers that have been studied in patients with GC need to be mentioned (Table 2). These are the fetal sulfoglycoprotein antigen (FSA) and the carcinoembryonic antigen (CEA). Both are tumor-associated, but not tumor-specific antigens [22] and both have been purified and immunochemically characterized to a considerable degree [24]. The FSA is detectable in the gastric juice of 96% of patients with GC [14, 22, 12]. However, there is no correlation between FSA-concentrations and tumor stage, and FSA is also present in about 14% of patients with non-neoplastic gastric disease [14, 22, 12].

The other tumor marker, CEA, thus far has primarily been used for the detection of recurrences or metastases in patients with colon cancer [17]. The normal range of CEA in human serum or plasma, as determined by radioimmunoassay, is 0 – 2.5 ng/ml [8]. As is evident from the data presented in Fig. 1, approximately 10% of healthy human subjects have values above 2.5 ng/ml, indicating that the CEA assay is not a qualitatively specific cancer test. However, 73% of patients with colon cancer show a significant increase of CEA levels, frequently higher than 10 ng/ml. In contrast, only about 54% of patients with GC disclose pathological values (Fig. 1). The CEA isolated from GC is chemically and immunologically identical to CEA present in colon cancer [20]. Yet, the amount of CEA extractable from gastric tumors is much lower than that isolated from colon carcinomas [16]. This might explain why patients with GC less frequently disclose pathological CEA levels.

Nevertheless, at present, the use of the CEA assay for the postoperative follow-up of patients with GC is under study in many parts of the world. Some preliminary results obtained in the Department of Surgery I in Ulm, are depicted in Fig. 2. The data shown represent preoperative serum-CEA-concentrations of 34 patients with GC, as related to tumor stage (determined by TNM-classification). In addition, the surgical treatment performed (curative or palliative) is indicated. As expected, a fair number (n = 12) of patients with GC exhibits no

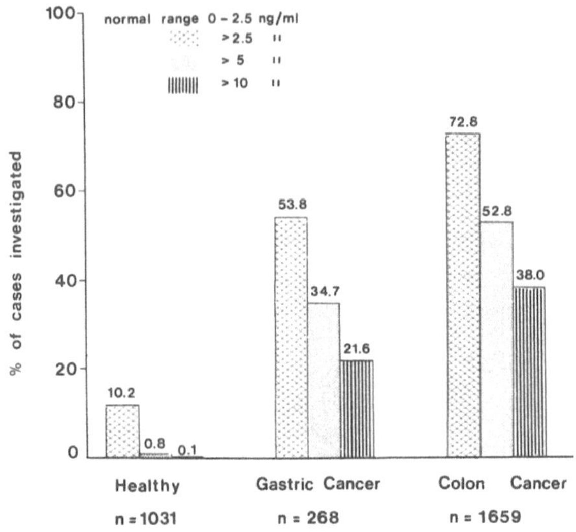

Fig. 1. Serum-CEA-concentrations in healthy subjects, patients with gastric cancer and patients with colon cancer, as determined by radioimmunoassay

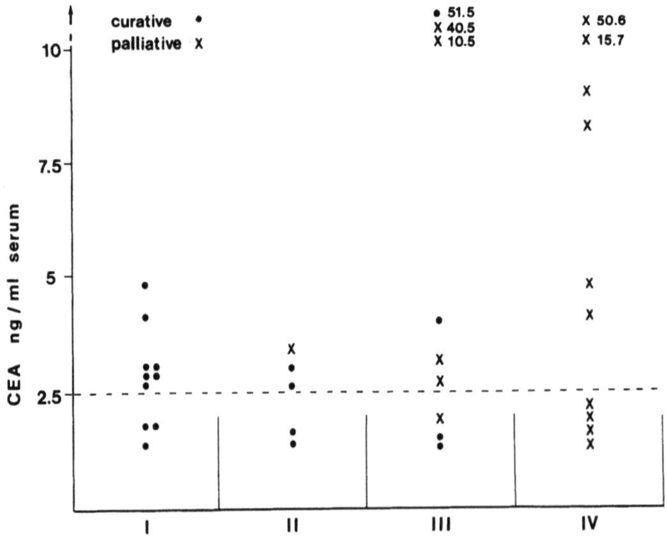

Fig. 2. Preoperative serum-CEA-concentrations in 34 patients with gastric cancer, as related to stage (based upon TNM-classification), and treatment (curative or palliative)

increase of the CEA level (Fig. 2). However, the remaining 22 patients disclosing pathological CEA values – at least as a trend – do show a correlation between preoperative CEA level and tumor stage. While CEA concentrations in patients of stages I – II, undergoing curative treatment, in general are low, CEA concentrations in patients of stages III – IV, receiving palliative treatment only, tend to be significantly increased (Fig. 2). Nevertheless, a considerable overlap of values is evident. Therefore, a sequential determination of pre- and postoperative CEA levels is required in order to improve the diagnostic significance of the assay.

Conclusion

No specific biological markers are currently available that permit a reliable preoperative staging of GC. However, tumor-associated antigens, such as CEA, CSAp [18], or others may well turn out to be useful for the postoperative follow-up of many patients with GC. A clear cut staging of GC by biological markers should not be expected, since the detectability of such markers in most instances is also dependent on factors unrelated to tumor spread.

References

1. Björklund, B.: Tissue polypeptide antigen; review of physical chemistry and clinical application. In: Clinical application of carcinoembryonic antigen assay. Krebs, B. P., Lalanne, C. M., Schneider, M. (eds.), pp. 59 – 63. Amsterdam, Oxford: Excerpta Medica 1978
2. Bone, G., Lauder, I.: Cellular immunity, peripheral blood lymphocyte count and pathological staging of tumours in the gastrointestinal tract. Cancer *30*, 215 – 221 (1974)
3. Bone, G., Appleton, D. R., Venables, C. W.: Cutaneous delayed hypersensitivity responses to 2 – 4 dinitrochlorobenzene – a prognostic guide in malignant disease. Br. J. Surg. *60*, 906 (1973)
4. Costanza, M. E., Das, S., Nathanson, L., Rule, A., Schwartz, R. S.: Carcinoembryonic antigen. Cancer *33*, 583 – 590 (1974)
5. Daver, A., Wafflart, J., Ben Boueli, A., Minier, J. F., Larra, F.: β_2-microglobulin (β_2-micro) and carcinoembryonic antigen (CEA) in intestinal cancers – a correlation with stage of disease. In: Clinical application of carcinoembryonic antigen assay. Krebs, B. P., Lalanne, C. M., Schneider, M. (eds.), pp. 460 – 465. Amsterdam, Oxford: Excerpta Medica 1978
6. Fuks, A., Banjo, Ch., Shuster, J., Freedmann, S. O., Gold, P.: Carcinoembryonic antigen (CEA): Molecular biology and clinical significance. Biochem. Biophys. Acta *417*, 123 – 152 (1974)
7. Hamasaki, K.: Cell-mediated immunity against digestive organ cancers: leukocyte migration inhibitory factor activity as an immunological parameter. Acta Med. Okayama *31*, 147 – 159 (1977)
8. Hansen, H. J., Snyder, J. J., Miller, E., Vandevoorde, J. P., Miller, O. N., Hines, L. R., Burns, J. J.: Carcinoembryonic antigen (CEA) assay. Hum. Pathol. *5*, 139 – 147 (1974)
9. Henle, W., Henle, G., Gunvin, P., Klein, G., Clifford, P., Single, S.: Patterns of antibodies to Epstein-Barr-Virus induced early antigens in Burkitt's lymphoma. Comparison of dying patients with long-term survivors. J. Natl. Cancer Inst. *50*, 1163 (1973)
10. Johnson, M. W., Maibach, H. I., Salmon, S. E.: Skin reactivity in patients with cancer. Impaired delayed hypersensitivity or faulty inflammatory response? N. Engl. J. Med. *284*, 1255 – 1257 (1971)
11. Klein, G.: Tumour antigens. Biochem. Soc. Trans. *4*, 8 – 9 (1976)

12. Lamerz, R., Fateh-Moghadam, A.: Carcinofetale Antigene. III. Andere Carcinofetale Antigene. Klin. Wochenschr. *53*, 403 – 417 (1975)
13. Lamerz, R., Fateh-Moghadam, A.: Carcinofetale Antigene. I. Alpha-Fetoprotein. Klin. Wochenschr. *53*, 147 – 169 (1975)
14. Lehmann, F. G.: Serologische Tumordiagnostik. Internist (Berlin) *16*, 214 – 222 (1975)
15. Lehmann, F. G.: Kongreßbericht: 5th meeting of the International Research Group of Carcino-Embryonic Proteins (IRGCP). Inn. Med. *4*, 388 – 390 (1977)
16. Lo Gerfo, P., Pennington, G.: Current status of carcinoembryonic antigen. Prog. Clin. Cancer *6*, 65 – 71 (1975)
17. Martin, E. W., James, K. K., Hurtubise, P. E., Catalano, P., Minton, J. P.: The use of CEA as an early indicator for gastrointestinal tumor recurrence and second-look procedures. Cancer *39*, 440 – 446 (1977)
18. Pant, K. D., Dahlman, H. L., Goldenberg, D. M.: A putatively new antigen (CSAp) associated with gastrointestinal and ovarian neoplasia. Immunol. Commun. *6*, 411 – 421 (1977)
19. Pappas, A., Scheurlen, P. G.: Lymphocyte transformation in malignant diseases. Communication II: Results in reticulo- and lymphoproliferative diseases as well as in carcinomas. In: Applied tumor immunology. Götz, H., Bücherl, E. S. (eds.), pp. 305 – 331. Berlin, New York: de Gruyter 1975
20. Rapp, W., Matzku, S., Wurster, K. H.: Stand der Isolierung CEA-ähnlicher Substanzen aus menschlicher Tumormagenschleimhaut. In: Tumorantigene in der Gastroenterologie. Lehmann, F. G. (ed.), pp. 39 – 43. Gräfelfing: Demeter 1976
21. Staab, H. J., Anderer, F. A., Stumpf, E., Fischer, R.: Second-look surgery of gastrointestinal carcinoma and the potential value of CEA monitoring. In: Clinical application of carcinoembryonic antigen assay. Krebs, B. P., Lalanne, C. M., Schneider, M. (eds.), pp. 94 – 100. Amsterdam, Oxford: Excerpta Medica 1978
22. Stillman, A., Zamcheck, N.: Recent advances in immunologic diagnosis of digestive tract cancer. Digest. Dis. *15*, 1003 – 1018 (1970)
23. Trejdosiewicz, L. K., Dykes, P. W.: Anti-tumour monocyte activity in gastric carcinoma patients receiving intra-tumoral C. parvum. In: The macrophage and cancer. James K., McBride, B., Stuart, A. (eds.), pp. 426 – 437. Edinburgh: Econoprint 1977
24. Vuento, M., Ruoslahti, E., Pihko, H., Svenberg, T., Ihamäki, T., Siurala, M.: Carcino-embryonic antigen-like substance in gastric juice. Immunochemistry *13*, 313 – 316 (1976)
25. Zöller, M., Matzku, S., Lernhardt, W., Schulz, U.: Evaluation of different antigen sources for leukocyte migration testing of gastrointestinal cancer patients. In: Clinical application of carcinoembryonic antigen assay. Krebs, B. P., Lalanne, C. M., Schneider, M. (eds.), pp. 155 – 160. Amsterdam, Oxford: Excerpta Medica 1978

Typing, Grading, and Staging of Gastric Carcinoma

P. Hermanek

Histological Classification (Typing and Grading)

The histological classification of stomach cancer is still done today in a wide variety of ways; different systems were and are being used. The *WHO classification* [6], which appeared in 1977, is an attempt at achieving international uniformity. It is our personal conviction to adhere to the WHO classification for each type of tumor which it includes, whether or not we consider the classification appropriate, for the simple reason that we want to make an effort to describe our cases in such a way that they can be compared internationally. Additional classifications, which we use, are included in parentheses in the individual cases.

Table 1 shows the WHO classification as far as it applies to stomach cancer. In the classification of cancers, the handling of tumors, which show several different structures, is disputed. It is, especially, in stomach cancer – mostly in advanced cases – where we frequently see many different structures in a single tumor. In regard to these pluriform tumors, the WHO system is based on the principle of classifying according to the dominant picture. Since the appearance of the WHO classification, we have used it to classify 167 stomach cancers (some, retrospectively). The frequency of occurrence of the individual types is shown in Table 1.

Each of our stomach cancers is classified according to Laurén [4] and Ming [5] along with the WHO classification. The *intestinal type according to Laurén* [4] is a compact tumor with well-demarcated margins; in most cases, glandular lumina are well developed and the epithelial elements resemble intestinal columnar cells. In contrast, in the *diffuse type,* poorly cohesive cells are scattered as solitary cells or in small clusters. The spread is dispersed with wide and diffuse infiltration and the tumor margins are poorly demarcated. Depending on the stage of the tumor, we find varying amounts of diffuse type. In the case load of the Surgical Clinic of the Erlangen University from the time period June 15, 1977 through Oct. 31, 1978, (total of 167 cases), we found the diffuse type in three early gastric cancers (17%), 33 of 100 resected advanced cancers (33%), and 28 of 49 nonresected cancers (57%).

According to the Laurén classification, a certain percentage of cases cannot be classified; of his group, it was 14%, in ours, it was 17%. This deficiency can be rectified by using the *Ming classification.* In this case, the pattern of spread is viewed as the most important feature, while the cell type moves into the background. The expanding type is characterized by growth en masse and by

Table 1. Histological classification of gastric carcinomas according to WHO (Oota 1977)

Tumor types	Frequency distribution Surgical Clinic Erlangen 15 June 77 – 31 October 78 (n = 167)
A. Adenocarcinoma	
I. Papillary	–
II. Tubular	79 (47%)
III. Mucinous	–
IV. Signet-ring cell carcinoma	32 (19%)
1. Adenocarcinoma, well-differentiated	26 (16%)
2. Adenocarcinoma, moderately differentiated	33 (20%)
3. Adenocarcinoma, poorly differentiated	20 (12%)
B. Adenosquamous carcinoma	1 (1%)
C. Squamous cell carcinoma	–
D. Undifferentiated carcinoma	52 (31%)
E. Unclassified carcinoma	2 (1%)

expansion, while the infiltrative type shows growth by individual penetration. We prefer the Ming classification. The differences from the Laurén classification are, in practice, not great and are mainly confined to classifying those tumors which the Laurén system cannot.

In summary, we recommend today the use primarily of the WHO classification, including the determination of the grade of differentiation of adenocarcinomas which it encompasses, for the histological classification of stomach cancers. However, in addition, the classification systems of Laurén and Ming should be applied.

Staging

Here, as well, relative uncertainty prevails in regard to stomach cancer as compared to tumors of other organs. The UICC mentioned in its comprehensive review of the TNM classification in 1974, two recommendations for stomach cancer: its own and that of the American Joint Committee for Cancer Staging [1] from 1972. In addition, there is the AJC classification of 1977 which is different again.

The varying *T classifications* are shown in Table 2. The crucial point is that in former classifications, T 1 meant only mucosa infiltration and T 2 grouped tumors together with infiltration of the submucosa, muscularis propria, and subserosa. This subdivision stands in contradiction to the fact that the crucial biological borderline lies between the submucosa and muscularis propria which is shown by the frequency of lymphatic metastases.

In the *N classification* (Table 3), the systems of the UICC and the AJC differ mainly in their definition of N 1 und N X + a, respectively. According to the AJC classification, N 1 means the involvement of the perigastric lymph nodes within a distance of 3 cm from the primary tumor; metastases in perigastric lymph nodes farther away fall under N 2. On the other hand, the UICC classifies

Table 2. T classifications of gastric carcinoma: correlation to the frequency of regional lymph node metastases

T classifications			Frequency of regional lymph node metastases	
AJC 1972 UICC 1974	Depth of infiltration	AJC 1977	Yoshida et al. 1977	Surgical Clinic Erlangen 1 May 69 – 31 October 78
T 1	Mucosa	T 1	3% (n = 120)	9% (n = 46)
T 1	Submucosa	T 1	11% (n = 136)	11% (n = 56)
T 2	Muscularis propria Subserosa	T 2	46% (n = 110)	50% (n = 232)
T 3	Serosa Contiguous structures	T 3 T 4	78% (n = 260)	85% (n = 279)

Table 3. N classifications for gastric cancer

UICC 1974		AJC 1977		Postsurgical treatment – pathological N classification (AJC 1977) Surgical Clinic Erlangen 15 June 77 – 31 October 1978
N X	No histological information	N X	Not determined	pN X 4 (3%)
N X –	No metastases to nodes	N 0	No metastases to regional lymph nodes	pN 0 40 (34%)
N X + a	Perigastric nodes only involved	N 1	Involvement of perigastric lymph nodes within 3 cm of the primary tumor along the lesser or greater curvature	pN 1 27 (23%)
N X + b	Involvement of other nodes which are removable at operation	N 2	Involvement of regional lymph nodes farther than 3 cm from the primary tumor, which are removed or removable at operation	pN 2 37 (31%)
N X + c	Involvement of nodes which are not removable at operation, e.g., those located along the abdominal aorta, or the mesenteric, or iliac arteries	N 3	Involvement of other intra-abdominal lymph nodes, such as the paraaortic, hepatoduodenal, retropancreatic, and mesenteric nodes	pN 3 10 (9%)

all perigastric lymph nodes, regardless of the distance from the primary tumor, as N X + a. Since June 1977, we have been classifying all stomach cancers according to the guidelines set down by the AJC in 1977. The results are illustrated in Table 3.

The AJC also introduced an *R classification* in its staging system of 1977: R 0: no residual tumor following surgical treatment, R 1: microscopic residual tumor, R 2: macroscopic residual tumor. This R classification is of special importance for gastric cancer because it is taken into consideration in *staging* (Fig. 1). We have been using this type of staging since June 1977. Among 118 surgically treated gastric cancers, 12 (10%) were stage I, 27 (23%) stage II, 48 (41%) stage III, and 27 (23%) stage IV. In four cases (3%), staging was not possible because local excision of the tumor or polypectomy did not yield regional lymph nodes for histological examination.

The greatest objection to the TNM classification and staging – that is, to the UICC system as well as to the AJC which is the more preferable system of the two for the above discussed reasons – is that neither classification takes into account the *definition of early cancer* as presented by the Japanese Society for Gastroenterologic Endoscopy in 1962. However, this term has, regardless of theoretical and linguistic reservations, proven itself in clinical practice and has been accepted in centers the world over. The AJC stage I coincides with early gastric cancer without metastases, which means it includes only part of what we refer to as early gastric cancer. A small number of early gastric cancers show lymphatic metastases. According to the AJC, they would come under stage III, despite the fact that they have a good prognosis as opposed to the poor prognosis of the rest of the group. Because this stands in contradiction to clinical reality, we proceeded in staging the stomach cancer which has been removed operatively as shown in Table 4.

In the evaluation of surgically removed tumors, the terms *curative and noncurative* have great meaning. Despite linguistic objections, they have been accepted worldwide. A curative procedure is assumed to be present if surgeon and pathologist both regard the tumor to be removed in its entirety and there is

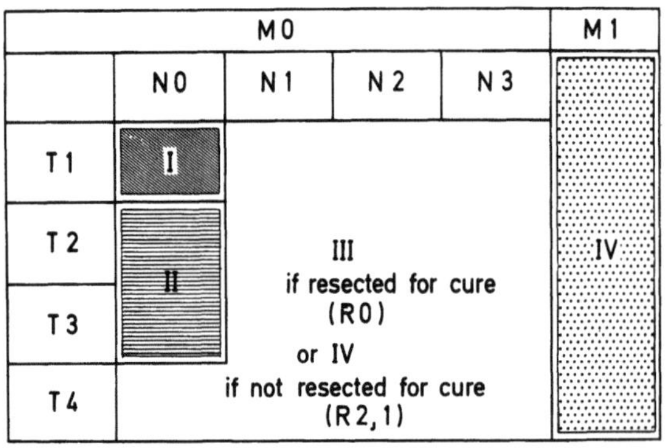

Fig. 1. Gastric carcinoma. Stage grouping according to AJC (1977)

Table 4. Staging of gastric carcinoma, procedure as performed by the Department of Surgical Pathology, University Erlangen-Nürnberg

1. Early gastric carcinoma
   a) Mucosa/submucosa
   b) pN Classification[a]
   c) R Classification[a]
2. Advanced gastric carcinoma
   a) pT Classification (T 2, 3, or 4)[a]
   b) pN Classification[a]
   c) M Classification[a]
   d) R Classification[a]
   (a–d: AJC stage II – IV[a])
   If R 0: absolute or relative curative resection

[a] According to AJC 1977

no indication of residual, local or distant metastases. According to the AJC nomenclature, a curative resection would be one with the R classification R 0.

Within these curative procedures, a distinction can also be made between *absolute and relative curative resections* for gastric cancer. This was first proposed by the Japanese Research Society for Gastric Cancer in 1963. The system developed by that society is rather complicated and cannot be described in detail within the scope of this presentation. It is probably too sophisticated to be practicable in western countries. Therefore, we have tried to simplify it without changing the basic Japanese concept. The marginal lymph node of each region of lymphatic drainage is especially examined. This is the lymph node of one area of drainage which is located farthest from the tumor and closest to the resection line. If separate histological examinations are carried out on marginal lymph nodes of all regions of lymphatic drainage, a distinction can be made between absolute and relative curative radical operations. The procedure in which the marginal lymph nodes of all lymph drainage regions are free of tumor is considered absolute curative. Of 114 (subtotal and total) gastrectomies, 29 (25%) were palliative and 85 (75%) were curative – of them, 54 (48%) absolute and 31 (27%) relative curative.

Importance of Typing, Grading, and Staging

Exact typing, grading, and staging are essential prerequisites in modern oncology. Depending on which organ is involved, their influence on the choice of therapy varies. However, in all organs, precise typing, grading, and staging are essential for accurate statistical evaluation of end results. Therefore, protocols of controlled clinical trials on therapy of tumors should deal with pathohistological techniques and systems of typing, grading, and staging to be used.

We must keep in mind that considerable personnel is required to do the necessary work on the tumor specimens. In a total gastrectomy, about 14 blocks of tumor and surrounding tissue as well as the resection lines, in addition to 60 lymph nodes in 20 – 25 blocks must be examined histologically. In early gastric carcinoma, it is considerably more. However, such efforts are absolutely necessary in large medical centers. They are the prerequisites for a valid and sufficiently accurate analysis of therapeutic results based on tumor morphology and tumor spread.

References

1. AJC (American Joint Committee for Cancer Staging and End-Results Reporting): Manual for staging of cancer. American Joint Committee, Chicago 1977
2. Japanese Research Society for Gastric Cancer: The general rules for the gastric cancer study in surgery. Jpn. J. Surg. *3*, 61 – 71 (1973)
3. Japanese Study for Gastroenterological Endoscopy. Cited by Murakami, T.: Pathomorphological diagnosis, definition and gross classification of early gastric cancer. In: Early Gastric Cancer. Murakami, T. (ed.). Tokyo: University of Tokyo Press 1971
4. Laurén, P.: The two histological main types of gastric carcinoma: Diffuse and so-called intestinal-type carcinoma. Acta Pathol. Microbiol. Scand. *64*, 31 – 49 (1965)
5. Ming, S.-Ch.: Gastric carcinoma. A pathobiological classification. Cancer *39*, 2475 – 2485 (1977)
6. Oota, K.: Histological typing of gastric and oesophageal tumours. Geneva: WHO 1977
7. UICC (Union Internationale Contre le Cancer): TNM Classification of Malignant Tumours. 2nd ed. Geneva: UICC 1974
8. Yoshida, K., Ikeuchi, H., Oshibe, M., Machida, T., Hoshi, H., Takahashi, M.: Surgical treatment and adjuvant chemotherapy of gastric cancer on the basis of pathological findings. Tohoku J. Exp. Med. *122*, 113 – 120 (1977)

Summary: Diagnostic Procedures for Gastric Cancer

One decisive factor for improving the prognosis of gastric cancer is the apprehension of the tumor at an early stage. The percentage of early gastric cancer among all gastric cancers in Europe is quoted at 15% to date. Japanese results with up to 40% early gastric cancers have yet to be achieved.

Although early cancer can by all means be detected using X-ray air-contrast methods, the crucial breakthrough was obtained by the routine performance of endoscopic methods of examination. This has the further advantage of securing the cancer diagnosis bioptically.

In the course of the operations, the surgeon is frequently confronted with the difficulty of localizing small carcinomas. In this case, endoscopic ink markings provide valuable assistance. Whereas small carcinomas can generally be considered operable, this is no longer certain of carcinomas with a diameter of over 2 cm. In order to further determine the extent of the cancer preoperatively, a number of additional examination procedures are recommended, such as ultrasonography, computerized tomography, scintigraphy, and peritoneoscopy. Biological markers, which would allow preoperative staging of the gastric cancer, are not yet available. Although with a careful radiological and endoscopic examination, the extent of the tumor, and with additional methods, the metastases can be relatively securely ascertained, an exploratory laparotomy should be projected. It is possible that even for a metastasizing gastric cancer, at least a subjective improvement of the patient can be achieved via palliative resection.

An impeccable, organ-specific typing, grading, and staging of the tumor in question is crucial. The internationally accepted classifications (WHO, TNM according to AJC or UICC) should be used for this. An additional division of carcinomas into those of the intestinal and those of the diffuse type should prove advantageous. Although the expenditure for such examinations is not inconsiderable, it is an indispensible necessity for any serious and internationally viable effort in oncology.

6 Prognostic Factors of Gastric Cancer

Cancer of the Stomach – Prognosis, Independent of Therapy

P. Schmitz-Moormann, H.-A. Heider, and C. Thomas

The prognosis of the gastric carcinoma is given a 5-year survival rate. After a period of 5 years, the survival rate of people with and without cancer of the stomach is equal, so that this period of control is sufficient. The overall survival rate of the gastric carcinoma ranges from 1.4% to 27.7%, the mean value is 11.9%. The prognosis is influenced not only by the therapy, but also by many other factors, independent of therapy. These factors are properties of the tumor and the carrier of the tumor, and factors produced by an interaction between the tumor and its carrier.

Properties of the Tumor Carrier

Age

Gastric cancer can occur as early as the third decade of life. The peak lies in the 7th decade. The mean ages are 54.5 (male) and 54.7 (female) in Japan and 65.0 and 62.1 in the United States.

The 5-year survival rate is low during the third decade, it rises during the following years, and decreases beyond the 55th year of life [8]. But the postoperative mortality increases with aging to about 300% in males and 600% in females. That means the postclinical development is more disadvantageous in younger patients than in older ones. Moreover, a relative 5-year survival rate shows a marked improvement of the prognosis beyond 75 years.

Sex

The data over sex distribution of gastric cancer ranges between 1 : 1 and 1 : 4 with predomination of men. On the average, 68% of gastric carcinomas was found in men, and 32% in women. The 5-year survival rates present only insignificant differences (Table 3) [3, 5, 13, 18, 21, 19, 29, 47].

Properties of the Tumor

Localization

Most frequently, the gastric carcinoma will be found in the antrum (mean value 62.0%). The carcinomas of the body (17.5%) are mainly localized at the lesser curvature; 10% are cardia cancer, 7.7% are diffuse.

The prognosis of the cancer is nearly equal for the lower and the intermediate third of the stomach, it is markedly worse in the upper third. In a more specific classification the worst prognosis was found by most authors for the cardia carcinoma (Tables 4 and 5) [4, 10, 15, 17, 21, 23, 28, 30, 35].

Macroscopic Appearance

For the macroscopic classification of gastric cancer, the scheme of Borrmann [6] is generally accepted:

Type 1: Circumscribed solitary polypoid cancer without ulcerations.
Type 2: Ulcerative carcinoma with elevated borders and sharp limitations.
Type 3: Ulcerative carcinoma with a mixture of elevated borders and diffuse spreading.
Type 4: Diffuse carcinoma.

Type 1 and type 2 present the best prognosis present with a mean 5-year survival rate of 34% and 38%, respectively. The mean value of type 3 is 19%, of type 4, only 10%. Furthermore, the size of the tumor is a good macroscopic indication. The maximal diameter of the gastric cancer measures 0–2 cm in about 10%. In about 15%, it was 2–4 cm, respectively, 4–6 cm, in 40% 6–9 cm, and in 20% more than 9 cm.

The prognosis and the maximal diameter of the gastric cancer show a good correlation. For a diameter of less than 2 cm there is a 5-year survival rate of 70%, between 2 cm and 5 cm about 33%, and between 5 cm and 10 cm about 17% [26, 35, 45, 62].

Microscopic Appearance

Microscopic classification of the gastric cancer can be based on the histological type and on the degree of differentiation. The histological classifications from various publications are different. Therefore, a comparison of the published results is often difficult or impossible. Ekers and Efskind [18] most frequently found a glandular adenocarcinoma. The best prognosis showed the carcinoma simplex and the papillary adenocarcinoma, while the prognosis of the solid and undifferentiated carcinoma was extremely poor (Table 1). Distinguishing

Table 1. 5- and 10-Year survival rate, dependent on the histological type (Eker and Efskind, 1960)

Type	Relative	Survival-Rate	
	Frequency	5-year	10-year
Carcinoma simplex	10.6%	54.8%	33.7%
Papillary adenocarcinoma	2.1%	61.9%	33.2%
Glandular adenocarcinoma	49.8%	26.4%	23.5%
Mucoid carcinoma	8.1%	20.5%	12.8%
Scirrhous carcinoma	19.5%	11.9%	7.9%
Solid carcinoma	1.8%	13.2%	0%
Undifferentiated carcinoma	7.4%	12.2%	0%

between the diffuse and the intestinal type, the latter revealed a distinctly favorable prognosis [35, 36, 44].

In the classification based on the differentiation of the carcinomatous tissue, the criteria of Broders [7] are generally accepted:

Grade 1: 75% – 100% of the carcinomatous tissue are differentiated.
Grade 2: 50% – 75% are differentiated.
Grade 3: 25% – 50% are differentiated.
Grade 4: 0% – 25% are differentiated.

In cancer of the stomach, 58% of cases corresponded to grade 1, 20% to grade 2, 30% to grade 3, and 45% to grade 4 [16, 20, 21, 45, 58, 64, 68, 71, 76]. The prognosis of the gastric cancer decreases with the grade of the dedifferentiation. The most extreme decrease is visible between grade 2 and grade 3 (Table 2).

Spread

Three forms of spreading are discernible:

1. Local infiltration of the tumor.
2. Metastasing in the lymphatic system.
3. Blood-borne metastasing.

Only 5% of the gastric cancers are limited to the mucosa and submucosa. About 20% invade the muscularis propria, and 75% infiltrate the serosa [11, 45, 53, 55, 58, 63]. The infiltration of the serosa is accompanied by a distinct worsening of the prognosis with a shortening of the 5-year survival rate from about 48% to 17% (Table 3). A further decrease is visible as soon as the cancer invades adjacent organs [18, 61, 63].

Metastases of regional lymph nodes occurred in 60% of cases. The mean survival rate decreased from 39% to 14% with the development of such lymph node metastases (Table 4). The prognosis worsened with the number of affected lymph nodes as well as with the number of affected groups of lymph nodes (Tables 5 and 6).

Table 2. Grade-dependent 5-year survival rate

Year	Author	Number	Grade (Broders)			
			1	2	3	4
1948	Steiner et al.	60	86.2%	58.8%	30.2%	23.3%
1952	Anderson et al.	117	66.6%	46.7%	16.7%	6.1%
1952	Berkson et al.	9620	56.8%	56.8%	31.4%	22.8%
1956	Gage et al.	384	66.7%	60.4%	43.9%	32.3%
1960	Eker and Efskind	1314	91.0%	70.0%	11.0%	9.0%
1962	Laurén et al.	153	32.0%	32.0%	28.0%	18.0%
1964	Dockerty		100.0%	45.5%	29.4%	20.9%

Table 3. Stage-dependent 5-year survival rate

Year	Author	Without serosal invasion	With serosal invasion
1953	Remine et al.	44.1%	–
1962	Laurén et al.	44.0%	16.0%
1965	Inberg et al.	46.8%	19.6%
1967	Yanagisawa	50.0%	15.0%
1968	Ichikawa	50.0%	20.0%
1972	Öhman et al.	33.0%	20.0%
1973	Hermanek	50.0%	17.5%
1973	Inberg et al.	50.0%	15.8%
1973	Priesching et al.	67.8%	30.1%
1976	Burkhardt et al.	46.2%	4.5%

Table 4. 5-Year survival rates, dependent on the affection of lymphatic glands

Year	Author	Without affection	With affection
1948	Moore et al.[a]	42.9%	5.1%
1951	Thomas et al.[a]	36.0%	9.0%
1952	Berkson et al.[a]	48.5%	18.6%
1952	Brown and Kane	–	19.0%
1952	Jemerin and Colp[a]	45.0%	19.0%
1952	Schrek[a]	42.7%	15.9%
1953	Anthun	14.0%	4.0%
1953	Walters and Berson[a]	48.5%	18.6%
1954	Marshall and Uram	9.3%	5.1%
1955	Cohart and Muller	13.0%	6.0%
1955	Ochsner et al.[a]	57.0%	12.0%
1956	Shahon et al.	57.1%	14.5%
1959	Urban and McNeer	71.0%	29.0%
1961	Hoerr[a]	55.3%	17.6%
1963	Zacho et al.	38.0%	35.0%
1965	Hoerr[a]	62.5%	22.4%
1965	Keller and Kinsey	23.0%	3.0%
1967	Goldenberg et al.	25.0%	4.0%
1971	Cantrell	45.7%	8.1%
1971	Lempinen	37.4%	20.0%
1973	Lempinen et al.	39.0%	13.0%

[a] After surgery

Table 5. 5-Year survival rate, dependent on the number of metastases in lymph nodes

Percentage of affected lymph nodes	5-Year survival rate
0%	50.6%
1% – 24%	24.1%
25% – 49%	12.3%
50% – 74%	2.9%
75% – 100%	2.9%

Table 6. 5-Year survival rate, dependent on the number of affected groups of lymph nodes

Number of groups	Eker and Efskind (1960)	Maruta and Shida (1968)
None	48.9%	38.6%
1 Group	19.2%	40.3%
2 Groups	8.5%	16.7%
3 Groups	6.3%	–

Interactions between Tumor and Tumor Carrier

The morphological signs of tumor defense seem to be of value for prognostic predictions. McCarty [54] saw a distinct increase of the survival time with growing intensity of lymphocytic infiltration, fibrosis, and hyalinization. Fley [24] found a rising percentage of long-time survivors with growing intensity of lymphocytic stromal infiltration. Inokuchi [37] described a clear increase of the 5-year survival rate with growing intensity of the lymphocytic stromal reaction of the primary tumor and of the metastases.

Up to now, the viewpoint of this paper would be merely monofactorial. All statements about the prognosis was done on the premise that only one factor change and that the effects of the remaining factors would cancel each other out. This kind of view is surely wrong. Rather, it is most probable that all the studied factors influence each other. This mutual influence is very easily recognizable for the different forms of spreading. The number of lymph node metastases increases with the size of the tumor [14, 25, 38, 58, 61 67]. These relations are the basis of a clinical stage system, as introduced by the *Union Internationale Contre le Cancer* [4]. In this staging system, all authors found a worsening of the prognosis with rising stage [4, 29, 40, 42, 53, 59].

But also the remaining factors, influencing the prognosis, often depend upon each other.

Thus, there is an age dependency of the prognosis, but no sex linkage. But considering the dependency from both, age and sex, a sex linkage becomes visible with an improvement of the prognosis for older women and younger men [18]. Similarly, every factor can be plotted against each other. Regarding age and frequency of metastases, there is a decrease of metastases with growing age (Table 7). Considering age and histological type, scirrhous cancer predominates between 20 and 30 years, whereas adenocarcinoma prevails in older people [21]. With regards to the frequency of metastases and the macroscopic type or the

Table 7. Age-dependent frequency of metastases

Age (years)	Number	With metastases	Without metastases
20 – 39	39	71.8%	28.2%
40 – 49	130	71.5%	28.5%
50 – 59	303	71.3%	28.7%
60 – 69	438	63.2%	36.8%
70 and older	253	56.9%	43.1%

histological differentiation, the frequency of metastases increases from type 1 to type 4 of Borrmann or from grade 1 to grade 4 of Broders [14, 17, 21, 25, 46, 56, 58].

As a matter of course, all these relations influence the prognosis, too. Thus, the adenocarcinoma shows an overall 5-year survival rate of 26.4%, the scirrhous carcinoma, 11.9%. But the survival rate of adenocarcinoma, localized in the antrum is 33.9%, and of scirrhous carcinoma of the antrum 25.4% [18, 21]. Even the prognosis, dependent upon the reaction of the tumor carrier against the tumor is influenced by the histological type. Thus, the 5-year survival rate of the intestinal type is 35.1%, of the diffuse type 26.1%. But regarding simultaneously the stromal reaction, the diffuse type shows much better prognosis than the intestinal type, when combined with a strong stromal reaction [36].

These examples thus elucidate, that an addition to the prognosis of the particular factors cannot result in the prognosis of the special combination of influencing factors. A well-founded prognosis can only be obtained from the different factors by a multifactorial evaluation with modern computer technique. In our experience, such multifactorial evaluations cannot be done in a

Table 8. Factors independent of therapy, influencing the prognosis (5-year survival rate)

Age	25 – 34	35 – 44	45 – 54	55 – 64	65 – 74	75 and older
Percentage [a]	16.8%	23.6%	22.6%	15.7%	16.7%	21.8%
Sex	No significant dependency					
Site	Lower	Intermediate		Upper third of the stomach		
Percentage	24.9%	23.0%		9.8%		
Macroscopic type (Borrmann)	Type	I	II		III	IV
Percentage		33.8%	37.8%		18.7%	9.8%
Size (∅)	5 cm	5 – 10 cm	10 cm			
Percentage	32.5%	17.5%	0%			
Histological type	Intestinal	Diffuse				
Percentage	35.1%	26.1%				
Grade of differentiation (Broders)		1	2		3	4
Percentage		71.3%	52.9%		25.8%	18.9%
Extension		T 1	T 2		T 3	T 4
Percentage		61.7%	38.5%		18.0%	7.8%
Metastases of lymph nodes		N 1	N 2		N 3	N 4
Percentages		33.0%	12.0%		10.0%	0%
Lymphocytic infiltration	0	1	2		3	4 grade
Percentage	9.0%	19.0%	32.0%		23.0%	17.0%

[a] Relative 5-year survival rate

retrospective study, but only in a prospective investigation. Perhaps such a multifactorial evaluation will give precise extrapolated 5-year survival rates of every factor, so that an addition or a multiplication of these values gives the precise prognosis of the special combination of factors influencing the prognosis.

Summary

The prognosis, independent of therapy, is influenced by different factors, such as age, sex, macroscopic, and microscopic appearance, spread, and stromal reaction (Table 8). But these factors are not independent from each other. Therefore, a monofactorial analysis of the prognosis is insufficient. Only a simultaneous multifactorial analysis will give valid data for a more precise prognosis.

References

1. Anderson, A. D., Dockerty, M. B., Gray, H. K.: A clinical and pathological study of the significance of malignant pyloric obstruction on postresection prognosis. Surg. Gynecol. Obstet. *95*, 85–92 (1952)
2. Anthun, O.: Carcinoma of the stomach. Acta Chir. Scand. *104*, 1–13 (1953)
3. Berkson, J.: Statistical summary. In: Cancer of the Stomach. Re Mine, Priestley, Berkson (eds.), pp. 207–236. Philadelphia, London: Saunders 1964
4. Berndt, H., Gummel, H., Wittig, G.: Statistische Untersuchungen über das Magenkarzinom. II. Lokalisation, Morphologie, Prognose. Dtsch. Gesundheitsw. *19*, 13–20 (1964)
5. Blalock, J. Ochsner, A.: Carcinoma of the stomach. Ann. Surg. *145*, 726–737 (1957)
6. Borrmann, R.: Geschwülste des Magens und Duodenums. In: Hdb. der speziellen pathologischen Anatomie und Histologie, hrsg. F. Henke und O. Lubarsch. Bd. IV/1, pp. 865–1054. Berlin: Springer 1926
7. Broders, A. C.: 1. Carcinoma: grading and practical application. Arch. Path. *2*, 376–381 (1926)
8. Brookes, U. S., Waterhouse, J. A. H., Dowell, D. J.: Carcinoma of the stomach: A 10-year survey of results and of factors affecting prognosis. Br. Med. J. *1965 1*, 1577–1586
9. Brown, C. H., Kane, C. F.: Carcinoma of the stomach: Review of 406 cases seen from 1940 to 1945: Operability, resectability and curability. Gastroenterology *22*, 64–79 (1952)
10. Burian, J., Bittmann, O., Siroky, J.: Analyse des langjährigen Überlebens von 1370 wegen Magen- und Kardiakrebs operierten Kranken. Zentralbl. Chir. *88*, 638–648 (1963)
11. Burkhardt, K., Peitsch, W.: Therapie und Prognose der Kardiakarzinome. Chirurg *47*, 615–621 (1976)
12. Cantrell, E. G.: The importance of lymph nodes in the assessment of gastric carcinoma at operation. Br. J. Surg. *58*, 384–386 (1971)
13. Cohart, E. M., Muller, C.: Socioeconomic distribution of cancer of the gastrointestinal tract in New Haven. Cancer *8*, 379–388 (1955)
14. Coller, F. A., Kay, E. B., McIntire, R. S.: Regional lymphatic metastases of carcinoma of the stomach. Arch. Surg. *43*, 748–761 (1941)
15. Denck, H., Helmer, F.: Zur Prognose des Magenkarzinoms. Chirurg *29*, 289–294 (1958)
16. Dochat, G. R., Gray, H. K.: Carcinoma of the stomach: prognosis based on a combination of Dukes' and Broders' methods of grading. Am. J. Clin. Pathol. *13*, 441–449 (1943)
17. Dockerty, M. B.: Pathologic aspects of primary malignant neoplasms of the stomach. In: Cancer of the Stomach. Re Mine, W. H., Priestley, J. T., Berkson, J., (eds.), pp. 173–206. Philadelphia, London: Saunders 1964
18. Ederer, F., Cuttler, S. J., Eisenberg, H., Keogh, J. R.: Survival of patients with cancer of the stomach, Connecticut, 1935–54. J. Natl. Cancer Inst. *25*, 1005–1021 (1960)

19. Eisenberg, H., Sullivan, P. D., Foote, F. M.: Trends in survival of digestive system cancer patients in Connecticut 1935 to 1962. Gastroenterology *53*, 528 – 546 (1967)
20. Eker, R., Efskind, J.: Investigations on the intramural spread of gastric carcinoma. Acta Pathol. Microbiol. Scand. *30*, 371 – 383 (1952)
21. Eker, R., Efskind, J.: The pathology and prognosis of gastric carcinoma. Based on 1314 partially and totally resected cases. Acta Chir. Scand. (Suppl.) *264*, 1 – 182 (1960)
22. Ferguson, L. K., Nusbaum, M.: Survival after surgical treatment of carcinoma of the stomach. Ann. Surg. *158*, 51 – 55 (1963)
23. Flood, C. A., Wells, J., Harvey, H. D.: Prognosis in cancer of the stomach. Am. J. Dig. Dis. *7*, 420 – 431 (1962)
24. Fley, O. A., Dockerty, M. B., Waugh, J. M.: Metastasis to the regional nodes of the splenic hilus from carcinoma of the stomach. Surg. Gynec. Obstet. *102*, 279 – 286 (1956)
25. Fujimaki, M.: The lymphatic spread of gastric carcinoma in surgical specimens. Acta Med. Biol. *8*, 83 – 108 (1960)
26. Gage, R. P., Comfort, M. W., Priestley, J. T., Dockerty, M. B., Weber, H. M.: The favourable outlook for the patient with small gastric cancer. Gastroenterologia (Basel) *86*, 474 – 484 (1956)
27. Goldenberg, I. S., Cohen, J. M., Skinner, D. G.: A study of survival patterns in patients with gastric carcinoma. Surg. Gynecol. Obstet. *124*, 241 – 250 (1967)
28. Goldsmith, H. S., Gosh, B. C.: Carcinoma of the stomach. Am. J. Surg. *120*, 317 – 326 (1970)
29. Gummel, H., Wittig, G., Berndt, H.: Therapieresultate und Prognose des Magenkarzinoms. Arch. Geschwulstforsch. *29*, 274 – 292 (1967)
30. Hawley, P. R., Westerholm, P., Morson, B. C.: Pathology and prognosis of carcinoma of the stomach. Br. J. Surg. *57*, 877 – 883 (1970)
31. Hermanek, P.: Frühdiagnose und Frühbehandlung des Magenkrebses aus der Sicht der chirurgischen Pathologie. Munch. Med. Wochenschr. *115*, 1509 – 1512 (1973)
32. Hoerr, S. O.: Carcinoma of the stomach. Am. J. Surg. *101*, 284 – 291 (1961)
33. Hoerr, S. O.: Malignant lesions of the stomach. An analysis of fifty-four five year survivors. Am. J. Surg. *109*, 14 – 20 (1965)
34. Ichikawa, H.: A modified proposal on T-classification for gastric carcinoma. Tokio: Igako Shoin 1968
35. Inberg, M., Laurén, P., Viikari, S.: Factors influencing survival after radical operation for gastric cancer. J. Int. Coll. Surg. *44*, 682 – 686 (1965)
36. Inberg, M. V., Laurén, P., Vuori, J., Viikari, S. J.: Prognosis in intestinal-type and diffuse gastric carcinoma with special reference to the effect of the stromal reaction. Acta Chir. Scand. *139*, 273 – 278 (1973)
37. Inokuchi, K., Inutsuka, S., Furusawa, M., Soejima, K., Ikeda, T.: Stromal reaction around tumor and metastases and prognosis after curative gastrectomy for carcinoma of the stomach. Cancer *20*, 1924 – 1929 (1967)
38. Iwanaga, T., Taniguchi, H.: Klinische Pathologie des Magenfrühkarzinoms. Leber Magen Darm *3*, 54 – 59 (1973)
39. Jemerin, E. E., Colp, R.: Gastric carcinoma. Statistical study based on 344 cases from 1938 through 1947. Surg. Gynecol. Obstet. *95*, 99 – 112 (1952)
40. Katsura, S., Kaneko, Y.: The current status of operation for gastric carcinoma in Japan and some suggestions for improvement of operative results. Tohoku J. Exp. Med. *102*, 195 – 206 (1970)
41. Keller, J. W., Kinsey, D. L.: Gastric cancer. A survey of five hundred and seventy-four cases. Ohio State Med. J. *61*, 1083 – 1088 (1965)
42. Kennedy, B. J.: TNM classification for stomach cancer. Cancer *26*, 971 – 983 (1970)
43. Kurokawa, T., Saito, T., Yonemura, H., Kayaba, M., Tada, K., Uruga, K., Sagara, M., Ishioka, K.: Cytological diagnosis of gastric cancer. Tohoku J. Exp. Med. *3*, 208 – 224 (1960)
44. Laurén, P.: The two histological main types of gastric carcinoma: Diffuse and so-called intestinal-type carcinoma. An attempt at a histo-clinical classification. Acta Pathol. Microbiol. Scand. *64*, 31 – 49 (1965)
45. Laurén, P., Viikari, S., Hyttinen, A., Autio, U.: Pathological features of gastric cancer affecting survival after curative resections. Ann. Chir. Gynaecol. Fenn. *51*, 342 – 350 (1962)
46. Lawrence, W., jr.: Carcinoma of the stomach. CA *23*, 286 – 304 (1973)
47. Lempinen, M.: Carcinoma of the stomach. III. Prognosis and some prognostic factors. Ann. Chir. Gynaecol. Fenn. *60*, 145 – 150 (1971)

48. Lempinen, M., Hjelt, L., Paile, A.: Prognostic factors in carcinoma of the stomach. Ann. Chir. Gynaecol. Fenn. *62*, 354 – 360 (1973)
49. Lumpkin, W. M., Crow, R. L., Hernandez, C. M., Cohn, I.: Carcinoma of the stomach. Review of 1035 cases. Ann. Surg. *159*, 919 – 937 (1964)
50. Maimon, S. N., Palmer, W. L., Kirsner, J. B.: Prognosis in gastric cancer: A study of five-year survivors. Am. J. Med. *5*, 230 – 236 (1948)
51. Marcus, G. H., Lill, H.: Über den Magenkrebs. Wien. Med. Wochenschr. *102*, 801 – 805, 825 – 831, 849 – 852 (1952)
52. Marshall, S. F., Uram, H.: Total gastrectomy for gastric cancer: Effect upon mortality, morbidity, and curability. Surg. Gynecol. Obstet. *99*, 657 – 675 (1954)
53. Maruta, K., Shida, H.: Some factors which influcence prognosis after surgery for advanced gastric cancer. Ann. Surg. *167*, 313 – 318 (1968)
54. McCarty, W. C.: Factors which influence longevity in cancer. Ann. Surg. *76*, 9 – 12 (1922)
55. Monafo, W. W., Krause, G. L., jr., Medina, J. G.: Carcinoma of the stomach. Morphological characteristics affecting survival. Arch. Surg. *85*, 754 – 763 (1962)
56. Moore, J. R., Morton, H. S.: Gastric carcinoma: A statistical review of 427 cases of carcinoma of the stomach from 1941 through 1950. Ann. Surg. *141*, 185 – 192 (1955)
57. Moore, G. E., State, D., Hebbel, R., Trelohr, A. E.: Carcinoma of the stomach. Surg. Gynecol. Obstet. *87*, 513 – 518 (1948)
58. Muto, M., Majima, S., Yoshida, K., Karube, K., Teshima, T., Yamaguchi, I.: The pathological aspects of stomach cancer in 1988 surgical cases. Tohoku J. Exp. Med. *81*, 143 – 162 (1963)
59. Nielsen, S. A. I., Amdrup, E., Christiansen, P., Fenger, C., Jensen, H. E., Lindskov, J., Nielsen, J.: Carcinoma of the stomach. An analysis of 385 cases treated 1955 to 1964. Acta Chir. Scand. *140*, 313 – 320 (1974)
60. Ochsner, A., Blalock, J., Sucre, A.: Carcinoma of the stomach. Am. Surg. *21*, 1 – 16 (1955)
61. Öhman, U., Wetterfors, J., Moberg, A.: Primary gastric cancer and its prognosis. Acta Chir. Scand. *138*, 378 – 383 (1972)
62. Öhman, U., Wetterfors, J., Moberg, A.: Histologic grading of gastric cancer. Acta Chir. Scand. *138*, 384 – 390 (1972)
63. Priesching, A., Wagner, O., Funovic, F.: Subseröse Magenkarzinome. Wien. Med. Wochenschr. *123*, 135 – 140 (1973)
64. Remine, W. H., Priestley, J. T.: Late results after total gastrectomy. Surg. Gynecol. Obstet. *94*, 519 – 525 (1952)
65. Remine, W. H., Dockerty, M. B., Priestley, J. T.: Some factors which influence prognosis in surgical treatment of gastric carcinoma. Ann. Surg. *138*, 311 – 319 (1953)
66. Remine, W. H., Gomes, M. M. R., Dockerty, M. B.: Long-term survival (10 to 56 years) after surgery for carcinoma of the stomach. Am. J. Surg. *117*, 177 – 184 (1969)
67. Rueff, F. L., von Bary, S., Silbernagel, A.: Das Magenkarzinom. Eine statistische Analyse. Munch. Med. Wochenschr. *115*, 410 – 415 (1973)
68. Schindler, R., Steiner, P. E., Smith, W. M., Daley, M. E.: The classification of gastric carcinoma. Surg. Gynecol. Obstet. *73*, 30 – 39 (1941)
69. Schrek, R.: Fifty per cent survival time as a measure of prognosis in cancer. Am. J. Clin. Pathol. *26*, 172 – 174 (1956)
70. Shahon, D. B., Horowitz, S., Kelly, W. D.: Cancer of the stomach; an analysis of 1152 cases. Surgery *39*, 204 – 221 (1956)
71. Slungaard, U., Weber-Laumann, A.: Prognosis of gastric carcinoma. Acta Chir. Scand. *129*, 425 – 433 (1965)
72. Steiner, P. E., Maimon, S. N., Palmer, W. L., Kirsner, J. B.: Gastric cancer: Morphologic factors in five-year survival after gastrectomy. Am. J. Pathol. *24*, 947 – 969 (1948)
73. Thomas, W. D., Waugh, J. M., Dockerty, M. B.: Prognosis of gastric carcinoma. Arch. Surg. *62*, 847 – 855 (1951)
74. Urban, C. H., McNeer, G.: The relation of the morphology of gastric carcinoma to long and short term survival. Cancer *12*, 1158 – 1162 (1959)
75. Walters, W., Berkson, J.: An improvement of 180 per cent in the five-year-survival rate of patients with carcinoma of the stomach. Ann. Surg. *137*, 884 – 891 (1953)
76. Walters, W., Gray, H. K., Priestley, J. T.: Prognosis and endresults in the treatment of cancer of the stomach. Arch. Surg. *46*, 939 – 943 (1943)

77. Yanagisawa, F.: Die Prognose des Magenkarzinoms nach der chirurgischen Behandlung im Hinblick auf die pathologisch-anatomische Untersuchung. Bruns Beitr. Klin. Chir. *214*, 356–357 (1967)
78. Zacho, A., Fischermann, K., Sørensen, B. L.: Prognostic role of breach of lymph node capsule in nodal metastases from gastric carcinoma. Acta Chir. Scand. *125*, 365–369 (1963)

Prognostic Significance of Stromal Reaction in Gastric Carcinoma

W. Schachenmayr and O. Haferkamp

Postoperative survival of a patient with gastric carcinoma essentially depends on the tumor extension at the time of therapy estimated by a pathological-anatomical staging. Surprisingly variable, however, is the progress of patients with the identical tumor development. Accordingly, attempts were made to refine the pattern of prognostically relevant morphological parameters. In addition to the typing of carcinoma, the histopathological tumor-grading has provided other prognostically useful information. In tumor-grading, no consideration is given to the tumor-stroma. The significance of stromal changes has been a matter of contention since the beginning of histopathological studies on tumor tissues [7]. Whereas one group of workers interpreted inflammatory infiltrates of certain cancers as a defense mechanism against tumor progression, others denied their prognostic importance and regarded them as an unimportant symptom of tumor extension.

New light has been thrown upon this problem following experimental tumor immunology during the last 15 years. There has been growing evidence of specific immune mechanisms directed against the seemingly autonomous tumor tissue. This host reaction includes the production of tumor-specific antibodies, the appearance of cytotoxic T-lymphocytes, and antibody-dependent "killer"-cells and the destruction of tumor cells by activated macrophages [1]. Moreover, a neutrophil-mediated tumor cytotoxicity caused by the peroxidase system could be demonstrated [4]. Under these considerations, it seems justifiable to look for morphological equivalents of these in vitro demonstrated antitumoral cell activities in histological slices of a carcinoma and to correlate their presence or absence with the progress of the disease.

A classical study of this kind was presented by Berg [2] who showed that in breast cancers a striking plasma cell infiltration of tumor stroma was found much more often among patients surviving 5 years or more than among those who died earlier. Other workers confirmed the prognostically favorable effect of lympho-plasmacellular stromal reaction not only in breast carcinoma [3], but also in cancers of other organs, including the stomach [5, 6]. This applies especially to the type of gastric carcinoma with lymphoid stroma described by Watanabe and co-workers [9]. In contrast to the usual picture of carcinoma with cellular infiltration of the surrounding stroma, the stromal reaction with masses of lymphocytes and plasma cells here, is much more pronounced than the tumor cells. So it seemed reasonable to analyse the morphology of stromal reaction in a retrospective pilot study on 49 cases of resected gastric cancers with known postoperative history and to examine the prognostic usefulness of various histological parameters. The patients originated from a consecutive series of Dr. Bell, former Chairman of the Department of Surgery, University of California, Medical Center, San Francisco, United States. A group of 19 patients who made favorable progress, i. e., having a survival time of 5 years or more, was separated from another group of 30 patients, who had died from carcinoma after an average of 3 years, postoperatively.

As expected, first of all, the depth of penetration by the carcinoma in the stomach wall influenced the course of the disease; in the majority of favorable cases, the muscularis propria was not penetrated by the tumor. Even more pronounced was the prognostic effect of proved lymph node metastases. Only 26% of the favorable cases had lymph node involvement, in contrast to 56% of the fatal cases. The histological type of carcinoma seemed to have no clear influence on the prognosis.

An analysis of the tumor stroma showed roughly five histological types of stromal reaction which had also previously been found in a series of large bowel cancers [8], namely, an aggressive granulocytic reaction, an aggressive lymphocytic reaction, a granulomatous histiocytic reaction, a mixed-cellular reaction, and a desmoplastic reaction. An example of the aggressive granulocytic stromal reaction is given by the gastric carcinoma of a 68 year old female, which had already broken into the liver. Histological sections of this tumor showed polymorphonuclear leukocytes penetrating massively from the stroma into the carcinomatous glands (Fig. 1). The patient survived 24 years after operation without a recurrence. The large diversity of stromal reaction is demonstrated by the following examples of a massive lymphocytic infiltration of the tumor stroma (Fig. 2), of a granulomatous-histiocytic reaction around tumor glands (Fig. 3), of a balanced infiltration of mixed granulocytes, lymphocytes, and plasma cells (Fig. 4) and, finally, of a massive increase of collagenous tissue characteristic of desmoplastic stromal reaction (Fig. 5). Because this classification into five types of stromal reaction was not suitable for a statistical analysis, since transitional forms occurred, the density of cellular infiltrates for each cell type and the

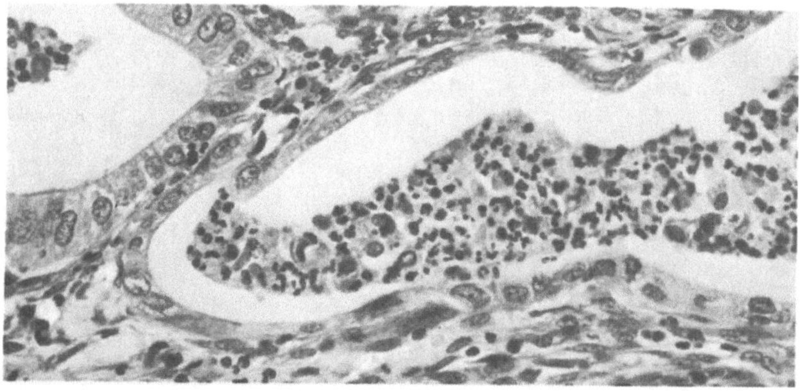

Fig. 1. Adenocarcinoma of the stomach with aggressive granulocytic infiltration into tumor glands (HE × 350)

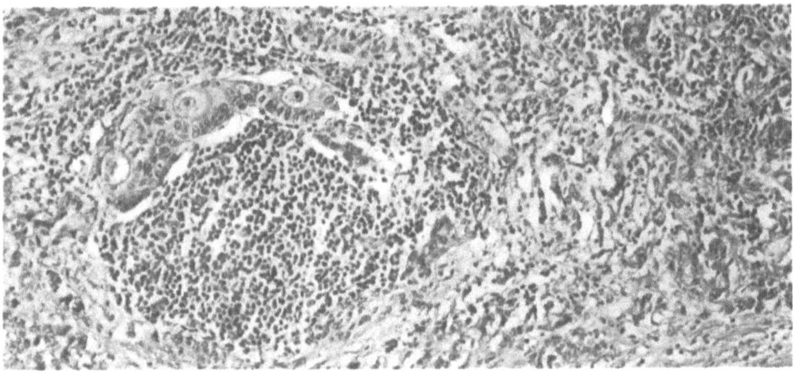

Fig. 2. Adenocarcinoma of the stomach with aggressive lymphocytic stromal reaction (HE, × 140)

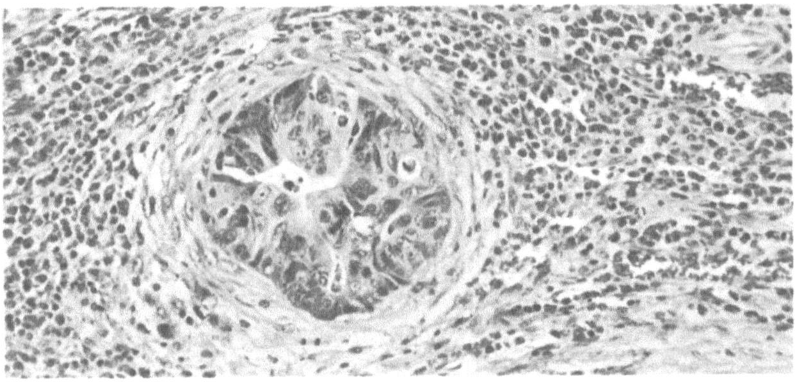

Fig. 3. Granulomatous-histiocytic stromal reaction around a tumor gland of gastric adenocarcinoma (HE, × 220)

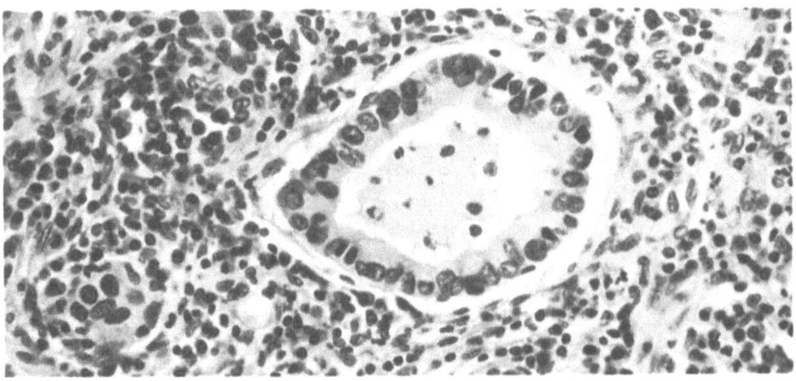

Fig. 4. Adenocarcinoma of the stomach with mixed-cellular stromal infiltration (HE, × 350)

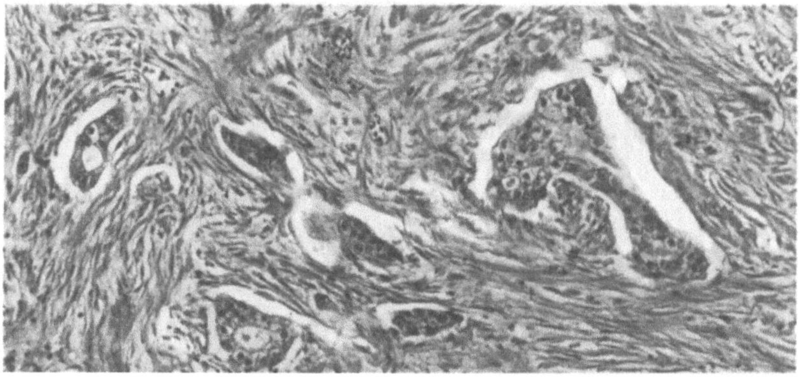

Fig. 5. Massive stromal fibrosis in gastric adenocarcinoma (HE, × 140)

amount of fibrosis in the tumor stroma of all 49 carcinomas were evaluated semiquantitatively without knowledge of the individual's further case history. The results showed some interesting tendencies (Table 1). Polymorphonuclear leukocytes infiltrated aggressively into carcinomatous glands preponderantly in favorable cases. In this group also a markedly larger proportion of carcinomas with massive stromal infiltrates of lymphocytes, plasma cells, and macrophages was found as compared with the unfavorable cases; this difference being sta-

Table 1. Stromal reaction and prognosis in 49 cases of gastric carcinoma

Stromal reaction	Favorable cases (19)	Unfavorable cases (30)
PMN leukocyte infiltrate		
None or slight	10 (53%)	18 (60%)
Moderate	3 (16%)	8 (27%)
Massive	–	1 (3%)
In tumor glands	6 (31%)	3 (10%)
Lymphocytic infiltrate		
None or slight	2 (11%)	7 (23%)
Moderate	11 (58%)	19 (64%)
Massive	6 (31%)	4 (13%)
Plasma cell infiltrate		
None or slight	3 (16%)	11 (37%)
Moderate	9 (47%)	13 (43%)
Massive	7 (37%)	6 (20%)
Macrophage infiltrate		
None or slight	9 (48%)	23 (77%)
Moderate	4 (21%)	4 (13%)
Massive	6 (31%)	3 (10%)
Fibrosis		
None or slight	9 (48%)	12 (40%)
Moderate	5 (26%)	4 (13%)
Massive	5 (26%)	14 (47%)

tistically significant for stromal macrophages. The unfavorable cases, in contrast, had more carcinomas with massive stromal fibrosis. The presence of this desmoplastic reaction was also significantly correlated with deeper tumor penetration of the stomach wall and lesser plasmacellular stromal infiltration, which underlines the prognostically unfavorable effect of this type of stromal reaction.

Conclusion

1. Irrespective of the question whether there are morphological equivalents of tumor-immunologic mechanisms, a scale of changes can be observed in tumor stroma. These may be divided roughly into an aggressive granulocytic reaction, an aggressive lymphocytic reaction, a granulomatous-histiocytic reaction, a mixed-cellular reaction, and a desmoplastic stromal reaction. Transitional forms may occur.

2. Semiquantitative differences of stromal reaction may be demonstrated when comparing favorable with unfavorable cases of operated gastric carcinoma. Pronounced occurrence of macrophages, lymphocytes, and plasma cells within the tumor stroma and the invasion of polymorphonuclear leukocytes into tumor glands may be regarded as prognostically favorable signs. The desmoplastic reaction, in contrast, should rather be regarded as an unfavorable sign.

3. As a résumé, in addition to the known significance of tumor extension in the prognosis of an operated gastric carcinoma, the type of stromal reaction should be considered and these preliminary results followed up in a prospective study.

References

1. Allison, A. C., Ferluga, J.: How lymphocytes kill tumor cells. N. Engl. J. Med. *295*, 165–167 (1976)
2. Berg, J. W.: Inflammation and prognosis in breast cancer. A search for host resistance. Cancer *12*, 714–720 (1959)
3. Black, M. M., Barclay, T. H. C., Hankey, B. F.: Prognosis in breast cancer utilizing histologic characteristics of the primary tumor. Cancer *36*, 2048–2055 (1975)
4. Clark, R. A., Klebanoff, S. J.: Neutrophil-mediated tumor cell cytotoxicity: Role of the peroxidase system. J. Exp. Med. *141*, 1442–1447 (1975)
5. Hawley, P. R., Westerholm, P., Morson, B. C.: Pathology and prognosis of carcinoma of the stomach. Br. J. Surg. *57*, 877–883 (1970)
6. Inokuchi, K., Inutsuka, S., Furusawa, M., Soejima, K., Ikeda, T.: Stromal reaction around tumor and metastasis and prognosis after curative gastrectomy for carcinoma of the stomach. Cancer *20*, 1924–1929 (1967)
7. Paile, A.: Morphology and prognosis of carcinoma of the stomach. Ann. Chir. Gynecol. Fenn. (Suppl.) *175*, 1–56 (1971)
8. Schachenmayr, W., Haferkamp, O., Rosenau, W., Bell, H. G.: Carcinoma of the large intestine: Stromal reaction, local extension, and prognosis (unpublished)
9. Watanabe, H., Enjoji, M., Imai, T.: Gastric carcinoma with lymphoid stroma. Its morphologic characteristics and prognostic correlations. Cancer *38*, 232–243 (1976)

A Statistical Trial on Evaluation for Prognosis of Gastric Cancer

Hiroaki Nakazato, Kimiyuki Kato, Masashi Goto, and Yoshihiro Matsubara

It is difficult to evaluate effectiveness of surgery and its adjuvant therapies on patients with curatively resected gastric cancer. Usually, survival time expressed in terms of months has been used as a scale to assess the performance of the therapies.

In an ideal clinical trial, such as a controlled therapeutic trial in phase study, it is desirable that some prognostic variables are selected prior to random assignment of each treatment to be compared; evaluation of the results is then given by the aid of observed survival time. However, the variables conceivable beforehand are so many that it is difficult to settle and stratify them in advance.

A model of our observational study is shown in Table 1. The first step is to predict postsurgical prognosis of the patients on some variables, that is, to reduce the variables into a prognostic factor, and then the possibility of its prediction is evaluated by a regression analysis. In addition, the prediction is tried for some cases.

By using such a model, we were able to establish a method of estimation of the therapeutic effects.

Imanaga's group, under a cancer research project organized by the Ministry of Health and Welfare, has carried out a survey as part of the project for

Table 1. A model of our observational studies for curatively resected gastric cancer patients

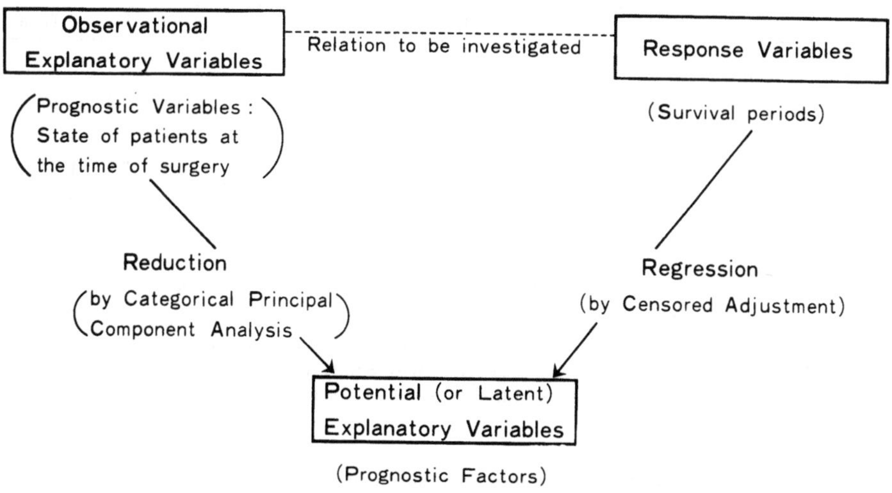

evaluating adjuvant chemotherapy on patients with curatively resected stomach cancer.

The cases undergoing the analysis were 430 in total. As shown in Table 2, follow-up study has been performed almost more than 8 years, and the number of patients who survived more than 8 years are nearly equal between both treated and control groups.

Table 3 shows prognostic variables which are mainly observed at the time of surgery and the categories which were used in this analysis. In the first step, a categorical principal component analysis was adopted by using nine variables with the exception of a chemotherapeutic one. The patient's state of illness, which is a prognostic factor to postsurgical survival period, was reduced from the 9 variables by the analysis, and the factor was characterized as a model of survival period.

The results are shown in Table 4. A categorical weight is given for each category of prognostic variables. A principal score for each patient can be calculated by adding the corresponding categorial weights from the table. The reduction rate of prognostic variables into the first principal component is about 64.7%.

Secondly, the possibility of the prediction in the analysis is evaluated. For this purpose, a regression line was estimated and its contribution evaluated. The estimation was proceeded by regression of postsurgical survival months on the prognostic factor, and the patients were divided into two groups, treated and control groups, because of the influence of the chemotherapeutic factor on survival period.

Figure 1 shows the estimated regression line and plots of 231 cases in the control group. The correlation coefficient between the factor and survival months is 0.48; this is significant. The contribution ratio is 0.23, so about 23%

Table 2. Patients number of curatively resected gastric cancer in the statistical study

	Postsurgical Period (years)										
	~1	~2	~3	~4	~5	~6	~7	~8	~9	9~	Total
Treated Group											
Dead	24	22	14	5	4	4	6	1	0	0	80
Censored	0	0	0	0	0	1	2	5	41	70	119 (111)*
Total	**24**	**22**	**14**	**5**	**4**	**5**	**8**	**6**	**41**	**70**	**199** (111)
Control Group											
Dead	35	32	26	9	6	3	4	3	3	3	124 (6)
Censored	0	0	0	0	0	0	0	0	40	67	107 (107)
Total	**35**	**32**	**26**	**9**	**6**	**3**	**4**	**3**	**43**	**70**	**231** (113)

Data from Imanaga's group under the W-I Study organized by the Ministry of Health and Welfare in Japan (Jan. 1965 ~ June 1966)
Follow-up in Dec. 1974.

* ( ) : The number of patients who survived more than 8 years.

Table 3. Factors and categories mainly used in analysis of prognosis on gastric cancer patients

Factors	Categories	Factors	Categories
1. Sex	Male Female	6. Size of Lesion	~5 cm 6~9 cm 10~ cm
2. Age	~39 yr. 40~59 yr. 60~ yr.	7. Metastases to Lymph Nodes	n_0 n_1 $n_2+n_3+n_4$
3. Extent of Resection	Total Distal Proximal	8. Serosal Invasion	s_0 s_1 s_2+s_3
4. Location	Cardia Median Antrum	9. Borrmann Type	0 1+2 3 4+5
5. Postsurgical Complication	+, −	10. Adjuvant Chemotherapy	+, −

Table 4. Categorical weight of "prognostic factors" in categorical principal component analysis

Factor	Category	Frequency (per cent)	Weight	Range
Sex	Male	285 (66)	0.220	0.652
	Female	145 (33)	− 0.432	
Age	~39	45 (10)	0.225	1.033
	40~59	206 (47)	0.454	
	60~	179 (41)	− 0.579	
Extent of Resection	Total	75 (17)	− 3.915	5.100
	Distal	342 (79)	1.014	
	Proximal	13 (03)	− 4.086	
Location	C	44 (10)	− 3.217	6.953
	M	136 (31)	0.228	
	A	231 (53)	0.970	
	All	19 (04)	− 5.983	
Postsurgical Complication	+	127 (29)	− 2.763	3.921
	−	303 (70)	1.158	
Size of Lesion	~5	205 (47)	1.800	5.312
	6~9	179 (41)	− 1.159	
	10~	46 (10)	− 3.512	
Metastases to Lymph Nodes	n_0	211 (49)	1.456	3.443
	n_1	117 (27)	− 0.893	
	$n_2+n_3+n_4$	102 (23)	− 1.987	
Serosal Invasion	s_0	228 (53)	1.612	4.158
	s_1	90 (20)	− 0.915	
	s_2+s_3	112 (26)	− 2.546	
Borrmann Type	0	99 (23)	3.193	5.753
	1+2	154 (35)	− 0.075	
	3	122 (28)	− 1.342	
	4+5	55 (12)	− 2.560	

among the variations of postsurgical survival periods are explained by the variation of the prognostic factor.

One more result may be pointed out from this figure. The discrimination between good and poor prognoses is possible to distinguish from the positive or negative score on the prognostic factor. Thus, a postsurgical period corresponding to zero point on the factor can be reflected to about 67 months. This fact means an appropriate evaluation for prognosis of gastric cancer, because good or poor prognosis has been clinically and empirically understood to be discriminated between nonsurvival and survival cases at a point of 5 years.

From the above-mentioned studies, the possibility of predicting the prognosis of the patients was evaluated. However, in practical survival study, the survival months of those patients do not provide a thorough evaluation because of censored observation. When prediction of survival months itself is carried through, a reasonable adjustment may be needed for an estimated regression formula.

Figure 2 shows the comparison of two formulas in which one is adjusted by censored observation and the previously mentioned regression formula in the control group. The two ellipses are those of 95% rejection for the two groups, short-term death and long-term survival, which were classified by the period of 67 months.

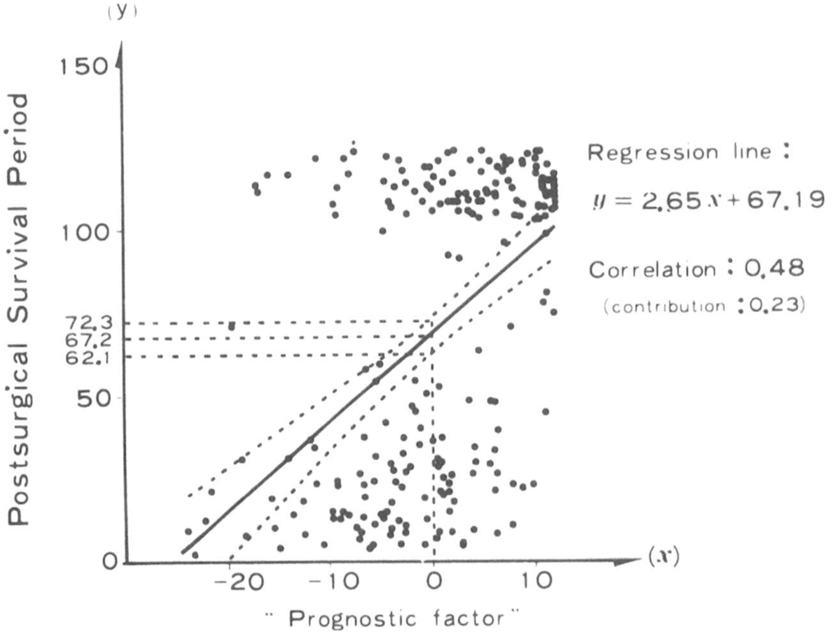

Fig. 1. Regression of the postsurgical survival period on the "prognostic factor" (control group n = 231)

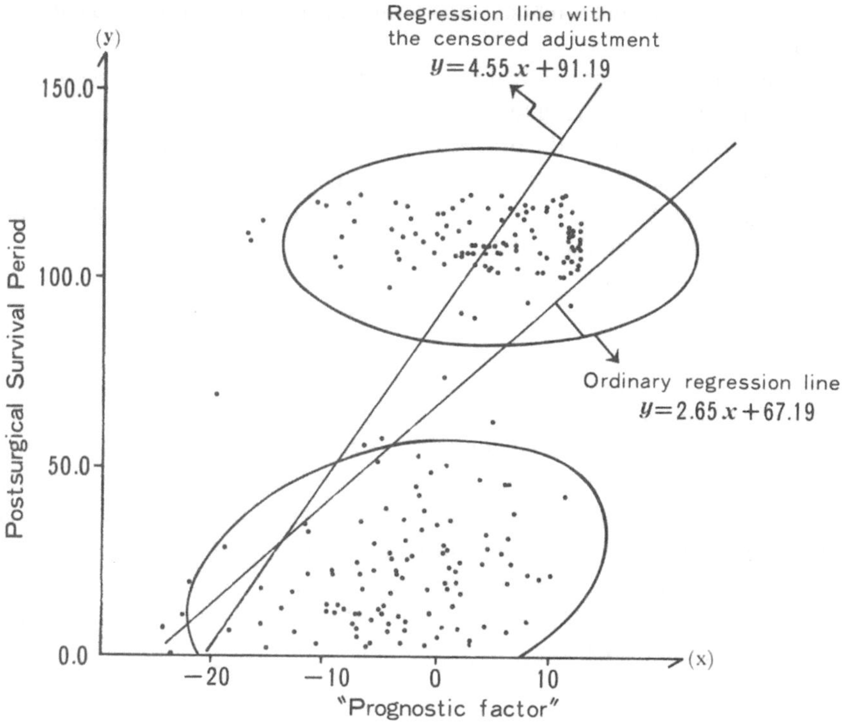

Fig. 2. Comparison of the regression with the censored adjustment and the ordinary regression for control group

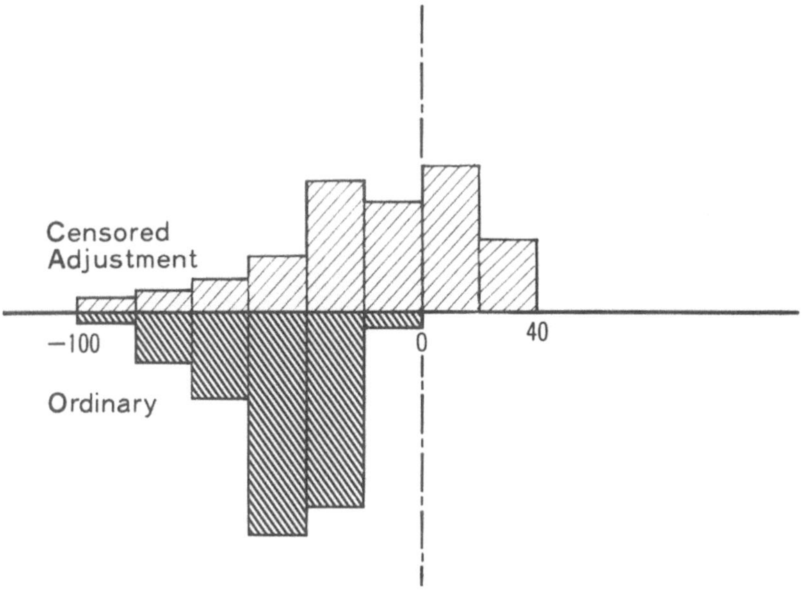

Fig. 3. Comparison of the regression with the censored adjustment and the ordinary regression on the deviations between the predicted values and the actual censored observations

The conventional regression line is drawn as if the line discriminates the two groups, while the line after censored adjustment passes in the middle of the long-term survivors.

This indicated that survival time may be predicted if the regression line, after censored adjustment, is taken into consideration.

In order to compare the practical meaning of the two regression analyses, survival time was exponentially predicted for the censored cases. As seen in Fig. 3, the regression analysis after censored adjustment can be compared favorably with the conventional analysis.

Conclusion

By using nine prognostic variables which were mainly observed at the time of surgery, a possibility of prediction for prognosis was evaluated for the curatively resected gastric cancer patients. A prognostic factor was reduced from the nine variables and it was favorable to predict survival period of those patients by regression analysis. The analysis after censored adjustment is more suitable for prediction than that of the conventional analysis. We hope the observational study may be carried on for further evaluation for prognosis of the patients and for therapeutic response.

Summary: Prognosis of Gastric Cancer

Patients with gastric cancer, who have survived the disease for 5 years, generally have the same life expectancy as persons of the same age without a tumor. However, only about 10% of all gastric cancer patients to date survive for 5 years. The chance of recovering from gastric cancer at present depends on whether a radical excision of the tumor is possible or not. Beyond this, the prognosis of the ailment is determined by a multitude of factors independent of therapy. Surgical mortality increases with increasing age. Tumors of the proximal third of the stomach, probably partially due to the increased surgical mortality in this group, have a poorer prognosis than those of the distal third of the stomach. Well-differentiated polypous tumors can be considered prognostically more favorable than dedifferentiated, diffusely infiltrating carcinomas. Cancers of the intestinal type have a more favorable prognosis than those of the diffuse type. Tumor infiltration of the serosa or lymph node metastases significantly impair the 5-year survival rate for the same histological tumor type. Aside from the local extent of the tumor, the stromal reaction is of prognostic significance, whereby the presence of macrophages, lymphocytes, and polymorphonuclear leukocytes in the tumor is considered a positive sign, and the desmoplastic reaction an extremely unfavorable one.

All these factors are not independent of each other. Only a simultaneous multifactorial analysis of all contingents can lead to statements of prognostic significance. All of these various prognostic factors need to be considered in planning an inquiry about therapeutic approaches, so that uniformly relevant statements about different models of therapy may be gained.

7 Surgical Therapy

Value of the Gastrectomy "*de Principe*"

R. Pichlmayr and H.-J. Meyer

Introduction

For gastric cancer, the only method of treatment at present available is surgery; the results so obtained, however, are far from satisfactory (Table 1). The reason for this lies not so much in the type of operation performed as in the stage of tumor development of most gastric cancers at the time of diagnosis and treatment, most being so advanced, that they are no longer curable surgically. Nevertheless, it is possible to cure this type of cancer with surgery as shown by the excellent results with early gastric cancer as well as a certain measure of success even with advanced gastric cancer. For this very reason, the question must be raised time and time again – particularly taking into account new developments or information from the diagnostic or pathomorphological fields – if there has been a recurrence of the carcinoma at the primary site of operation, that is, a locally recurrent tumor: was the operation sufficiently extensive? These tumors show a high morbidity as well as a high mortality rate. Perhaps most significant for the subsequent question up for discussion, the site of origin in up to 60% of cases was the gastric wall, in 30%, the perigastric lymph node tissue, and in approximately 10%, the duodenum (Table 2). The appearance of these locally recurrent tumors does, of course, in no way mean that more radical surgery could decisively reduce their frequency. It is, however, a reason and an obligation to test this possibility. This can be done either by carrying out very precise surgery appropriate to the stage of tumor development or by performing radical surgery as a matter of principle, that is, the gastrectomy *"de principe"*. While basically, preference should be given to that method of therapy which exactly fits individual requirements, this is difficult to put into practice. In the following text, the various aspects of a gastrectomy *de principe* will be presented.

Gastrectomy "*de Principe*"

It is true that a more extensive operation automatically means a greater danger of early and late postoperative morbidity and mortality. This must and can be accepted when the tumor stage is advanced; it is not justifiable, or only to a limited degree, with tumors which can also be treated satisfactorily in a less drastic manner. The standard performance of a gastrectomy, however, also encompasses these cases – at least to a certain extent. As a result, supporters of

Table 1. Prognosis of gastric cancer, 5-year survival rate (literature review)

	Cancer of the stomach n	5-Year survival rate %
Hegemann (1968)	1085	10.5
Gilbertsen (1969)	1983	10.2
Kennedy (1970)	1241	15.0
Schwemmle (1973)	1145	8.6
Rueff (1973)	673	11.2
Moritz (1973)	605	10.2
Pothe (1974)	1838	4.7
Inberg (1975)	2590	5.8
Desmond (1976)	1363	8.9
Wolff (1976)	672	11.1

Table 2. Locally recurrent gastric carcinoma after distal subtotal gastrectomy (literature review)

	Recurrence in the gastric stump	Recurrence in the perigastric lymph nodes
Kuru (1943; 1952)	49%	21.7%
McNeer (1958)	62.2%	25.7%
Hamaguchi (1959)	65.4%	19.2%
Inuzuka (1960)	45.5%	13.6%
Berne (1961)	78.6%	10.7%
Schreiber (1964)	65.9%	34.1%
Koga (1969)	64.5%	22.5%

the gastrectomy *de principe* were or are few in number. Leading the field as early as 1950, were Lahey as well as Lortat-Jacob, Ribet, and Giuli, and in the beginning also Longmire [6, 9, 10, 11].

At the 1976 German Surgical Congress in Munich and several times since then, we pointed out the value of a gastrectomy and also explained that many of the misgivings about total gastrectomy were no longer valid [18, 19, 20]. The use of liberal criteria for gastrectomy is also recommended by many other centers today as well [3, 7, 13, 17]. The more theoretical arguments, however, are used mainly in support of the performance of a gastrectomy rather than concrete evidence. Indications that clinical results after gastrectomy are better have been demonstrated above all by the teams of Giuli and McNeer. Thus, Giuli [6] was able to show a 5-year survival rate after gastrectomy *"de nécessité"* of only 20%, whereas the rate after a gastrectomy *de principe* was 40%. McNeer [12], on the other hand, obtained a better rate of survival after the performance of an elective total gastrectomy, above all when the tumor was located in the distal third of the stomach. These results cannot be used as evidence, however, as they were not controlled studies and the types of cases naturally differed. The studies do show, however, that a gastrectomy can lead to good, perhaps surprisingly good results.

The necessity for radical surgery when the gastric walls are involved is obvious from the frequent occurrence of tumors at this location. That radical dissection of the lymph nodes even when they contain metastases is also of use was and is debatable, although Japanese investigators point out very clearly that it is this very procedure which gives rise to better survival rates [8, 14, 15].

Thus, the current situation has been depicted. According to theoretical considerations, the gastrectomy *de principe* must be the appropriate procedure; according to clinical data, it may be appropriate. However, clinical evidence, one way or the other, is lacking.

Postoperative Mortality and Morbidity

First of all, it is crucial that the shortcomings of a gastrectomy be eliminated. The operative mortality and long-term morbidity are the two most important factors.

Practically all reports published in previous decades gave very high mortality rates and thus, provided the main argument against setting too liberal criteria for gastrectomy (Table 3). Only Lahey [9] was able, as early as 1950, to lower the mortality rate from 34.6% to 9.4%, thus, entitling him to perform a gastrectomy *de principe* – even with early cancers. This generally high mortality rate may on the one hand, depend on a far from optimal operating technique – the use of too restrictive criteria prevents the individual surgeon from gaining experience and there are unavoidable risks attached to an esophageal anastomosis; on the other hand, it may be conditional on a negative choice of patients when the criteria for gastrectomy *de nécessité* are used for selection. Accordingly, the teams, which in recent years have been able to reduce the mortality, are those which have been able to gain greater personal experience and which also to some extent had patients with a more favorable prognosis. The mortality is of course particularly low when the patient selection is positive. Thus, for a gastrectomy "of choice," the postoperative mortality rate is between 10% and 20%, for a gastrectomy *de nécessité*, between 20% and 35%. In any case, the reduction of the mortality rate to approximately 10% as been shown in several reports is certainly one of the decisive advances in this field [17, 18, 19, 21]. The main argument against the gastrectomy is thereby at least substantially weakened. Resection procedures are also encumbered with a mortality rate of approximately this value; on the other hand, a strict comparison in this regard is not possible.

Morbidity and the long-term well-being of the patients depend primarily on the severity of the esophageal reflux. They are much less dependent on the abolition of the reservoir and digestive function of the stomach remnant. Both the esophageal reflux and the function of the substitute stomach depend on the kind of surgical reconstruction used after total gastrectomy of the stomach. In general, however, it can be stated that these problems, in particular, the grave reflux problem, can be solved in a satisfactory fashion using several procedures. Thus, at the present time, the two main objects – a high mortality rate and frequent, severe reflux complaints – have to a large extent been refuted. True, it must be emphasized that particularly good results have been obtained by teams which are intensively involved with gastrectomy and that in the final analysis

Table 3. Postoperative mortality after total gastrectomy (literature review)

	Total	Postoperative mortality	
	n	n	%
Lahey (1950)	127	31	24.4
Gütgemann (1963)	64	21	32.0
Hegemann (1968)	113	34	30.0
Gilbertsen (1969)	123	30	24.4
Giuli (1972)	151	51	33.8
Schreiber (1972)	113	38	32.8
Bünte (1973)	200	61	30.5
McNeer (1974)	94	16	17.0
Wolff (1976)	95	30	31.6
Peiper (1978)	74	10	13.5
Average	1154	322	27.9
Own cases (1977)	216	27	12.5

even an excellent operating technique will doubtlessly not prevent the risk attached to a gastrectomy which always lies somewhat higher than that of an equally well-performed subtotal distal resection. Only if the advantages to be gained by performing the more radical operation outweigh the obligatory increase in the accompanying dangers, should a gastrectomy *de principe* be given preference over another procedure.

At the present time, we can only state – but this "only" is already a great advance – that reductions in mortality and morbidity entitle the use of liberal criteria for gastrectomy, that is, the performance of a gastrectomy *de principe* is at least justified.

Criteria for a Gastrectomy *"de Principe"* and Operative Procedures

On the basis of the considerations given here, we have increasingly come to the point of view – particularly since 1974 – that a gastrectomy *de principe* should be a standard procedure, whereby the criteria shown in Table 4 are used.

Table 4. Treatment of cancer of the stomach

Advanced and early gastric cancer	Gastrectomy "de principe" Extensive lymph node dissection Splenectomy, resection of the greater and lesser omentum
Exceptions:	
Prepyloric localization	Distal subtotal gastrectomy Extensive lymph node dissection without splenectomy Resection of the distal omentum
High operative risk	Individual indications

The operating procedure for a gastrectomy consists of the removal of the greater omentum. When the tumor is located in the posterior wall of the stomach, it is also necessary to resect the posterior wall of the bursa omentalis above the pancreas. The gastrectomy must be carried out from the distal to the proximal side. The lymph node dissection and splenectomy must be performed en bloc. In order to ensure that an exact lymph node dissection is carried out, it seems particularly important to us that the A. hepatica communis as well as the upper margin of the pancreas are skeletonized. In our procedure, the paraaortal lymph nodes are retained, despite the otherwise extensive lymph node dissection. In particular, attention should be drawn to the possibility of carrying out an extensive lymph node dissection up to the cardia using the described technique even with a distal subtotal resection.

The correctness of performing a splenectomy as part of the standard procedure is again currently under discussion [1, 5]. On the one hand, even with distal gastric cancers, metastases are to be found in the splenic hilus lymph nodes (according to Bengmark [16] in 7% – 23% of cases) and their removal is only possible together with a splenectomy; on the other hand, the spleen may play a greater role in the continuing anti-cancer defense mechanisms [8] or in long-term morbidity than was taken in account in recent years. Thus, Orita [16] found that there was an improvement in the long-term results after a splenectomy only for early tumor stages.

Table 5. Cancer of the stomach (own material: 1. May 1968 – 31. December 1977)

Total	Resections	Early gastric cancers
n = 786	n = 531 = 67.6%	n = 58 = 7.4% of n total = 10.9% of n resections

Table 6. Cancer of the stomach (excluding early cancers). Methods of operation and postoperative mortality (own material: 1. May 1968 – 31. December 1977; total n = 728)

	Total		Postoperative mortality	
	n	%	n	%
Without resection:	255	35.0	68	26.7
Laparotomies	148	20.3	38	25.6
Palliative bypasses	42	5.8	11	26.2
Implantation of tubes	65	8.9	19	29.2
Resections:	473	65.0	68	14.4
Distal subtotal gastrectomies	190	26.1	27	14.2
Total gastrectomies	216	29.7	27	12.5
Proximal subtotal gastrectomies	67	9.2	14	20.9

Own results

In the period 1968 – 1977, 786 patients were operated for gastric cancer (Table 5 and Fig. 1). The resection quota was approximately 70%, whereby the operating procedures shown in Table 6 were used. Since 1974, the reconstruction in our procedure is carried out almost exclusively using a jejunal interposition. As to be expected, the actuarial survival curve [4] after 235 gastrectomies shows a dependence on the tumor stage [2]. With 22 gastrectomies carried out at tumor stage I and showing an operative mortality of 4.5%, the 5-year survival rate was 95%, at tumor stage II, 30%, at stage III, 16%, and at stage IV, no patient survived the second postoperative year; altogether, the 5-year survival rate was 26% (Fig. 2).

If one examines the relationship between the survival rate and the type of operation selected by the surgeon (curative/palliative), as to be expected, the survival after palliative gastrectomy is low. In our procedure, we often deliberately perform a noncurative gastrectomy. After the so-called curative resection, however, a relatively favorable 5-year survival rate of 37% was obtained in 104 patients without early gastric cancer (Fig. 3). This is slightly lower than the rate obtained by Giuli for the gastrectomy *de principe*. In all cases reported here, a gastrectomy *de principe* was carried out, so it does not represent a controlled study and thus does not permit an exact comparison between different procedures.

Conclusions

1) At present, it is not possible to pass judgement as to the value of the gastrectomy *de principe* as opposed to other procedures (Fig. 4).

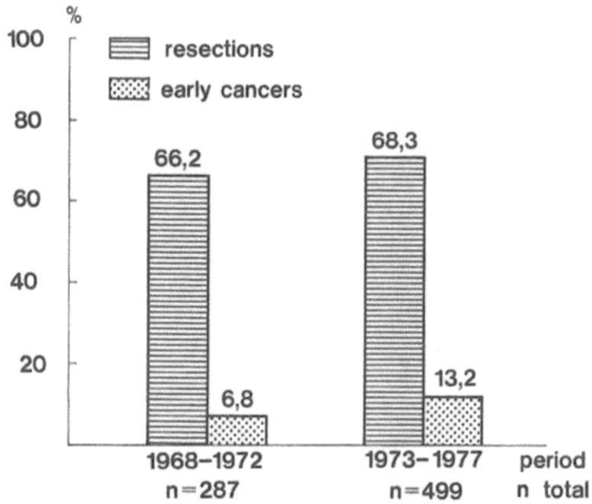

Fig. 1. Resection rates and number of early gastric cancers (own material: 1. May 1968 – 31. December 1977)

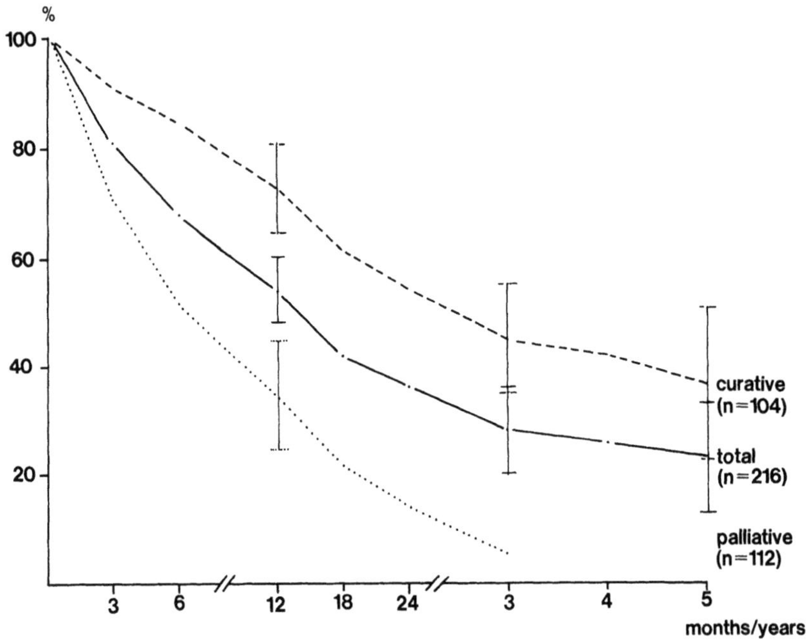

Fig. 2. 5-year survival rate (actuarial method) after total gastrectomy (own material: 1. May 1968 – 31. December 1977; total n = 235)

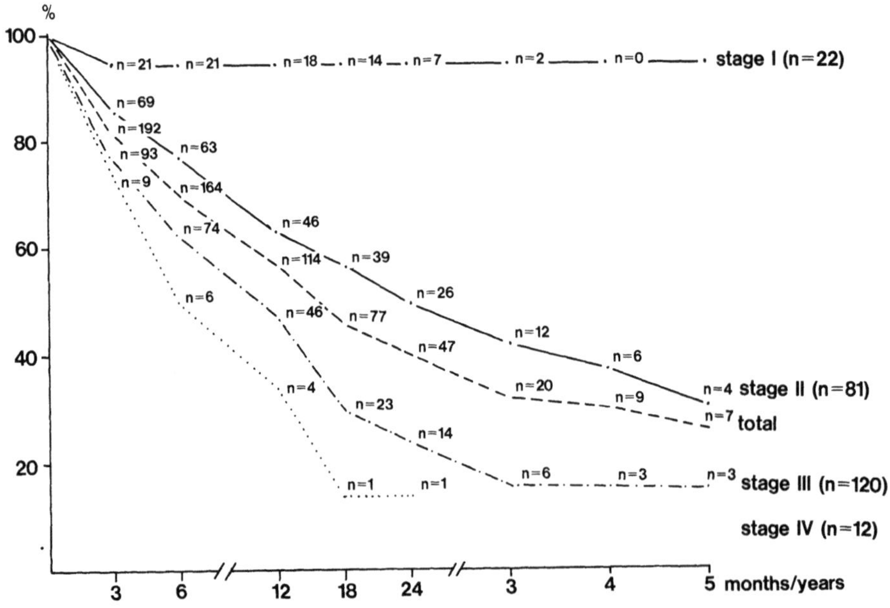

Fig. 3. 5-year survival rate (actuarial method) after total gastrectomy (own material: 1. May 1968 – 31. December 1977; total n = 216)

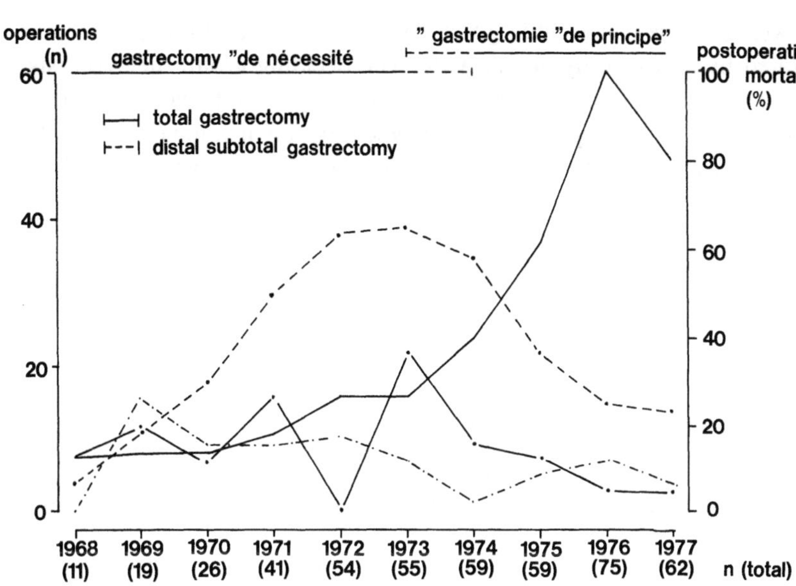

Fig. 4. Distal subtotal – and total gastrectomy: number of operations and postoperative mortality (own material: 1. May 1968 – 31. December 1977)

2) There are significant arguments in favor of the gastrectomy *de principe*. These increase in importance when one takes into account the advances made in recent years in reducing the number of major problems associated with a gastrectomy. Thus, the use of liberal criteria for a gastrectomy can be justified.

3) Perhaps the most important effect of a gastrectomy *de principe* is the extensive lymph node dissection. Apart from the splenic hilus lymph nodes, this can be carried out to the same extent as with a subtotal distal gastrectomy.

4) One should not set one's expectations, as to the effectiveness of a gastrectomy, too high. Most gastric cancers are so advanced by the time they are to be treated that surgery alone cannot affect a cure. A small number of patients can be treated by partial resection. That group of patients which can only be treated by gastrectomy is not large and it is unlikely that this will produce a statistically significant difference in the overall results. In our opinion, it is rather a matter of benefiting the individual, perhaps very few patients. The gastrectomy *de principe* could greatly increase in importance if the advances in chemotherapy prove the principle of maximal tumor reduction to be correct.

5) How can the value of the gastrectomy *de principe* be fully clarified? As no striking differences in the overall results are to be expected, comparisons between different clinics as well as between different methods of treatment used by the same team should bring no significant findings. This raises the question of the necessity of a controlled study. Such a study should be confined to cancers of the distal and middle third of the stomach. The inoperable cases would be eliminated

as well as those which undergo palliative resection and those which can only be treated by gastrectomy *de nécessité*. The deciding group then consists of those patients to be treated randomly either by distal partial gastrectomy or gastrectomy *de principe*. The tumor type must be histologically classified; either before selection of the kind of operation or at least, postoperatively.

References

1. Bengmark, S., Domellöf, L., Olsson, A. M.: The Role of splenectomy in stomach cancer operations. Digestion *4*, 314–320 (1971)
2. Berndt, H., Gummel, H.: Erfahrungen mit der Stadieneinteilung des Magenkrebses. Arch. Geschwulstforsch. *30*, 42–52 (1967)
3. Brünner, H.: Indikationen zur Gastrektomie beim Magenkrebs. Therapiewoche *26*, 6619–6626 (1976)
4. Cutler, S. J., Ederer, F.: Maximum utilization of the life table method in analyzing survival. J. Chronic. Dis. *8*, 699–713 (1958)
5. Fujimaki, M., Soga, J., Wada, K., Tani, H., Aizawa, O., Kawaguchi, M., Ishibashi, K., Maeda, M., Kanai, T., Omori, Y., Muto, T.: Total gastrectomy for gastric cancer. Cancer *30*, 660–664 (1972)
6. Giuli, R., Estenne, B., Clot, Ph., Faure, J. C., Hay, J. M., Richard, C. A., Lortat-Jacob, J. L.: Résultats éloigués de 482 interventions d'exérèse pour cancer gastrique. Ann. Chir. *26*, 1283–1296 (1972)
7. Häring, R., Kotlorz, H., Xanthakos, D.: Hat die Gastrektomie oder Kardiaresektion als 'Ultima-ratio-Eingriff' beim fortgeschrittenen Magenkrebs noch ihre Bedeutung? Langenbecks Arch. Klin. Chir. *320*, 126–136 (1968)
8. Jinnai, D.: Evaluation of extended radical operation for gastric cancer, with regard to lymph node metastasis and follow-up results. Gan. *3*, 225–231 (1968)
9. Lahey, F. H., Marshall, S. F.: Should total gastrectomy be employed in early carcinoma of the stomach? Ann. Surg. *132*, 540–560 (1950)
10. Longmire, W. P., Jr.: Total gastrectomy for carcinoma of the stomach. Surg. Gynecol. Obstet. *84*, 21–30 (1947)
11. Lortat-Jacob, J. L., Giuli, R., Estenne, B., Clot, P.: Intérêt de la gastrectomie totale pour le traitement des cancers de l'estomac. Chirurgie *101*, 59–67 (1975)
12. McNeer, G., Bowden, L., Booher, R. J., McPeak, C. J.: Elective Total Gastrectomy for Cancer of the Stomach: End results. Ann. Surg. *180*, 252–256 (1974)
13. Merkle, P.: Ausdehnung und Taktik bei der operativen Therapie des Magencarcinoms. Klinikarzt *7*, 381–385 (1978)
14. Mine, M., Majima, S., Harada, M., Etani, S.: End results of gastrectomy for gastric cancer: Effect of extensive lymph node dissection. Surgery *68*, 753–758 (1970)
15. Okajima, K.: Surgical treatment of gastric cancer with special reference to lymph node removal. Acta Med. Okayama *31*, 369–382 (1977)
16. Orita, K., Konaga, E., Okada, T., Kunisada, K., Yumura, M., Tanaka, S.: Effect of splenectomy in tumor-bearing mice and gastric cancer patients. Gan. *68*, 731–736 (1977)
17. Peiper, H. J., Siewert, R.: Magenersatz. Chirurg *49*, 81–88 (1978)
18. Pichlmayr, R., van Alste, H. E.: Die totale Gastrektomie als Regeloperation beim operablen Magencarcinom. Langenbecks Arch. Chir. *345*, 595 (1977)
19. Pichlmayr, R., Meyer, H. J., van Alste, H. E.: Die Gastrektomie als Standardoperation beim Magencarcinom. 10th Internat. Magensymposium: Magenkarzinom – Frühdiagnostik und Therapie, Berlin,Stuttgart: Thieme. (In press)
20. Pichlmayr, R., Meyer, H. J.: Verfahrenswahl und Ergebnisse der operativen Behandlung von Krebsrisikoerkrankungen und Frühcarcinomen des Magens. Chirurg *49*, 479–484 (1978)
21. Schreiber, H. W., Eichfuss, H. P., Schumpelick, V.: Magenersatz. Chirurg *49*, 72–80 (1978)

On the Problem of "Stage-Appropriate" Treatment of Gastric Carcinoma

A. Priesching

The "stage-appropriate" operation constitutes an attempt to adapt the extent of resection to the carcinoma situation. This is to observe a *principle of clinical oncology:* to apply a treatment designed for *maximal survival time* while the patient enjoys an *optimal quality of life.*

The many different clinical and oncological facets of gastric carcinoma make it necessary to limit the scope of our subject:

1) We confine ourselves to surgery and assume that radical surgery could not be replaced by any other type of treatment.

2) Reference is only made to those cases where we do a resection or gastrectomy for curative purposes; in other words, to cases where there are no organ metastases or no histologically verified metastases outside the celiac region.

3) Whatever we are going to say does not apply to penetrating carcinomas (with the exception of invasion toward the colon and into the liver which have no impact on the extent of resection of the stomach and of the gastrolymphatic drainage areas).

4) We assume that we are not forced to limit the *radical* extent of the operation. Such limitations would imply that:

a) We deviate from the originally established strategy (which should be defined in a *descriptive* manner) because we suppose that the required surgical intervention would not be compatible with the patient's general condition – i.e., the risk would be too great. Such typical limitations would be: distal resection instead of gastrectomy, purely abdominal approach rather than additional thoracotomy, foregoing zone splenectomy, and refraining from adenectomy in the region of the hepatoduodenal ligament, of the vestibulum bursae omentalis, and of Haller's tripod.

b) Despite these limitations there is neither macroscopic nor microscopic (positive cutting edges) evidence of any tumor tissue left behind.

In about one-third of the patients undergoing "curative" surgery, it is necessary to limit the radical nature of the operation. With the type of patients who come to us for clinical surgery, this suggests that whatever we have to say in the following paper only applies to about 30 of 100 patients who leave our hospital with the diagnosis of "gastric cancer".

There can be no question that problems of the extent of resection can only be studied in a controlled clinical trial. The first step would consist of an estimate of the number of patients needed for such a trial. In order to study surgical alternatives, such as resection versus gastrectomy – provided the total duration of trial is 5 years and the work is based on practical hypotheses with regard to the difference in results – about 10 clinics in a position to admit 100 patients annually have to work together. The work done has to be identical both in terms of tactics and technique. What we can and must do now is to draw up working hypotheses on which sensible questions for multicentered studies may be based.

Those who regard local differences in the extent of radical extirpation as significant, start with the hypothesis that tumorous tissue left behind will cause *clinically significant recurrences.* This is the case whenever the local recurrences (gastric stump, anastomosis, regional lymph nodes) are the only manifestations or precede other recurrences or are at least concomitant in regard to pathogenesis.

Nobody wants to sacrifice more organs than are necessary for the benefit of the patient. Trends towards being more radical in surgery – such as extended gastrectomy performed as a matter of principle and without considering the stage of the tumor – are understandable because of *three aspects of uncertainty* involved in trying to establish the actual stage of the tumor for the purpose of a stage-appropriate approach: uncertainty regarding the preneoplastic area of the stomach, the outlines of the primary tumor, and the presence of lymphogenic metastases.

Preneoplastic Area

As a rule not the entire stomach, but only part of it is in the preneoplastic stage. In this region, carcinomas do occur more frequently than in other regions. The area of the primary tumor constitutes the epicenter. Surface spread occurs mostly by neoplastic transformation of the adjacent epithelium. This holds true in about 6% of early carcinomas and histologically this is confirmed in about 20% of the cases by the presence of multiple foci at the time of diagnosis. These foci are grouped around the epicenter and are located within the preneoplastic area; only in exceptional cases – such as in multiple polypous carcinoma of pernicious anemia patients – are these foci distributed at random over the entire stomach. From this, we have to conclude:

1) During endoscopy, we have to search for multiple foci. This holds particularly true for the early stages where partial rather than total gastrectomy is more likely to be performed. In addition, an attempt should be made to outline preneoplastic areas by endoscopy, by multiple biopsy, and by resorting to the help of a pathologist. Whether partial or total gastrectomy is preferred in the case of diffuse distribution will depend on several factors.

2) A safety zone is to be maintained between the carcinomatous tissue farthest away in the oral and aboral directions on the one hand, and the resection line on the other; 5 cm seems to be adequate.

3) Patients having undergone resection and not showing any signs of recurrence should be integrated into an endoscopic follow-up program.

Growth of Invasion

There is a difference between the macroscopic and microscopic outlines of a carcinoma; this difference increase with the degree of malignancy [11]. As a *consequence,* a *safety distance* should be put between the macroscopic outlines and the resection line. These requirements vary greatly and range between 3 and 12 cm. In practice, we find that the distance from the tumor to the resection line, as established by the pathologist, decreases with the more upward site of the tumor, with its growing size, and the more diffuse nature of its outlines. Tumor-positive resection lines may be reduced to practically zero if the following procedure is adopted:

1) In the case of diffuse invasive carcinoma – a visual diagnosis – no attempt should be made to establish the outlines of the tumor macroscopically since in an unusually large number of cases this results in tumor-positive resection lines [10]. Rather, a gastrectomy should be performed. If the diffuse invasive carcinoma approaches the pylorus and is visible even with a macroscopic diagnosis, then in operable cases, a duodenal invasion of 25 – 300 mm has to be expected; this requires appropriate duodenal inroads, taking along the entire periduodenal tissue. If by macroscopic, X-ray, or endoscopic methods such a carcinoma is shown to reach the cardia, *esophagogastrectomy* has to be resorted to even if multiple biopsies in the cardia region disclose negative results; in these cases, the lower third of the esophagus, together with the entire peri-esophageal tissue, should also be removed.

2) In case of a tumor with diffuse outlines, a safety margin of 5 cm should be added; in tumors where macroscopic methods reveal proximity to the pylorus, a margin of 3 cm is adequate [3, 7, 13].

3) In about 70% of all tumors, including the diffuse types [6], the difference between the outlines of the tumor assessed macroscopically and those established under the microscope is less than 3 cm. In most polypous and ulceropolypous neoplasms, this difference is less than 1 cm. If there are no lymph node metastases – as it happens in 50% of cases – then a safety margin of 5 cm is definitely too much if it would mean gastrectomy. It would be desirable to change this recommendation of a safety zone of 5 cm for these tumors if they belong to the "intestinal type". However, this would have to be based on the certainty that there is no lymph node involvement – something that is not yet possible to achieve in practice.

Lymphogenic Metastases

Intraoperative inspection and palpation cannot confirm or preclude the presence of lymph node metastases with the precision required for surgery. Even the diagnosis of "advanced lymphogenic metastases" is incorrect in more than 20% of cases, that of metastases in the curvatures in more than 40%; even the definite statement that no metastases exist had to be corrected for about 25% of the patients [10]. These results require a change of tactics and the use of the frozen section diagnosis.

1) Lymphogenic metastases spread in the direction of the flow; this is the decisive fact. Metastases are formed at different levels in the drainage zones which correspond to the site of the tumor. First, the lymph nodes close to the tumor and only later those distant from it are affected. Adjacent nodes may be left out through by-passing ("jumping metastases"). This is a rare phenomenon and not of clinical significance if it occurs within the celiac region. Atypical lymph flow and detours because of metastatic blocks hardly constitute a tactical problem because they occur only in the advanced stages.

From the tactical point of view these problems are eliminated by extirpating the lymph regions adjacent to the collection area V en bloc with the primary tumor (see below).

2) If the extent of resection does not only depend on the type of tumor and its site, but also on the extent of lymphogenic involvement, it is impossible to act without the help of a pathologist. Of course, the decisions based on a frozen section test result are also subject to error; however, they are better than those based on inspection and palpation alone. The question to be put to the pathologist is the following: are there metastases? This question is asked if we are confronted with either of these two different intraoperative situations:

a) We are convinced that we are dealing with lymphogenic metastases. If this knowledge has considerable impact on the surgical approach, such as enlarging the area to be removed or leaving in the tumor altogether, then our assessment should be confirmed or corrected by the pathologist.

b) We cannot arrive at a clinical decision, and presence or absence of lymphogenic metastases would lead to a different scope of resection.

The lymph node group affected (i. e., the range of involvement is between one and all nodes in the group) will be more easily identified, the more involvement there is within the group, the more lymph nodes are examined, the more sections per node of equal size are studied, and the better the strategy of selection for removal turns out to be [6, 9, 10].

If cancer treatment is merely regarded as a *local problem*, one might react to the uncertainties involved in its spread as follows:

1) Within the preneoplastic field, about which we know little, the tumor itself merely constitutes the epicenter. Without gastrectomy, subsequent eruptions are merely a matter of time.

2) It is impossible to identify the outlines of the primary tumor during the operation. The greater the extent of resection, the greater the certainty of having eliminated it.

3) Lymphogenic metastases cannot be precluded. In the course of every resection, lymph drainage areas are left in place. Since the probability of all lymphogenic metastases during surgery increases (for a given area of resection) as the involved area decreases in size, radical lymphatic tissue extirpation seems particularly indicated in the early stages.

4) The radical approach complies with the established oncological rule that in case of doubt a procedure should be selected which promises the best chance of complete tumor extirpation.

One thing is certain: At present, we are not in a position to make a diagnosis sufficiently accurate to allow us to perform stage-appropriate surgery. *We have to include safety margins.* However, the simple strategy of the maximal degree of radical surgery has severe drawbacks:

1) Incidence and fatal nature of complications increase with the extent of the intervention. Even if the mortality rate of extensive gastrectomy could be lowered to that of resection, this is no argument in its favor unless we are forced to resort to it for oncological reasons. The fact that survival rates following *'gastrectomie de principe'* are better than following stage-appropriate gastrectomy and in particular, better than following *'gastrectomie de nécessité'* cannot be considered an argument in favor of *gastrectomie en principe*, since these survival rates include cases with a favorable prognosis which might have been served by resection.

2) The quality of life of gastrectomized patients is inferior to those who have undergone resection. Gastrectomized persons are more vulnerable to life's general adversities and they are less likely to enjoy their retirement.

3) Good results with early cases were primarily obtained by resection and not by gastrectomy. The question arises whether in early gastrectomy – quite apart from the quality of life – the survival rate may be either raised or lowered by a stage-appropriate approach (see below).

4) Local recurrence of malignant tissue at the gastric stump and lymph node, recurrence in the area surrounding the stomach, for practical purposes, no longer occur as only or primary manifestation of recurrence – provided the method we describe below is used. The patients die of hematogenic, peritoneal, pleural, and other tumors and have lymph node metastases. All this is not prevented by local radical extirpation – but possibly stimulated.

5) Local improvement may be achieved in the majority of patients even without extreme enlargement of the area to be extirpated:

a) Local recurrence at the gastric stump may be avoided by safety zones which are adapted to the type of carcinoma.

b) In case of multifocal events, the safety distances should be measured from the foci at the two extreme ends. Also, the risk of secondary tumors is usually overestimated. In the course of endoscopic check-ups, taken at regular intervals they may be diagnosed as early carcinomas.

c) Safety zones in the lymph drainage areas are created by extirpating the drainage regions close to the tumor (including collection zone V) and by examining the distant zones with the frozen section method. If the result is negative, there need be no extension of extirpation into the stomach (esophagus) and into the lymphatic ducts. However, for reasons of safety, radical extirpation is applied more often than necessary in these cases.

Assessment criteria with regard to the extent of partial gastrectomy:

1) Incidence of recurrence or secondary carcinoma at the gastric stump and recurrence of lymph node malignancy within the celiac region

a) as the only recurrence,
b) as primary manifestation with ensuing generalization,
c) as concomitant manifestation.

2) *Survival rates:* Within homogeneously structured groups of patients, we check differences due to the methods applied.

3) If two methods are identical in terms of oncology, the one resulting in a better *quality of life* should be given priority.

Determining the Required Extent of Resection

In order to properly determine the safety zones in the digestive tract and the lymph system, we need criteria for decisions which may be applied during surgery. In addition to the criterion of degree of invasion, the characteristics of tumor malignancy, tumor site, and the microscopic findings of lymph node involvement (frozen section) have proved to be of value.

Tumor Malignancy

From the scale of prognoses, it is easy to recognize the two extremes, i.e., early carcinoma on the one hand, and advanced diffuse invasive carcinoma on the other. In selecting the safety zones, these two extremes should be compared with all other cases.

Early Carcinoma

If an early carcinoma is suspected on the basis of X-ray and endoscopic findings, prior to surgery site and extent have to be determined by endoscopy and an examination for multiple primary foci must be carried out. In early neoplasms of the mucosa, we may expect 5% lymph node metastases at the most; if the submucosa too has been invaded, the expected figure is about 15%. Mainly nodes adjacent to the tumor are affected; however, we should refrain from probing for lymph nodes close to the tumor because of the danger of iatrogenic dissemination.

Tactical conclusions: Except for special cases (malignant polyps, small mucosal neoplasms, etc.), early tumors are also operated in accordance with the rules of carcinoma surgery: extirpation is carried out in the healthy tissue en bloc (carcinoma and lymph drainage area) and against the direction of the lymphatic flow. The extent of resection is decided solely by the site of the tumor. In order to include the area subject to exposure, a 5 cm safety margin appears appropriate. The problem as to what extent this conventional safety zone could be reduced in favor of distal or proximal resection rather than of gastrectomy has not yet been solved. In addition, early carcinoma leaves us the following possibilities:

1) Distal resection based on the site of the tumor: Extirpation of lymph drainage zones I (extragastral), II, III, and V (see below).

2) Gastrectomy is required. If the carcinoma reaches the part of the stomach in the corpus-fundus region close to the spleen, gastrectomy with zonal splenectomy should be performed; in order to do this, the spleen, along with the lienal vessels, and the surrounding tissue have to be severed from the pancreas so that the entire zone IV is included. Otherwise, a simple gastrectomy including zones I, II, III, and V is carried out.

3) Proximal resection is possible depending on the site of the tumor: zones I and V are also removed, and zonal splenectomy is carried out if the tumor involves the part of the stomach close to the spleen.

Diffuse Invasive Carcinoma

The degrees of malignancy III [4] and IV [2] may be diagnosed with the naked eye if the carcinoma has invaded all layers of the wall. Then we know that [6]:

1) The outlines of the tumor cannot be identified by macroscopic methods (see above).

2) In more than 80% of cases, lymph node metastases in the tissue are removed during resection.

3) Frequently, three or all four lymph drainage zones are affected.

Tactical conclusions: Gastrectomy with radical lymph node extirpation (including zonal splenectomy or pancreatosplenectomy). If macroscopic observation shows the carcinoma to have reached the cardia, esophagogastrectomy is to be performed, i.e., surgery is extended to the lower third of the esophagus and the periesophageal tissue.

Carcinoma Location

If the case does not involve either an early carcinoma or a diffuse invasive one, the resection lines for nonpenetrating carcinomas are established on the basis of site and lymph node examination.

From the outlines of the tumor determined macroscopically and by palpation (perhaps by endoscopy), a safety margin of 5 cm each in the distal and proximal directions (measured in situ) is added. For tumors located close to the pylorus, a duodenal zone of 3 cm is sufficient [3, 6, 7, 12, 13].

Thus, a preliminary decision in favor of distal or proximal resection or in favor of gastrectomy is obtained. The definite decision must be made on the basis of the lymph node examination.

Lymph Node Examination

Designation of the drainage areas [5, 6, 10]:

I = Region of the left gastric artery.
II = Region of the right gastric artery.
III = Region of the right gastroepiploic artery and of the gastroduodenal artery.
IV = Region of the lienal artery.
V = Drainage area around Haller's tripod.

Tactical Approach: Drainage zones close to the tumor are extirpated without further examination (in addition to drainage zone V), lymph node groups distant from the tumor are examined by frozen section. If the result is positive, the corresponding zone is also extirpated.

I. On the basis of the location of the tumor, distal resection would be possible.

Without further examination, zones II and III are extirpated. Zone I (around the left gastric artery) and V (region of Haller's tripod) are examined.

Possibilities:

Zones I and V negative: Distal resection. Zone I (extragastric), II, III, and V are extirpated en bloc [10].

Zone I positive and V negative: Simple gastrectomy and extirpation of zones I, II, III, and V. If the carcinoma involves the part of the stomach close to the spleen or if the lymphatic involvement is extensive, gastrectomy with zonal splenectomy or pancreatosplenectomy should be resorted to when extirpating zone IV.

V positive (zone I positive or negative): Gastrectomy with radical extirpation of the lymphatic tissue (= with zonal splenectomy or pancreatosplenectomy).

Alternatives for the multicenter study:

I positive, V negative: Distal resection versus gastrectomy versus gastrectomy with zonal splenectomy versus gastrectomy with pancreatosplenectomy.

V positive (I positive or negative): same alternatives.

Frozen section test not available. Diagnostic and surgical decisions:

1) I and V (and IV) probably not involved: Distal resection also involving I (extragastral), II, III, and V.

2) I or V, but not IV probably affected: Gastrectomy including I, II, III, and V, perhaps also IV.

3) Extensive metastases within the celiac region probable: Gastrectomy with radical lymphatic tissue excision.

II. Location of tumor would make proximal resection possible.

Without further examination I and IV are extirpated (by zonal splenectomy or pancreatosplenectomy).

Zone III (lymph nodes around the right gastroepiploic artery) and V (region around Haller's tripod) are examined.

Possibilities:

III and V negative: Proximal resection with zonal splenectomy or pancreatosplenectomy, including zones I and V.

III or V positive: Gastrectomy with radical lymph tissue excision as esophagogastrectomy (extending to the lower third of the esophagus, including the periesophageal tissue).

Alternative for the multicenter study:

Zonal splenectomy versus pancreatosplenectomy.

Frozen section test not available:
1) Macroscopic techniques do not reveal any metastases: Proximal resection with zonal splenectomy en bloc with I and V.

2) Metastases likely, but II and III unaffected: Proximal resection with zonal splenectomy en bloc with I and V.

3) Extensive metastases likely: esophagogastrectomy with radical excision of lymphatic tissue.

III. Due to location of tumor, gastrectomy is indicated.

I, II, III, and V are extirpated. Zone IV has to be considered as the immediate drainage region (tumor extends into the body of stomach in the part proximal to the spleen), then gastrectomy is carried out, including a radical excision of the lymphatic tissue – without examining the lymph nodes. Otherwise: Examination of zone V.

Possibilities:
V negative: Simple gastrectomy (exception see above) including I, II, III, and V.

V positive: Gastrectomy with radical excision of lymphatic tissue.

Alternatives for the multicenter study:
I positive, V negative, and carcinoma in the part of the stomach where the lesser curvature is located. Simple gastrectomy versus gastrectomy with radical excision of lymphatic tissue.

Frozen section diagnosis not available:
Should the carcinoma be so extensive that gastrectomy is indicated, zone IV should also be extirpated when a zonal splenectomy or a pancreatosplenectomy is performed.

Summary

Stage-appropriate surgery presupposes a knowledge of the tumor situation sufficiently accurate for assessing the extent of resection. As yet, however, this is not possible. We have to include safety zones both in the stomach and in the lymph drainage area. Opinions differ as to the extent of these zones. In contrast to the principle of extended gastrectomy, it is suggested to differentiate between early and diffuse invasive carcinomas on the one hand, and all other cases in which site of tumor and lymph node involvement (frozen section) may serve as decision aids when determining the required extent of resection. Several surgical alternatives of the above proposals are discussed.

References

1. Berne, C. J., Freedman, M. A.: Local recurrence following subtotal gastrectomy for carcinoma. Am. J. Surg. *82*, 5 – 7 (1951)
2. Broders, A. C.: Grading of carcinoma. Minn. Med. *8*, 726 – 730 (1925)

3. Castleman, B.: Extension of gastric carcinoma into the duodenum. Ann. Surg. *103*, 348–352 (1936)
4. Chiari, H.: Zur Histologie des Magenkarzinoms. Wien. Klin. Wochenschr. *64*, 861–864 (1952)
5. Coller, F. A., Kay, E. B., Mc Intyre, R. S.: Regional lymphatic metastases of carcinoma of the stomach. Arch. Surg. *43*, 748–761 (1941)
6. Eker, R., Efskind, J.: The pathology and prognosis of gastric carcinoma. Based on 1314 partially and totally resected cases. Acta Chir. Scand. (Suppl.) *264*, 1–182 (1960)
7. Fodden, J. H.: The duodenal spread of pyloric carcinoma. Br. J. Cancer *2*, 239–249 (1948)
8. Güttgemann, A., Schreiber, H. W.: Das Magen- und Kardiakarzinom. Stuttgart: Enke 1964
9. Hermanek, P., Bünte, H.: Die intraoperative Schnellschnittuntersuchung. München, Berlin, Wien: Urban & Schwarzenberg 1972
10. Priesching, A.: Die Therapie des Magenkarzinoms. München, Berlin, Wien: Urban & Schwarzenberg (in press)
11. Verbrugghen, A.: Intramural extension of gastric carcinoma. Arch. Surg. *28*, 566–579 (1934)
12. Wilkinson, E. J., Hause, L.: Probability in lymph node sectioning. Cancer *33*, 1269–1274 (1974)
13. Zinninger, M. M., Collins, W. T.: Extension of carcinoma of the stomach into the duodenum and esophagus. Ann. Surg. *130*, 557–566 (1949).

Local Excision – A Therapeutic Procedure in Early Gastric Carcinoma?

P. Hermanek

A small, early gastric carcinoma can occasionally be removed totally by endoscopic polypectomy. Histological examination with step sections must prove that the resection lines are free of tumor. In such cases, we must ask whether or not this polypectomy is a sufficient therapeutic procedure. The same is true for local surgical excision, in contrast to subtotal or total gastrectomy, where the tumor is removed with wide margins of safety, together with the regional lymph nodes.

The key to the problem is the frequency of regional lymph node metastases. Local excision and polypectomy are insufficient if the tumor has already spread to nodes. According to a summary of reports (Hermanek, 1978), about 3% of early gastric carcinomas, limited to the mucosa, have spread to the regional lymph nodes. This frequency is influenced by the macroscopic type of tumor and its histology. The localization of the carcinoma must be also taken into consideration. Especially in tumors near the cardia, the risk of radical surgery (proximal partial or total gastrectomy) is higher than the risk of lymphogenous metastases which remain unremoved.

Table 1. Early gastric cancer. Curative polypectomy or local excision. Medical and Surgical Clinic Erlangen, Oct. 31, 1978

Patients:	11	
Tumors:	12	
Average age:	72 years	
Males:	6	
Females:	5	
Procedure:	Operative endoscopy	4
	Surgery	7
Localization:	Upper third	3
	Middle third	6
	Lower third	3
Average diameter:	23 mm	
Macroscopic type:	I	8
	IIa	4
Depth of infiltration:	Mucosa	5
	Submucosa	7
Histology:	Intestinal-type,	
	Well-differentiated	4
	Moderately differentiated	7
	Poorly differentiated	1

Up until Oct. 31, 1978, eleven patients with 12 early gastric carcinomas were treated curatively by endoscopic polypectomy (four patients) or by local surgical excision (seven patients). Endoscopic polypectomy was performed by the Medical Clinic (Head Prof. Dr. L. Demling), surgery by the Surgical Clinic (Head Prof. Dr. F. P. Gall), University of Erlangen. The clinical and pathological data are summarized in Table 1.

One patient died in the postoperative phase, four patients died later, free of tumor, six patients are alive. There were no cancer recurrences and no cancer deaths (average follow-up, 3.5 years).

Conclusion

Endoscopic polypectomy or local surgical excision can be taken into consideration as curative therapy in selected cases of early gastric carcinoma, especially, not very large polypoid tumors of the intestinal-type which are located near the cardia and are limited to the mucosa.

Reference

Hermanek, P.: Operative endoscopy as curative therapy for early stages of gastrointestinal cancer. In: Operative endoscopy. Demling, L., Koch, H. (eds.). Stuttgart: Schattauer (in press)

Influence of the Choice of Surgical Procedure in Gastric Cancer on the 5-Year Survival Time

P. Merkle, P. Schlag, and Ch. Herfarth

The choice of surgical procedure in the therapy of gastric cancer has in recent decades been distinguished by differing views with regard to the radicality of the surgical approach. The trend to total gastrectomy, particularly predominant in the United States during the 1950s, was followed by a period of disenchantment, since the effectiveness expected of increased radicality failed to materialize. The results produced by Longmire [2] and Gilbertson [1] did not show any improvement in the 5-year survival rate after total gastrectomy. Investigations by McNeer et al. [4] and by Lortat-Jacob et al. [3] conversely revealed more favorable prognostic results after total gastrectomy. Mine et al. [5] pointed out the significance of lymph node dissection.

The controversy concerning the extent of radical procedure continues up to this day. For this reason, we analyzed our own patient pool with a view to elucidating the question regarding the interdependence of 5-year survival rate and therapeutic procedure. This is a retrospective study with all the uncertainty factors typical for it, as are the investigations cited in the references.

A total of 464 patients with gastric cancer were surgically treated in our clinic from 1965 to 1972; for 179 of these, i.e., 39%, the operation could be considered "curative"; we were able to determine the further fate of 167 patients, or their 5-year survival time. In the following listing, the early gastric cancers will not be taken into account; they will later be analyzed separately.

Of the curatively operated patients, 83 were resected, on 84 a gastrectomy was performed. The choice of procedure depended, in retrospect, on the extent of the tumor, size, general condition of the patient and, last but not least, on the individual surgeon.

Following resection, the 5-year survival rate was 31%, and only 21% after gastrectomy. The fact that the patients with gastrectomy made a considerably poorer showing can definitely be attributed to a disproportionate distribution of stages, as Table 1 shows. Patients with stage T_3 or N_0 were predominantly resected, whereas the majority of patients with a gastrectomy had stage T_4 or N_1.

No significant conclusions can therefore be drawn on the basis of these figures. For this reason, the survival time after resection and gastrectomy was respectively correlated with the individual tumor stages. This resulted in the following (Table 2): no difference in the prognosis was determined with regard to the depths of infiltration T_2 through T_4, irrespective of resection or gastrectomy. There is the familiar decrease in the 5-year survival time with increasing depth of infiltration.

Table 1. Partial versus total gastrectomy in stomach cancer 1965 – 1972

	T 2	T 3	T 4	N 0	N 1	N 2
Partial gastrectomy	25	39	18	37	16	17
Total gastrectomy	12	26	45	23	40	19

Table 2. Gastrectomy and 5-year survival rate: tumor extent (T) 1965 – 1972

	Partial gastrectomy	Total gastrectomy
T 2	40% (10/25)	33% (4/12)
T 3	28% (11/39)	35% (9/26)
T 4	16% (3/18)	11% (5/45)

Correlating the 5-year survival rates with the lymph node involvement, we find that after total gastrectomy no difference can be observed between lack of lymph node involvement and involvement of the first lymph node station, whereas survival rates after resection are significantly reduced whenever lymph nodes of the first station were affected. It should be noted that no patient exhibiting lymph node involvement of the second station suvived (Table 3).

When the survival times were correlated with the stage of differentiation of the carcinoma (Table 4), distinct differences in the 5-year survival times for anaplastic and macroscopically scirrhous cancers became evident.

For the 29 cases of early cancer, which were analyzed separately [6], and in the treatment of which, 21 resections and eight gastrectomies were performed, no significant differences with regard to the 5-year survival times could be determined. The graphs of the mortality rates are practically parallel (Fig. 1).

Table 3. Gastrectomy and 5-year survival rate: lymph node-involvement (N) 1965 – 1972

	Partial gastrectomy	Total gastrectomy
N 0	46% (17/37)	31% (7/23)
N 1	19% (3/16)	36% (11/40)
N 2	0% (0/17)	0% (0/19)

Table 4. Partial versus total gastrectomy in poorly differentiated tumors: 5-year survival rate 1965 – 1972

Partial gastrectomy:	7.1% (1/14)
Total gastrectomy:	20% (5/25)

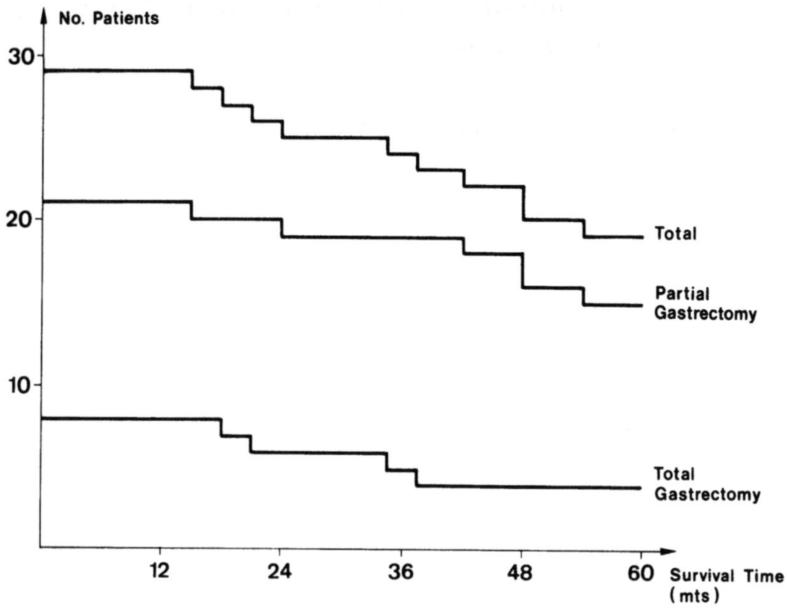

Fig. 1. Mortality rates by partial and total gastrectomy for early gastric cancer

Summary

In a retrospective study, an attempt was made to determine the significance of the choice of surgical procedure in the treatment of gastric cancer with regard to the 5-year survival time. The following statements can be derived:

1) In advanced gastric cancer with involvement of the first lymph node station or anaplastic gastric cancer, a better 5-year survival rate was found after gastrectomy with regional lymph node dissection when compared with the resections.

2) It seems important to note that no patient with proven involvement of the second lymph node station survived, whether or not a resection or a gastrectomy was performed.

3) The 5-year survival time for early gastric cancer is independent of partial or total gastrectomy.

References

1. Gilbertson, V. A.: Results of treatment of stomach cancer. Cancer *23*, 1305 (1969)
2. Longmire, W. P., Jr., Kuzma, J. W., Dixon, J. W.: The use of Triethylenethophosphoramide as an adjuvant to the surgical treatment of gastric carcinoma. Ann. Surg. *167*, 293 (1968)
3. Lortat-Jacob, J. L., Giuli, R., Estenne, B., Clot, P.: Intérêt de la gastrectomie totale pour le traitment des cancers de l'estomac. Chirurgie *101*, 59 (1975)
4. McNeer, G., Lawerence, W., Ashley, P., Pack, G. T.: End results in the treatment of gastric cancer. Surgery *43*, 897 (1958)
5. Mine, M., Majima, S., Harada, M., Etani, S.: End results of gastrectomy for gastric cancer: Effect of extensive lymph node dissection. Surgery *68*, 753 (1970)
6. Schlag, P., Meister, H., Merkle, P., Haferkamp, O., Herfarth, Ch.: Prognostische Aspekte des Magenfrühkarzinoms. Dtsch. Med. Wochenschr. **104**, 659 (1979)

Problems Associated with the Surgical Treatment of Cancer of the Gastric Stump

H.-J. Meyer, H. Ziegler, and R. Pichlmayr

Introduction

The occurrence of gastric cancer in patients with a history of gastric surgery has increased in frequency within the last three decades and thus increased in importance for the surgeon, even though it is not possible to decide whether the pathogenesis and incidence of these cancers depend on the previous illness or operation [2, 3, 4, 5, 6, 8]. Despite the advances made in diagnosis and operating technique, the long-term prognosis with this form of cancer – apart for a few individual cases – is extremely poor [1, 7, 10, 13].

Patients

Of 786 operations for gastric cancer between 1 May 1968 and 31 December 1977, 39 were cancers of the operated stomach, a relatively high frequence of approximately 5% (Table 1). The average period between the initial operation and the appearance of the carcinoma was 23.9 ± 11.1 years, whereby a subtotal resection with gastrojejunal anastomosis according to B II had been carried out 35 times and a gastroenterostomy four times (Table 2).

There was a clear predominance of males, the ratio of males to females being 18.5 to one. The average age of the patients was 63.0 ± 8.1 years, similar to the average age of the patients appearing in our clinic with primary cancers of the stomach (Table 3).

Table 1. Carcinoma occurring after gastric surgery for benign disease (1 May 1968 – 31 December 1977)

	Carcinoma of the anastomosis/stump (a) n	Carcinoma of the stomach (b) n	Ratio a/b %
Total	39[a]	786	5.0
Resections	18	531	3.4
Without resection	21	255	8.2

[a] Incl. 1 early cancer.

Table 2. Carcinoma occurring after gastric surgery for benign disease (1 May 1968 – 31 December 1977)

	n	Time interval (years)
Total	39	23.9 ± 11.1
Carcinoma of the gastric stump (first operation: B II)	35	23.3 ± 9.8
Carcinoma of the anastomosis (first operation: GE)	4	29.0 ± 21.3

Table 3. Carcinoma occurring after gastric surgery for benign disease. Sex ratio and mean age (1 May 1968 – 31 December 1977)

	n	Mean age (years)
Total	39	63.0 ± 8.07
Males	37[a]	62.4 ± 7.8
Females	2	74.0 ± 2.8

[a] Incl. 1 early cancer.

The list of symptoms was headed by pain in the upper abdomen and loss of weight in 67% and 62% of patients, respectively [7, 9, 13]. In all cases, the diagnosis was established using both X-rays and endoscopy plus the histological and cytological examinations of multiple tissue biopsies. Only once was an early cancer detected in this manner (histological conformation, postoperatively) [11, 12].

After the diagnosis had been made, a resection was carried out in a total of 18 patients (46.2%), whereby in 11 cases, it was necessary to perform an extended operation with removal of the pancreas, the transverse colon, or surgical intervention in two cavities. In 13 cases, a resection of the stomach remnant with an anastomosis according to Roux-Y, jejunal interposition, or esophagojejunostomy was performed; in five cases, a subtotal resection, again with a gastrojejunostomy, according to B II or Roux-Y.

The postoperative mortality was 27.8%; in no case, however, was a proximal anastomotic insufficiency the cause of death. This postoperative mortality was clearly higher than that after gastrectomy or subtotal distal resection for primary cancer, the differences being 18.9% and 7.2%, respectively.

After one gastrectomy of the stomach remnant and one subtotal resection – despite the fact that there was a safety distance from the tumor to the proximal

Table 4. Carcinoma occurring after gastric surgery for benign disease. Therapy and postoperative mortality (1 May 1968 – 31 December 1977)

	Therapy	Postoperative mortality	
	n	n	%
Resections	18	5	27.8
Total gastrectomy	13	4	30.8
Subtotal gastrectomy	5	1	20.0
Without resection	21	7	33.3
Laparotomy	12	5	41.7
Palliative bypasses	4	–	–
Implantation of tubes	5	2	40.0

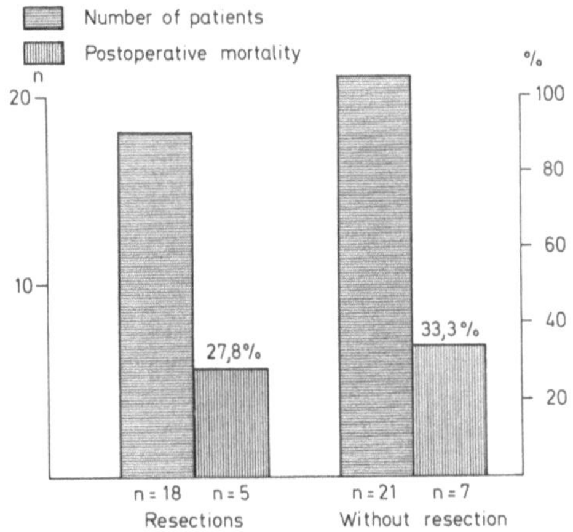

Fig. 1. Carcinoma occurring after gastric surgery for bening disease. Therapy and postoperative mortality (1 May 1968 – 31 December 1977)

resection line – there were two early recurrent carcinomas. After the second operation, an exploratory laparotomy, and gastrectomy of the stomach remnant, both patients died postoperatively.

In 21 cases only, a palliative operation could be carried out, in comparison with the primary cancer, the postoperative mortality was also higher, altogether 33.3% (Table 4 and Fig. 1).

In conformity with the high postoperative mortality rate accompanying cancer of the gastric stump, the long-term results were also depressing. After palliative operations, all patients died within a period of 4.9 ± 3.6 months. When the gastric stump was resected, six other patients died within an interval of 11.0 ± 7.7 months; only seven patients are still alive after an average period of observation up to 31.1 ± 21.4 months (Table 5).

Conclusions

1) As it is often difficult to diagnose cancer of the gastric stump – characteristic symptoms are lacking, and those symptoms present can easily be misinterpreted

Table 5. Carcinoma occurring after gastric surgery for benign disease. Survival time (1 May 1968 – 31 December 1977)

Survival time (mean: 31,6 + 21,4 months)		
After 4 weeks		n = 27
After 6 months		n = 13
After 1 year		n = 11
After 2 years		n = 3
After 5 years		n = 1[a]
	Total	n = 39

[a] Early gastric cancer.

as those associated with the operated stomach – cancer of the gastric stump is mostly at a very advanced stage by the time it is to be treated surgically (of our patients, over 80% were at tumor stage III and IV). Thus, it is only possible to perform a resection in half the cases, a curative operation is even more seldom feasible. It is therefore inevitable that the postoperative mortality and long-term results are extremely unfavorable.

2) An extended total gastrectomy is in most cases accompanied by a very high primary mortality (30.8% in our patients); therefore, one often aims for a subtotal resection. In most cases, however, we consider the gastrectomy to be the only curative operation, particularly as the best results in treatment of cancer of the gastric stump are at present obtained after this operation.

3) The prognosis for cancer of the gastric stump can certainly be improved, just as it improved for primary cancers once the diagnosis could be established at an early enough stage. The only long-term survivor in our group had an early cancer in the gastric stump.

References

1. Achatzy, R., Schönwalder, K., Bünte, H.: Chirurgie des Magenstumpfcarcinoms. Klinikarzt *6*, 7 – 12 (1973)
2. Böttcher, H., Hantschmann, N.: Das Magenstumpfkarzinom. Med. Klin. *68*, 175 – 179 (1973)
3. Clémencon, G., Baumgartner, R., Leuthold, E., Miller, G.: Das Karzinom des operierten Magens. Dtsch. Med. Wochenschr. *101*, 1015 – 1020 (1976)
4. Dahm, K., Rehner, M.: Das Carcinom im operierten Magen. Stuttgart: Thieme 1975
5. Griesser, G., Schmidt, H.: Statistische Erhebungen über die Häufigkeit des Karzinoms nach Magenoperationen wegen eines Geschwürleidens. Med. Welt *35*, 1836 – 1840 (1964)
6. Hilbe, G., Salzer, G. M., Hussl, H., Kutschera, H.: Die Carcinomgefährdung des Resektionsmagens. Langenbecks Arch. Klin. Chir. *323*, 142 – 153 (1968)
7. Kienzle, H. F.: Das Magenstumpfkarzinom. Med. Klin. *72*, 399 – 405 (1977)
8. Morgenstern, L., Yamakawa, T., Seltzer, D.: Carcinoma of the gastric stump. Am. J. Surg. *125*, 29 – 38 (1973)
9. Peitsch, W., Burkhardt, K.: Zur Pathogenese und Klinik des Magenstumpfcarcinoms. Langenbecks Arch. Klin. Chir. *341*, 195 – 203 (1976)
10. Radomsky, J., Lüders, K., Ungeheuer, E.: Chirurgische Behandlung des Magenstumpfkarzinoms. Munch. Med. Wochenschr. *120*, 557 – 560 (1978)

11. Rehner, M., Soehendra, N., Eichfuss, H. P., Dahm, K., Eckert, P., Mitschke, H.: Frühcarcinome im (Billroth-II-)Resektionsmagen. Dtsch. Med. Wochenschr. *99*, 533 – 534 (1974)
12. Rösch, W., Elster, K.: Gastrointestinale Präcancerosen. Baden-Baden, Brüssel, Köln, New York: Witzstrock 1977
13. Saegesser, F., Jämes, D.: Cancer of the gastric stump after partial gastrectomy (Billroth II principle) for ulcer. Cancer *29*, 1150 – 1159 (1972)

Summary: Surgical Therapy

The value of the gastrectomy *de principe* can not yet be estimated. The significant improvement of morbidity and mortality after total gastrectomy over the last few years, however, argues in favor of this procedure, since it allows an extensive removal of lymph nodes, and since it takes into consideration that a carcinoma has frequently intramurally infiltrated beyond the usual safety limit of 5 cm. An evaluation of the gastrectomy *de principe* will only then become possible, when those cases with advanced cancer requiring a gastrectomy *de nécessité* are excluded and when the survival rate for cancers of the antrum or corpus is tested in dependence of the radical extent of the surgical procedure. To this avail, further investigations are urgently required.

Those retrospective analyses are interesting in this context, which demonstrate good results for total gastrectomy as opposed to partial gastrectomy in those patients with dedifferentiated carcinomas or with lymph node metastases close to the stomach even in consideration of the postoperative mortality.

The stage-adapted surgery for gastric cancer offers interesting aspects. It seems most warranted for small, well differentiated polypous carcinomas of the antrum in the form of a partial gastrectomy. The multitude of surgical proposals, all of which are, however, based solely on general oncological-surgical and pathophysiological considerations and not on appropriate clinical studies, demonstrates the problem with stage-adapted surgery. The wealth of proposed individual alternatives of surgical approaches cannot be evaluated for their effectiveness.

As a rule, cancer of the gastric stump is diagnosed in a very advanced stage. Half of the patients can, however, be operated, if the surgery is as radical as possible. Due to the very poor long-term results, a curative effect cannot be achieved in the majority of cases. Aside from the necessity of an extended total gastrectomy in treatment of gastric stump cancer, the prognosis can only be improved by an early diagnosis via systematic examinations of all surgically treated gastric or duodenal ulcer patients.

In some cases with a small early carcinoma, its endoscopic removal by way of polypectomy becomes possible. This procedure is justified if the cancer is restricted to the mucosa. The type of tumor and its localization, under consideration of the surgical risk in case of more radical procedures, must be included in the calculation. An analysis of histological sections as proof of an excavation in healthy tissue is of absolute necessity. If these criteria are considered, the procedure of local tumor extirpation is justified for patients with extreme risk factors.

8 The Patient After Total Gastrectomy

Pathophysiological Consequences of Total Gastrectomy

Harald Goebell

Total gastrectomy is mainly performed in patients with gastric carcinoma. The 5-year survival rate of these patients ranges between 8% and 20% [5, 19, 20] and a recurrence of the carcinoma, together with the problems following the total loss of the stomach, may develop. Therefore, the sequelae of the operative procedure per se can be better evaluated in the relatively rare cases of Zollinger-Ellison Syndrome, with massive bleeding from the stomach or polyposis, who have had total gastrectomy performed. The most striking feature of these patients is weight loss [1, 6, 7, 4, 12, 15, 23]. Table 1 summarizes the findings of a patient with esophagojejunostomy 4 years after operation. Despite normal absorptive

Table 1. Clinical and metabolic data of a male patient 4 years after total gastrectomy with esophagojejunostomy and jejunojejunal anastomosis

Patient P. B. – 44 years	
1974	Total gastrectomy. Early cancer of stomach.
1974	Weight 90.0 kg – Height 183.0 cm
1978	Weight 60.0 kg
Problems: bile vomiting, reflux esophagitis with retrosternal pain, dumping	
Absorption studies:	
Serum total protein:	7.8 g%
Xylose-Test:	normal (5.6 g/5 h)
Lactose-Test:	normal increase blood sugar (75 → 150 mg%)
Fecal weight:	195 g/24 h
Fecal fat:	4.6 g/24 h (with 100 g oral load)
Glucose absorption:	70 → 170 → 35 mg%
(100 g orally)	(1 h) (2 h)
Calcium:	10.5 mg%
Chymotrypsin, feces:	175 µg/g feces (normal)
Hematological data:	
Hb:	12.1 g%
HB_E:	29.0 µµg
Serum iron:	71.0 µg%
Folic acid:	3.6 µg/ml (normal 3 – 20)
B_{12} (substituted):	364 pg/ml (normal 300 – 1000)
Schilling-Test:	severely impaired
Iron absorption after oral load:	71 → 135 µg%

function tests, a loss of 54% of his preoperative weight was observed. Adams [1], studying the weight of 20 patients with esophagojejunostomy without pouch in the 3rd postoperative month, found that only seven patients (38.8%) were always within "normal" limits, i.e., within the 5th and 95th centiles, whereas 60.2% were below this range. On the other hand, only nineteen (10.5%) of 182 patients cummulated in the literature regained "normal" weight [4]. Difficulties exist in defining the reference point. Bradley et al. [6] investigated ten patients without malignancy and observed that none gained his normal preoperative weight, but five were able to achieve 90% of the minimum standard of "ideal body weight" (optimum weight for height, sex, age: Metropolitan Life Insurance Company). Obviously, these patients stabilized their weight on a new level with time [1, 4]; the patients of Bradley averaging 15% lower than "ideal body weight". A further important point is that most of the patients reach the maximum of their weight loss before operation.

The fact that some patients are able to gain significant weight postoperatively demonstrates that this is physiologically possible after total gastrectomy. The problem of weight loss, encountered by many of these patients, implies somatopsychological features: physical weakness, tiredness, reactive depression, absence of hunger, anorexia. Factors which can further contribute to weight loss are the presence of malabsorption, insufficient intake nutrients, and immediate postoperative sequelae, such as dysphagia, reflux esophagitis, and dumping syndrome.

Malabsorption and Its Possible Causes

Although malabsorption of fat and protein occurs in about half of the patients [6, 3, 7, 12, 22, 23], its contribution to malnutrition in these patients obviously is only of minor importance. Table 2 summarizes some data on the fecal fat excretion. Adams [3] found elevated excretion of fat in 12 of 20 patients, which in eight patients did not exeed 15 g/day and in four others was between 15 and 20 g/day. Hays et al. [10] reported an excretion of 4–16 g/day in four patients with jejunal pouch and Bradley et al. [6] found in 6 of 7 patients with pouch, an

Table 2. Fecal fat excretion in total gastrectomy

Without jejunal pouch			With jejunal pouch		
20 patients		3 patients	4 patients	7 patients	
< 7 g/day	8	–	4–16 g/day	< 7 g/day	3
7–15 g/day	8	–		7–15 g/day	2
15–20 g/day	4	2		15–20 g/day	1
>20 g/day	–	1		>20 g/day	1
(Adams, 1967)		(Bradley et al. 1975)	(Hays and Clark, 1960)	(Bradley et al., 1975)	

excretion below 20 g/day. Schwartz et al. [22] observed a correlated rise of fat excretion with rising oral intake of fat in patients with total gastrectomy, whereas this was not observed in the same order of magnitude in normal persons. On the other hand, Bradley et al. [6] measured only a modest increase of fat excretion in three patients with doubling of oral fat intake from 50 to 100 g/day. With up to 100 g of oral intake, the assimilation usually takes place for 80 g (= 720 kcal) and more [17]. Bradley reported a mean coefficient of malabsorption of 17.1% (normal < 10%) for fat in ten patients [6]. Elevated excretion of nitrogen in feces was also observed in about 50% of patients [6, 3]. In Bradley's study, it ranged between 0.9 and 3.6 g/day (normal < 2.0 g) in ten patients, exceeding 2.0 g in five patients. Mean excretion was 2.3 g/day, the coefficient of malabsorption being 18.1% (normal < 15%).

Since patients after total gastrectomy usually show normal morphological jejunal pattern [6, 3, 15] and normal transit time [6], other causes for malabsorption of fat and nitrogen must be considered. One possible cause is *bacterial overgrowth* in the upper jejunum, which has been pointed out by Bradley et al. [6]. They observed significant anaerobic colonization of the jejunum in their patients, including *Bacteroides spurius, Clostridia, Veillonella* sp., and *Lactobacilli* in numbers ranging from 10^5 to 10^{10}, whereas in persons with normal gastric acid and unimpaired intestinal motility only small numbers of bacteria are found in the upper intestine. This bacterial overgrowth may well be responsible for some of the disturbed assimilation of fat and protein, as it is known from the blind loop syndrome.

As an other important cause for malabsorption, *pancreatico-cibal asynchrony* in patients with exclusion of the duodenum from contact with chymus has been claimed. This possibility has not been investigated in detail in patients with total gastrectomy. From a theoretical point of view, a poor mixture of biliary and pancreatic secretion with food in the jejunum and a loss of proper release of gastrointestinal hormones from duodenal mucosa (secretin, cholecystokinin, pancreozymin) must be considered. Bradley substituted pancreatic enzymes exogenously in one patient and could reduce fat excretion by 40% [6]. A similar observation has been made by Lundh [13] on patients with total gastrectomy.

Absorption Studies

Carbohydrate absorption has been studied for D-xylose, glucose, and lactose [3, 6]. The absorption of glucose usually shows the pattern of early hyperglycemia and of late hypoglycemia (Table 1) [3, 15, 6]. It reflects early absorption from the jejunum and excess release of insulin. Mildly abnormal D-xylose absorption has been found in four of ten patients by Bradley et al. [6]. They discuss bacterial use of D-xylose as a possible cause. Lactose splitting has been observed to be normal in our case (Table 1).

Low intake of calcium and vitamin D with food and impaired absorption because of steatorrhea can account for postoperative osteopathia. Hypocalcemia and elevated alkaline phosphatase are taken as signs for this disturbance of bone metabolism. Adams [3] reported radiologically detectable bone disease in 2 of 18 patients. Bradley et al. [6] observed positive total body balance of N, P, Ca, K, and Cl during a controlled study of intake and excretion in all of ten patients studied.

Hematological Problems

Total gastrectomy leads to megaloblastic anemia because of total loss of intrinsic factor. Without substitution of vitamin B_{12}, this type of anemia can probably develop within 2–3 years. Adams [2] measured serum vitamin B_{12} levels immediately after operation until 120 weeks. The level was falling progressively in order to stabilize on a new niveau after about 20 weeks between 100 and 200 pg/ml [2]. Iron deficiency has been found up to 90% [2]. Its causes are manifold: blood loss before and during operation, loss of iron into the RES because of tumor cachexia, malabsorption, and/or occult bleeding in the intestinal tract.

Role of Impaired Intake of Food

Only few dietary investigations in patients which total gastrectomy have been recorded [1, 6, 15, 10, 17]. All studies come to the conclusion that a least at certain times, the total intake of calories is too low and accounts for most of the weight loss in these patients. Adams [1] recorded the dietary histories of 14 patients with esophagojejunostomy. He found a daily caloric intake ranging from 1131 to 3075, demonstrating the wide margin between the patients. He interprets his data in the sense, that comparing them with recommended dietary allowances, only two patients had adequate intake of nutrients. A controlled study of food intake was carried out by Bradley et al. [6] on ten patients. He studied the patients in a hospital with voluntary access to food ("hospital smorgasbord intake"). He compared the values with recommended dietary allowances (RDA) and with the voluntary intake during 1 week at home. Table 3 shows the results. It was obvious that nine of ten patients approached or exceeded the RDA for calories when they were in the hospital. Back again at home, the caloric intake declined 29% from the value reached in the hospital. The daily caloric intake then reached only 85% of RDA and was less by 348 kcal/day.

Another controlled study was carried out on four patients with reconstructed pouch by Hays and Clark [10]. The daily spontaneous intake of food was absolutely in the range which was found in ten normal controls (Table 4).
The patients absorbed 81% of the ingested protein; the comparative figure in the controls was 87%. Fecal fat excretion was slightly elevated in the patients, resulting in absorption of 85% of the ingested fat compared to 95% in the controls.

In summary, these studies demonstrate that at least patients with a jejunal pouch are able to ingest more calories than they need for maintenance of ideal weight, even gaining weight again if they eat under controlled conditions in the hospital. On the other hand, these patients obviously eat less if they are at home under normal environmental conditions. The retrospective data of Adams [1] give some hint that perhaps patients without a pouch regularly eat less than they need according to recommended caloric allowance.

Table 3. Voluntary food intake in individual home environments compared to recommended diatary allowance (RDA) and hospital food intake (from Bradley et al., 1975)

Patient	Calories (kcal)			Carbohydrate (g)			Fat (g)			Protein (g)		
	RDA	Hosp.	Home	RDA	Hosp.	Home	RDA	Hosp.	Home	RDA	Hosp.	Home
MH	2406	2334	1627	333	263	171	94	103	67	56	89	67
AR	2355	3650	3762	295	404	353	103	178	154	59	121	138
JL	2700	3510	3396	383	368	238	105	182	181	56	115	174
WM	2388	2269	1883	333	230	180	93	123	85	56	67	99
WO	2605	3725	1254	320	460	168	100	160	47	65	116	44
CB	2818	1860	1183	260	254	104	100	67	55	65	61	49
BQ	1947	2862	1955	279	457	224	78	86	82	46	77	81
TS	1995	3053	1340	279	293	134	77	161	66	48	119	60
Mean	2402	2908	2050	310	341	197	94	133	92	56	96	89
Standard error	110	248	350	14	33	27	4	16	17	2	9	16
% of RDA	100	121	85	100	110	63	100	141	97	100	171	158

Table 4. Spontaneous food intake of 4 patients with total gastrectomy, esophagojejunostomy with pouch, and of 10 controls (from Hays and Clark, 1960)

	Protein	Fat	Carbohydrate	Calories
W. R.	72	73	495	2926
L. R.	100	100	549	3496
M.	100	100	576	3604
H.	102	140	421	3352
Controls (n = 10)	95	96	527	3345

	Total gastrectomy with jejunal pouch (n = 4)	Normal controls (n = 10)
Fat intake/24 h	103 g	96 g
Fat excretion/24 h	16 g	5 g
Assimilation	87 g = 85%	91 g = 95%
Protein intake/24 h	94 g	95 g
Protein excretion/24 h	17 g	11 g
Assimilation	77 g = 81%	84 g = 87%

Causes of Impaired Food Intake

The causes of inadequate food intake obviously are multifactorial and related to each other. Figure 1 tries to depict some of these factors which demonstrate the psychosomatic features of postoperative weight problems.

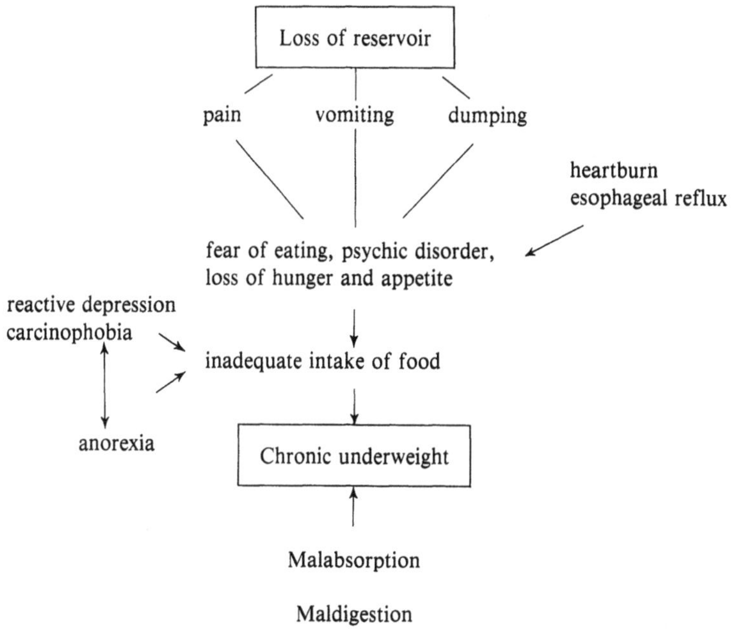

Fig. 1. Pathophysiological sequelae of total gastrectomy with loss of reservoir

Absence of hunger and anorexia were predominant features in 9 of 19 patients in Adams' study [1]. They were connected with reactive depression, fear of relapse of the carcinoma, and inability to work. Dysphagia was observed in up to 40% of patients [1], often together with heartburn and other symptoms of alkaline reflux into the esophagus. This problem was typical for esophagoduodenostomy in about 60% and esophagojejunostomy in about 30% [16] and was claimed to be no major problem after reconstruction of a pouch with esophagojejunoplication [24]. The loss of reservoir function without reconstructive procedures seemed to be a problem for the psychological state of patients with total gastrectomy. The capacity of the small bowel to accept food at a single meal has been found in these cases to be only 10% – 20% of the normal capacity [15]. This obviously has a direct influence on the patient's personal initiative to take in food. A dumping syndrome has been reported in about 50% of patients in Adams' series [1]. Other observers have seen it even more frequently. Diarrhea was usually no problem [1].

Is the Reconstruction of a Pouch Favorable?

This question is not easy to answer because of lack of controlled studies with and without a pouch. In an experimental study with rats using esophagojenunostomy, esophagoduodenostomy, and a Roux-Y-procedure, no differences of fat absorption were observed [25]. The patients studied by Adams [1, 2, 3] had had no reconstructive procedures. Bradley et al. [6] studied seven patients with a Hunt-Lawrence-pouch and three with esophagojejunostomy without pouch. They claimed no statistical differences between the two procedures concerning voluntary food intake, relation to ideal body weight, number of daily meals, anaerobic bacteria present, and intestinal transit time (Table 5), but found a decrease of early satiety without a pouch. Different procedures have been proposed to increase storage capacity and to improve nutrition after total gastrectomy [11]. Scott et al. [23] have followed eight patients with a Hunt-Lawrence-pouch for 3–5 years and found it favorable. Moreno [15] has compared five patients with a double lumen jejunal pouch interposed between the esophagus and duodenum with two patients with esophagojejunostomy. He found an increase of reservoir capacity from 20% to 80% of normal with the pouch, but did not observe statistical differences in postoperative weight gain or in fat and nitrogen absorption. Mainly positive results with reconstructive pouch procedures have been reported by German surgeons [20, 8, 20, 14]. Reflux esophagitis and dumping syndrome were no more a problem in these patients with [8, 20] and without duodenal passage of food [19, 14, 6]. Considerable weight gain has been seen by Brünner and Kempf following interposition of a jejunal loop with pouch between esophagus and duodenum according to Longmire-Gütgemann [8]. In summary, the reconstruction of a pouch seems to have positive consequences for the patients concerning prevention of dumping and alkaline reflux and a better acceptance of food with a single meal.

Role of Duodenal Passage

Some surgeons favor the passage through the duodenum [8, 20], other claim this to be of minor importance, favoring esophagojejunostomy [14, 6, 19]. Table 6

Table 5. Comparison of nutritional parameters in pouch versus nonpouch reconstruction (from Bradley et al. 1975)

	Type of Reconstruction	
	Hunt-Lawrence	No pouch
Number of Patients	7	3
Smorgasbord (% RDA)		
Caloric intake	125	130
Carbohydrate	172	275
Fat	148	158
Protein	181	175
Coefficient of malabsorption		
Fat	10.6%	31.0%
Protein	15.9%	23.3%
Daily protein balance (g)	+2.3	+1.6
Relation to ideal body weight	87%	81%
Dumping symptoms	3/7	0/3
Number of daily meals	4.7	3.6
Deconjugated bile salts present	7/7	3/3
Anaerobic bacteria present	7/7	3/3
Jejunal histology	Normal	Normal
Intestinal transit (min)	195	180

Table 6. Pathophysiological consequences of exclusion of the duodenum from normal passage of food

Exclusion of duodenum means	Impaired function	Relevance
Loss of absorptive capacity	Fe, Ca, vitamins, food stuffs	Low
No release of secretin by HCL	Water, bicarbonate secretion pancreas, bile	? Stimulation by bile acids in duodenum
No release of CCK-PZ	Gallbladder contraction enzyme secretion pancreas	? Vagal stimulation
Desintegrated mixture of biliary and pancreatic secretion with food	Digestion	Important

summarizes the pathophysiological consequences of exclusion of the duodenum. The loss of absorptive capacity is low with respect to food stuffs, minerals, and vitamins, since the jejunum is able to absorb them sufficiently. With total lack of HCL in the duodenum, the release of secretion should be impaired. On the other hand, it has been shown that bile acids entering the duodenum release considerable amounts of secretin leading to increased flow of bile and of pancreatic fluid [9]. The release of cholecystokinin-pancreozymin should be impaired if no food is entering the duodenum. But vagal stimulation can achieve pancreatic enzyme secretion. The most important point is the possible desintegration of the mixture of digestive juices with food in the jejunum. This has been discussed earlier in this paper. The exact role of this pancreatico-cibal asynchrony resulting in a relative pancreatic digestive insufficiency is not yet clear. It must be studied, therefore, whether it is favorable to substitute pancreatic enzymes exogenously. In summary, and having in mind the positive experiences with exclusion of the duodenum in the Billroth II procedure of gastric surgery, the reconstruction of duodenal passage after total gastrectomy obviously has no decisive advantages over the method of esophagojejunostomy.

References

1. Adams, J. F.: The clinical and metabolic consequences of total gastrectomy. I. Morbidity, weight and nutrition. Scand J. Gastroenterol. *2*, 137 (1967)
2. Adams, J. F.: The clinical and metabolic consequences of total gastrectomy. II. Anaemia, metabolism of iron, vitamin B_{12}, and folic acid. Scand J. Gastroenterol. *3*, 145 (1968)
3. Adams, J. F.: The clinical and metabolic consequences of total gastrectomy. III. Notes on metabolic functions, deficiency states, changes in intestinal histology, and radiology. Scand. J. Gastroenterol. *3*, 152 (1968)
4. Berndt, H.: Die Pathogenese der agastrischen Dystrophie. Chirurg *34*, 298 (1963)
5. Bünte, H., Döring, I.: Erfahrungen mit 200 totalen Gastrektomien beim Magenkarzinom. Bruns Beitr. Klin. Chir. *220*, 244 (1973)
6. Bradley, E. L., Isaacs, J., Hersh, Th., Davidson, E. D., Millikan, W.: Nutritional consequences of total gastrectomy. Ann. Surg. *182*, 415 (1975)
7. Brain, R. H. F.: Sequelae of radical gastric resections: Clinical and metabolic findings in 35 cases. Lancet *1951 1*, 1137
8. Brünner, H., Kempf, P.: Der Dünndarmersatzmagen. Klinik und Ergebnisse nach 51 jejunalen Interpositionen. Dtsch. Med. Wochenschr. *100*, 1044 (1975)

9. Hartmann, W., Goebell, H., Hotz, J., Hanssen, L. E.: Release of secretin and stimulation of bile flow during duodenal perfusion with bile acids in the cat. In: Biological effects of bile acids. Paumgartner, G. (ed.). Lancaster: MTP Press (in press)
10. Hays, R. P., Clark, D. A.: Nutrition in patients with total gastrectomy and a jejunal food pouch. Ann. Surg. *152*, 864 (1960)
11. Herrington, J. L.: Various types of pouch replacement following total gastrectomy: historical data and current throughts regarding total gastrectomy. Ann. Surg. *34*, 879 (1968)
12. Kelly, W. D., McLean, L. D., Perry, J. F. et al.: A study of patients following total and near-total gastrectomy. Surgery *35*, 964 (1954)
13. Lundh, G.: Intestinal digestion and absorption after gastrectomy. Acta Chir. Scand. (Suppl. 231) *1*, 51 (1958)
14. Merkle, P., Schlag, P., Krause, F.: Zur Frage der agastrischen Dystrophie nach Gastrektomie. Chirurg *47*, 380 (1976)
15. Moreno, A. H.: Studies on nutritional and other disturbances following operations for cancer of the stomach. With particular reference to the use of a jejunal pouch as a substitute gastric reservoir. Ann. Surg. *144*, 779 (1956)
16. Nakayama, K.: Evaluation of the various operative methods for total gastrectomy. Surgery *40*, 488 (1956)
17. Randall, H. Th.: Alterations in gastrointestinal tract function following surgery. Surg. Clin. North Am. *38*, 585 (1958)
18. Rush, F. B., Ravitch, M. M.: The evolution of total gastrectomy. Int. Abstr. Surg. *114*, 411 (1962)
19. Säuberli, H., Largiadèr, F.: Die totale Gastrektomie. II. Resultate von 71 eigenen Fällen. Bruns Beitr. Klin. Chir. *220*, 35 (1973)
20. Schreiber, H. W.: Radikalität und pathophysiologische Gesichtspunkte bei der Resektion des Magenkarzinoms. Langenbecks Arch. Klin. Chir. *314*, 213 (1966)
21. Schreiber, H. W., van Ackeren, H., Rehner, M.: Chirurgische Behandlung bösartiger Geschwulstkrankheiten des Magens. Chirurg *33*, 551 (1972)
22. Schwartz, M. K., Bodansky, O., Randall, H. T.: Metabolism in surgical patients. II. Fat and mineral metabolism in totally gastrectomized patients. Ann. J. Clin. Nutr. *4*, 51 (1956)
23. Scott, H. W., jr., Law, D. H., Gobbel, W. G. et al.: Clinical and metabolic studies after total gastrectomy with a Hunt-Lawrence jejunal food pouch. Ann. J. Surg. *115*, 148 (1968)
24. Siewert, J. R., Peiper, H., Jennewein, H. M., Waldeck, F.: Die Oesophago-Jejunoplication. Chirurg *44*, 115 (1973)
25. Wendelbo, O., Øystese, B., Helsingen, N.: Fat absorption after total gastrectomy. Acta Chir. Scand. *125*, 135 (1963)

Importance of the Duodenal Passage Following Gastrectomy

J. R. Siewert, G. Schattenmann, and R. Ebert

When dealing with the vast possibilities of reconstruction methods following total gastrectomy, two main principles seem to stand out. Some surgical procedures attempt to maintain duodenal passage through the interposition of variable forms of jejunal segments, other procedures do away with the duodenal passage and undertake a direct reconstruction in the form of an esophagojejunostomy. As a rule, the preservation of the duodenal passage is technically more complicated, since at least one more anastomosis is required. The value of preserving the duodenal passage for the patient is questionable. Prospective comparative studies on this problem have yet to be published. Initial studies (Troidl, Kiel, Alexander-Williams, Birmingham) have not proved duodenal continence to be advantagous.

Bradley's retrospective study, which incidentally also covered the necessity of constructing a pouch, likewise found no significant differences in the various surgical techniques.

In the evaluation of the method or reconstruction following gastrectomy, one needs to differentiate clearly between problems reflected by the underlying disease and those brought about by the surgical approach. That is why studies concerning the benefit of duodenal preservation should be restricted to patients with benign underlying diseases or to those patients with so-called early cancer.

Pathophysiological Aspects

The duodenum influences the chyme in the following manner:

1) The acidic chyme is neutralized; when leaving the duodenum, the duodenal contents are neutral. To this end, the duodenum must regulate the evacuation of the stomach in such a manner that the amount of acid received from the stomach at a given time should never exceed the amount neutralized in the duodenum. As an additional factor, the mucosa of the duodenum secrets secretin and cholecystokinin (CCK). These substances cause the pancreas and liver to secrete fluids rich in bicarbonates. Furthermore, small amounts of H-ions are absorbed by the mucosa of the duodenum. Following gastrectomy, this neutralization process ceases.

2) The duodenum regulates the osmotic pressure of the evacuated chyme. Particularly following gastrectomy, the contents of the substitute stomach and its osmotic pressure are directly dependent upon the type of food intake. In the

usual case, the equilibrium of osmotic pressure is produced by the regulation of the evacuation of the stomach and by direct supplementation of secretions.

The regulating effect of stomach evacuation on osmotic pressure ceases following gastrectomy. Ingested food immediately reaches the duodenum. An isotonic state is achieved solely by secretion supplementation. Even so, total equilibrium is not always achieved.

3) An important part of digestion begins in the duodenum. The secretion of CCK and secretion invokes a timed stimulation of the pancreas and a simultaneous supplementation of pancreas enzymes and bile. The segmental nature of the duodenum guarantees proper blending of the ingredients.

4) The absorption begins in the duodenum.

Glucose, galactose, and other monosaccharides, amino acids, and smaller polypeptides and free fatty acids can be absorbed by the duodenum.

The last two mentioned aspects are relevant following gastrectomy and represent strong arguments in the discussion of the necessity to preserve duodenal passage.

Tests and Findings

The following tests were utilized in the examination of seven patients who underwent esophagojejunoplication without duodenal preservation and six patients, who underwent an interposition procedure of the Seo-Longmire type:

- Absorption tests, i. e., glucose and insulin serum levels under glucose stress, (GTT).
- Tests of fat absorption, carotin serum levels, and feces fat.
- Bacterial analysis with the help of C^{14} glycocholate tests.
- Laboratory tests involving iron levels, total protein, and including albumin fraction, and body weight measurements.

Results

The results of the glucose, gastric inhibitory polypeptide (GIP), and insulin serum levels under glucose stress (GTT) are shown in Figs. 1 – 3. These figures show that in cases without duodenal preservation blood sugar levels reach higher values (max. 300 mg%) 60 min after oral glucose ingestion. Simultaneously, small amounts of GIP and insulin are secreted. When duodenal passage is maintained, blood sugar levels run to 235 mg%. This is the case even though GIP and insulin levels increase (GIP: max. value 4600 pg/ml in 30 min; insulin: 246.3 units/ml in 30 min). This implies markedly increased glucose absorption and synchronous metabolism due to simultaneous insulin secretion in cases where duodenal passage is maintained.

Carotin levels and feces fat were measured as criteria for fat absorption. Since carotin is liposoluable provitamin A, it can only be metabolized in the presence of adequate fat absorption. Independent of duodenal passage, the carotin level was pathologically decreased following gastrectomy, (46 ± 3.2

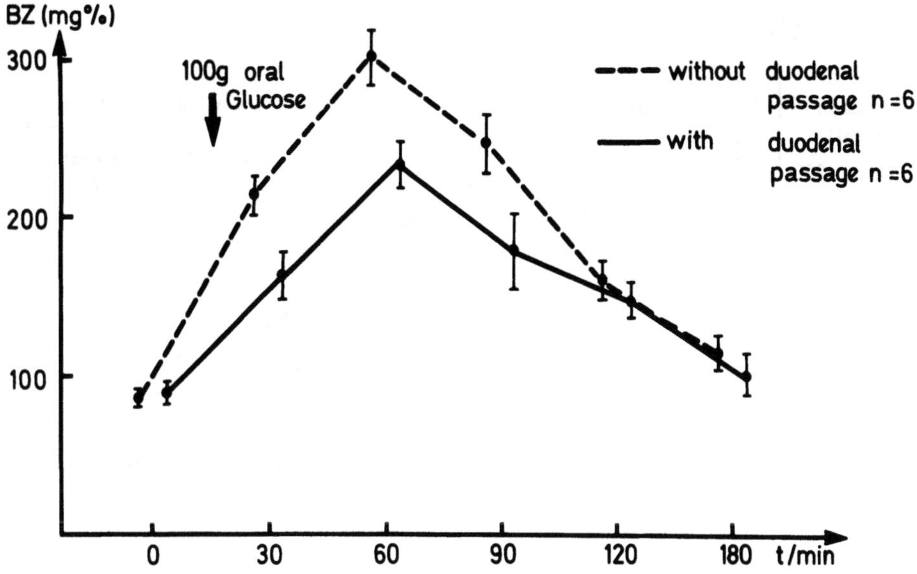

Fig. 1. GTT in patients with total gastrectomy with and without duodenal passage

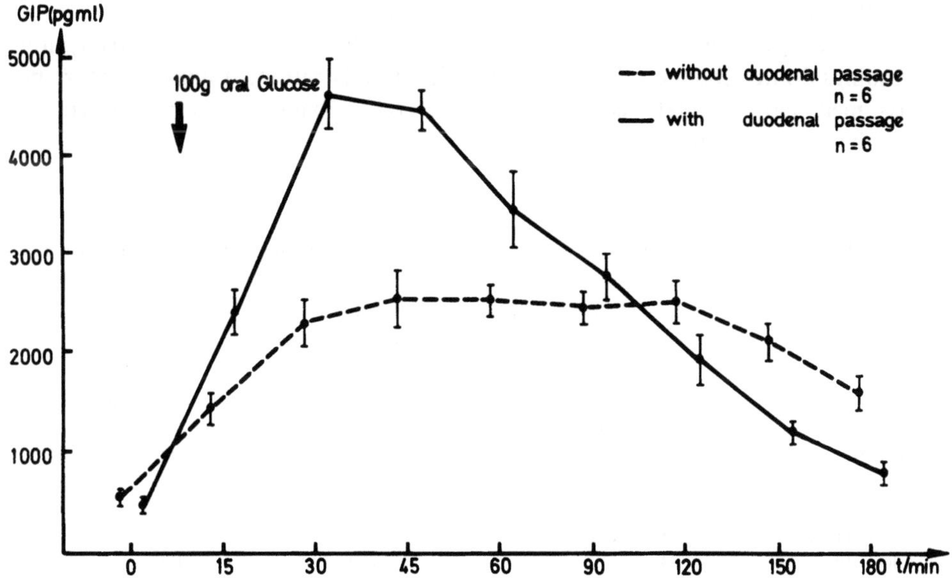

Fig. 2. GIP levels in patients with and without duodenal passage

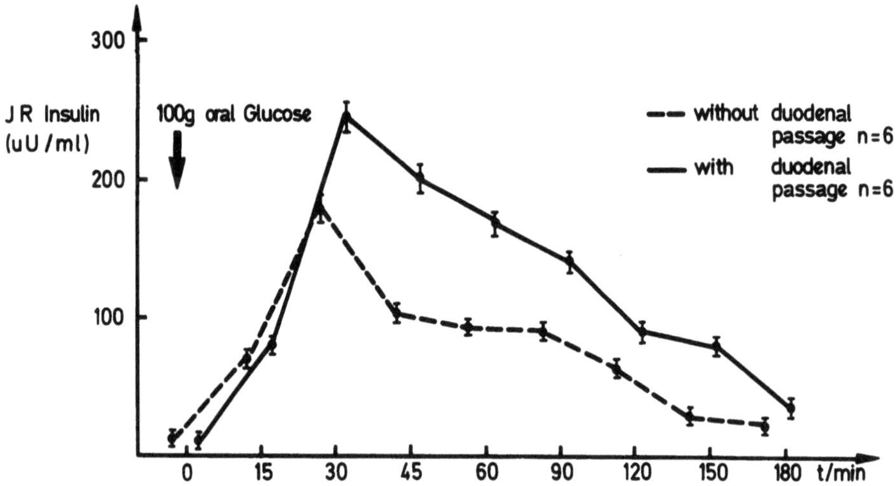

Fig. 3. Insulin values in patients with and without duodenal passage

without duodenal passage; 47.2 ± 4.4 with duodenal passage). Furthermore, feces fat values showed no significant difference between the two groups (14.5 ± 9.4 g without duodenal passage; 11.8 ± 7.3 g with duodenal passage) (Table 1).

In the literature, bacterial imbalance of the small bowel is quoted as being a probable cause of fat malabsorption following gastrectomy. Our findings showed a somewhat higher rate of pathological respiratory tests in patients without duodenal passage than in patients where it had been maintained. However, it must be said that the difference was not statistically significant, as the number of cases was inadequate. According to reports by Bradley [2, 3], malabsorption findings do not change following antibiotic administration. It must therefore be assumed that the relationship between bacterial imbalance and malabsorption has been overestimated.

Table 1. Comparative analysis of laboratory values in patients with and without duodenal passage

	Esophago-jejunoplication	Interposition (Seo-Longmire)	Normals
Total protein	6.8 + 0.4 g%	7.1 + 0.7 g%	6.2 – 8.0 g%
Albumin	57.9 + 6.7%	58.3 + 2.3%	57 – 68%
Serum iron	82.5 + 39.3 μg%	103.8 + 27.4 μg%	65 – 135 μg%
Carotin level	46 + 3.2 μg%	47.2 + 4.4 μg%	100 – 150 μg%
Feces fat	14.5 + 9.4 g/day	11.8 + 7.3 g/day	8 g/day
C^{14} inhalation	25% path.	15% path.	–
Ideal BW	84.2 + 14.3%	86.7 + 7.6%	100%
Glucose tol. test	+ + +	+ + +	–
	n = 8	n = 7	

Total protein and albumin in the serum are recognized laboratory criteria for the evaluation of nitrogen metabolism. Normal and comparable values were found to exist in both patient groups (6.8 ± 0.4 g%, i.e., 57.9 ± 6.7% albumin without duodenal passage; 7.1 ± 0.7 g%, i.e., 58.3 ± 2.3% albumin with duodenal passage). Body weight taken as a measure of nutrition did not show differences in the two groups. Irrespective of the existence of duodenal continence, the body weight of patients who have undergone gastrectomy falls to 15% below the calculated ideal body weight (Table 1).

Conclusion

The findings are still incomplete and need supportive research, but they are nonetheless consistent. All examined patients who underwent gastrectomy, suffered from malnutrition. This was reflected in the loss of about 15% of normal body weight. This malnutrition occurred in patients with as well as without duodenal continence and seemed to be the result of malabsorption as well as inadequate food intake, as studies by Bradley [2, 3] have shown. Signs of fat malabsorption were equally evident in decreased carotin levels and increased feces fat in both patient groups. On the other hand, nitrogen absorption seemed to undergo little pathological change, at least when reviewing laboratory values for total protein and albumin fraction, which were normal. An improved glucose absorption with maintained duodenal passage was of no more than superficial value, since it had no influcence on the nutritional status of the patient. These findings show that convincing arguments in favor of preserving duodenal passage have yet to be found.

References

1. Alexander-Williams, J.: Personal communication
2. Bradley, E. L.: Postsurgical syndromes after total gastrectomy. Blum, A. L., Siewert, R. (eds.).London: Saunders (in press)
3. Bradley, E. L., Isaacs, J., Hersh, Th., Davidson, E., Millikan, W.: Nutritional consequences of total gastrectomy. Ann. Surg. *181*, 415 (1975)
4. Peiper, H. J., Siewert, R.: Magenersatz. Chirurg *49*, 81 (1978)
5. Troidl, H.: Personal communication

Significance of the Duodenum for Carbohydrate Metabolism in Patients After Total Gastrectomy

R. Bittner and H. G. Beger

Nutritional problems which develop in patients following total gastrectomy are of sufficient severity and occur frequently enough to warrant detailed investigations of operative procedures which may obviate these symptoms. It is well documented that construction of a substitute gastric reservoir is of greatest importance in the attempt to relieve certain undesirable effects of total gastrectomy. However, there are only a few studies concerning the significance of the maintenance of the route of ingested foodstuff through the duodenum in contrast to bypassing this juncture. This is all the more astonishing as the mucosa of the duodenum is able to secrete several hormones which have an essential effect on the exocrine and endocrine pancreatic functions [9, 1].

The aim of the present study was to evaluate the significance of the preservation of the passage of the food through the duodenum on carbohydrate metabolism.

Patients and Methods

Two patient groups after total gastrectomy for cancer of the stomach and different forms of reconstruction were studied: one group of eight patients with end-to-side esophagojejunostomy (Graham) and exclusion of the duodenum, and a second group of four patients with transplantation of a long intestinal loop (jejunum) between the esophageal and duodenal remnants (Gütgemann-Schreiber). The clinical data of the patients are summarized in Table 1. There are no statistical differences between the two groups with respect to age, body weight, and height. No patient had a personal or family history of diabetes mellitus. The preoperative fasting glucose concentrations of each patient were within the normal range.

Table 1. Clinical data of the patients after total gastrectomy for cancer of the stomach and different forms of reconstruction

Reconstruction	n	Age (yr)	Body weight (kg)	Height (cm)
Without duodenal passage	8	62 ± 9	53.6 ± 13	164 ± 10
With duodenal passage	4	56.5 ± 10	55.5 ± 10	170.5 ± 8

On the average, 10 months after the operation in all patients, an oral glucose tolerance test (OGT) was performed. After an overnight fast, the patients received 1 g/kg body weight glucose as a 50% solution to be taken orally within 3 – 5 min. Blood samples were taken – in defined intervals after the oral glucose load from a plastic cannula inserted into a cubital vein.

Glucose was determined enzymatically with the God-Perid method. Insulin was measured according to the douple antibody radioimmunoassay method of Hales and Randle using the immunotest-kit of Sorin.

All the data in the figures are given as the median of eight or four patient values. The Mann-whitney U-test was employed for the statistical analysis.

Results

Figure 1 shows the medians of the glucose concentrations of both test groups before and after oral glucose load. It is remarkable that already the fasting glucose level in the patients with food passage through the duodenum is about 20 mg/100 ml lower than in the patients with exclusion of the duodenum. This difference is statistically significant ($P < 0.05$). Furthermore, the increase towards the peak concentration after the glucose load in the patients with the transplanted jejunal loop is with 1.4 mg/min significantly lower ($P < 0.02$) in contrast to the 2 mg/min of the patients without duodenum. In addition, in these patients, the peak glucose concentration is significantly lower ($P < 0.05$). The comparison of the individual peak concentrations of all the patients shows a much more pronounced difference between the two groups: in the patients with exclusion of the duodenum, the highest glucose peak is 238 mg/100 ml and the lowest peak is 146 mg/100 ml. On the other hand, in the patients with glucose passage through the duodenum, the highest glucose peak is 167 mg/100 ml and the lowest peak is 116 mg/100 ml only. In summary, preservation of the duodenum means that the peak glucose concentrations are about 40 – 70 mg/100 ml lower.

Figure 2 shows the corresponding insulin concentrations. In the patients with duodenum, insulin is higher at each measuring point. The peak is reached about 30 min earlier and is significantly higher ($P < 0.005$). In order to give quantitative evidence of these results, the areas below insulin and glucose concentration curves were calculated [8]. Figure 3 shows that in the patients with glucose passage through the duodenum, the insulin area is about 45% larger than in the patients with exclusion of the duodenum ($P < 0.05$). In addition, the "insulinogenic index" [5] – quotient of insulin area divided through the glucose area – which gives evidence of the secretory capacity of the β-cells is about three times greater.

Discussion

Since the first total gastrectomy by Carl Schlatter in 1897, more than 40 different forms of reconstruction of the digestive tract [4] have been published. This great

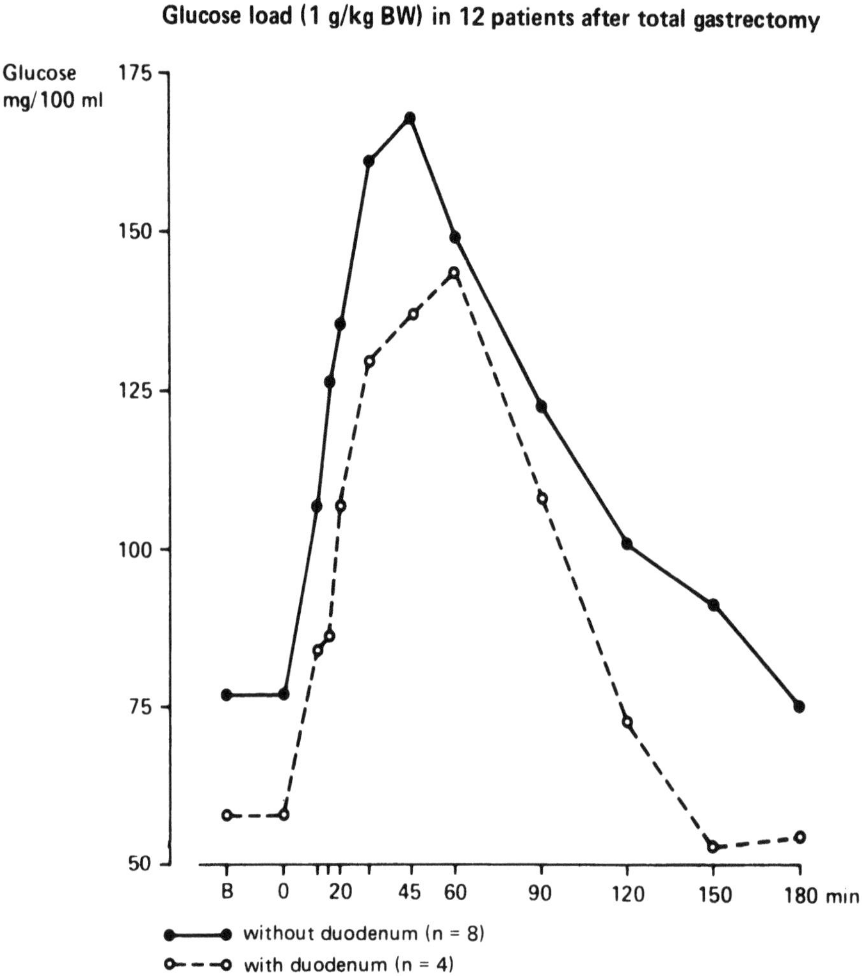

Fig. 1. Medians of glucose concentrations before and after oral glucose load in patients with and without food passage through the duodenum

number characterizes a common uncertainty in finding the best method. The lack of precise data concerning the digestive and the metabolic functions of the patients without a stomach is responsible for the difficulty the surgeon has in selecting one method over another. Therefore, it is not astonishing that there is also unclarity over the significance of preservation of the foodstuff passage through the duodenum. The present study about carbohydrate metabolism proves that patients with a transplanted jejunal loop and maintenance of the duodenum in the digestive tract have a significantly improved glucose tolerance. This may be explained as follows: by means of the jejunal pouch and the duodenum, the passage of glucose is delayed. Moreover, the glucose solution is diluted with the intestinal juice. According to these two beneficial effects, the absorption of the glucose is delayed, too. Therefore, a sudden overflowing of the organism with glucose is prevented. Furthermore, the measurements of insulin show also that the secretory capacity of the β-cells is significantly improved. Despite lower glucose

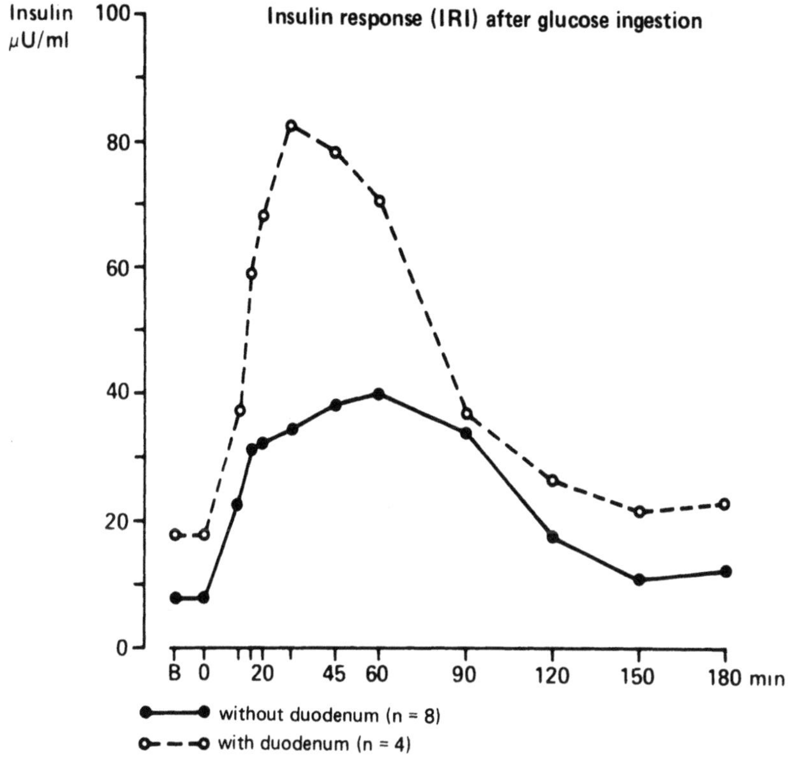

Fig. 2. Medians of insulin concentrations before and after oral glucose load

levels, the insulin secretion is about 45% larger than in the patients with exclusion of the duodenum. It is suggested that this better insulin response is caused by one or several hormones of the intestinal mucosa (predominantly of the duodenum and proximal jejunum) – secretin, pancreozymin, gastric inhibitory polypeptide (GIP), insulin releasing peptide (IRP) – which have a well-proven insulinotropic action [2, 3, 6]. So, it can be differentiated between a hyperglycemic and a alimentary stimulus of insulin secretion. In order to describe this interaction between glucose, intestinal hormones, and β-cells, Unger and Eisentraut [7] formed the term "entero-insular axis". In addition, if we think that there is not only an entero-endocrine interaction, but also an entero-exocrine and even an endocrine-exocrine pancreatic relationship [1], the preservation of the foodstuff passage through the duodenum seems to be extraordinarily important for an optimal course of the digestive functions.

Conclusion

In two groups of patients after total gastrectomy for cancer of the stomach and different forms of reconstruction, an investigation of glucose tolerance and insulin secretion was performed. One group (four patients) had a reconstruction with preservation of the food passage through the duodenum; the other group (eight patients) had a reconstruction with exclusion of the duodenum.

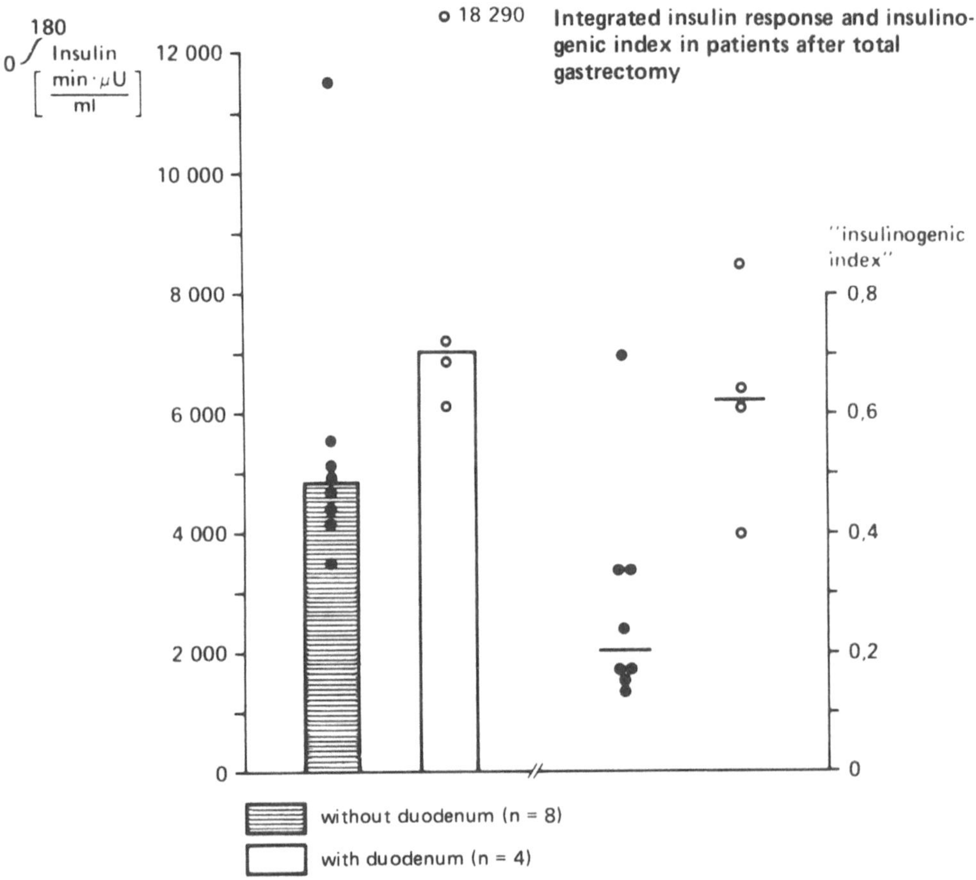

Fig. 3. Insulin areas below the concentration curves (*left*) and "insulinogenic index"(*right*) of patients with duodenum passage in contrast to the patients without duodenum

The results demonstrated that in the patients with preserved passage of the glucose through the duodenum, the glucose tolerance was significantly better and the secretory capacity of the β-cells was significantly improved.

References

1. Bank, S.: Pancreatic endocrine-exocrine relationship in health and disease. Scand. J. Gastroenterol. *7*, 503 – 507 (1972)
2. Creutzfeldt, W.: Insulin-releasing factors of the gastrointestinal mucosa (incretin). Gastroenterology *67*, 748 – 750 (1974)
3. Creutzfeldt, W., Ketterer, H.: Effect of gastrointestinal hormones on insulin and glucagon secretion. N. Engl. J. Med. *282*, 1139 – 1141 (1970)
4. Schreiber, H. W., van Ackeren, H., Rehner, M.: Chirurgische Behandlung bösartiger Geschwulstkrankheiten des Magens. Chirurg *43*, 551 – 558 (1972)

5. Seltzer, H. S., Allen, E. W., Herron, A. L., Jr., Brennan, M. T.: Insulin secretion in response to glycemic stimulus; Relation of delayed inital release to carbohydrate intolerance in mild diabetes mellitus. J. Clin. Invest. *46*, 323 – 335 (1967)
6. Turner, D. S., Etheridge, L., Marks, V., Brown, I. C., Mutt, V.: Effectiveness of the inestinal polypeptides, IRP, GIP, VIP and motilin on insulin release in the rat. Diabetologia *10*, 459 – 463 (1974)
7. Unger, R. H., Eisentraut, A. M.: Entero-Insular Axis. Arch. Intern. Med. *123*, 261 – 266 (1969)
8. Welborn, T. A., Rubenstein, A. H., Haslam, R.: Normal insulin response to glucose. Lancet *1966 1*, 280 – 284
9. Youngs, G.: Hormonal control of pancreatic endocrine and exocrine secretion. Gut *13*, 154 – 161 (1972)

Nutritional History in Gastrectomized Patients

W. Rösch

The term "agastric dystrophy" implies that following partial or total gastrectomy maldigestion with consecutive malabsorption causes severe impairment of the nutritional status. Henning et al. [2] could demonstrate in patients with Billroth II resection that 80% had fat malabsorption, 77% functional pancreatic insufficiency, 64% carbohydrate malabsorption, and 52% iron deficiency anemia. Further analysis of the pathophysiology of pancreatic secretion in these patients revealed that maldigestion phenomena were not due to inactivity atrophy of the pancreas, but rather due to a decreased release of secretin and pancreozymin from the jejunum [3]. In comparison with maximal exogenous stimulation, the endogenous release of these two hormones following food intake amounts only to 25% of the bicarbonate production and to 50% of the enzyme output. In addition, pancreatic asynchrony with rapid emptying of the stomach and delayed flow of the pancreatic juice contributes to the process of maldigestion.

The weight loss in gastrectomized patients exceeds that of partially resected patients. Careful analysis of the pre- and postoperative nutritional status showed a mean decrease in body weight of 14 kg. Meal frequency varied between 3 and 10. Of 10 patients, in whom subtile analysis of food intolerance was undertaken, only one was capable of performing his preoperative activities. Two patients did not receive vitamin B_{12} substitution, another only occasionally; all three were dystrophic. Most patients complained of hypotension, recurrent diarrhea, anorexia, nausea, and vomiting. The most commonly stated food intolerances were milk and milk products, wine and beer, vegetables, fruits, and juices. Three of ten gastrectomized patients did not tolerate meat or sausages (Table 1) [1].

Since most gastrectomized patients tend to eat "soft food," an inappropriate intake of protein and a deficit of electrolytes and vitamins is common. The above mentioned milk intolerance leads to a calcium deficiency which is further strengthened by an impaired calcium absorption. The basic principle of 6 – 8 small meals, avoiding hyperosmolar food, has to be supplement by life-long enzyme substitution in granulate form, monthly injection of 100 μg vitamin B_{12} and calcium as well as iron tablets.

References

1. Berg, G., Matzkies, F., Sailer, D.: Ernährung nach Gastrektomie. Fortschr. Med. *95*, 1869 – 1874 (1977)
2. Henning, N., Berg, G., Wüst, H., Zeitler, G.: Störungen nach Magenresektion. Dtsch. Med. Wochenschr. *91*, 843 – 851 (1966)
3. Tympner, F., Rösch, W., Domschke, W., Demling, L.: The function of the exocrine pancreas after exogenous and endogenous stimulation in Billroth II patients. Acta Hepatogastroenterol. (Stuttg.) *23*, 444 – 448 (1976)

Table 1. Nutritional history of 10 gastrectomized patients

Patient Age	Years post-op.	Height cm	Weight pre-op	Weight post-op	Difference	Meal/d	Vit. B_{12}	Complaints	Food intolerance
E. N. 33	4	167	58	56	− 2	10	+	Hypotension	Anemia meat, cereals, vegetables, fruit, coffee, wine
A. D. 41	5	185	90	87	− 3	3	+	Episodic tachycardia	Cereals, milk, fruits, beer
L. B. 49	6	170	70	50	−20	6	−	Dystrophy	Milk, vegetables, fruits, eggs, beer
J. G. 56	4	166	103	85	−18	6	+	Hypotension	Fruits, wine
G. G. 57	8	175	74	79	+ 5	6	+	None	Milk, wine
H. P. 57	5	180	64	51	−13	4	+	Diarrhea, Nausea, Vomiting, Anorexia	Cereals, milk, fruits, coffee, wine
J. M. 63	7	174	74	61	−13	8	+	Diarrhea	Milk, vegetables, fruits
A. B. 64	11	180	105	65	−40	6	−/+	Hypotension, Diarrhea, Weakness, Recurrent Fever	Meat, milk, cereals, vegetables, fruits, beer
J. O. 65	12	179	65	60	− 5	4	+	Diarrhea, Vomiting, Heart burn	Cereals, milk, fruits, coffee, wine, beer
J. H. 66	11	168	77	52	−25	6	−	Anorexia	Meat, fish, cereals, milk, wine, beer

Summary: The Patient After Total Gastrectomy

The lack of a food reservoir and the possibility of a continuous esophageal reflux of bile and pancreatic juices are the main consequences of a total gastrectomy. By using the small intestine to create a substitute stomach, either in the form of a long, interposed jejunal loop or in the form of a jejunal pouch, decisive improvements in the postoperative quality of life of stomachless patients were achieved. The so-called agastric dystrophy is thereby primarily reduced to a sufficient caloric intake and the necessary substitution of vitamin B_{12}.

The maintenance of the duodenal passage is of only subordinate importance to the future quality of life of these patients. There is, however, the possibility that a maintained duodenal passage furthers speedier adaptation to the condition of being without a stomach. Even if there is no duodenal passage, malassimilation syndromes are rare. Certain deviations of the insulin secretion can be determined for cases lacking duodenal passage, but these deviations do not significantly influence the regulation of the glucose metabolism. The release of gastrointestinal hormones in the stomachless patient with and without duodenal passage is at this time still uncertain. According to all previous information, however, this regulatory mechanism is of subordinate importance to the practical nutritional problems following gastrectomy. The intake of gastric enzyme and HCl-preparations is unnecessary, because even under physiological conditions, a very small portion of protein digestion is effected by gastric peptidases. The necessity of providing a stomachless patient with pancreatic enzymes needs to be determined for each individual case. Adding these enzymes to the ingested foods as soon as possible yields advantages, especially for deep enteroanastomoses, since foods blend with pancreatic juices at a relatively late stage in this case.

Reflux esophagitis, which also constitutes a severe encumbrance of gastrectomized patients, on the other hand, can only be controlled by means of suitable surgical procedures.

9 Experiences with Various Reconstructive Methods After Total Gastrectomy

Various Types of Reconstructive Methods After Gastrectomy

Introduction

The long-term development following gastrectomy is frequently agonizing, so that the term agastric dystrophy was coined. Severe reflux esophagitis, lack of appetite, and a sensation of fullness, an early and late postalimentary syndrome can result in such considerable subjective discomfort, that sufficient intake of nutrients with a satisfactory caloric substitution no longer becomes possible.

Our own examinations of patients, on whom a gastrectomy with simple esophagojejunostomy according to Graham had been performed between 5 and 11 years before, demonstrated that the subjectively debilitating consequences were above all responsible for creating increased suffering (Merkle et al., 1976). Malnutrition is a factor only until the small intestine, which is now connected to the esophagus, has sufficiently adapted to the increased volume of food. There is a reduction in weight over the first 1–2 years, which is compensated after this term if there is no recurrence of the cancer. Only 10%–25% of the patients remained underweight. Thus, malabsorption only seems to play a subordinate role. There was, for instance, no discrepancy found in the Vitamin A test as criterium for the digestion and absorption of fat. This is in accord with the investigations of Bradley et al. (1975), who calculated a loss of fat of 17%–69% and a nitrogen loss of 18%–45% after gastrectomy in the course of their reexaminations. This is equivalent to a caloric loss of 100–500 calories. If this loss of calories is compensated by an increased input after adaptation of the intestinal volume, an undue loss of weight can be avoided.

The most conspicuous and most excruciating complaint after gastrectomy is a severe reflux esophagitis caused by the neutralization of the anti-reflux mechanism. The complaints can lead to persistent anorexia. The early and late postalimentary syndrome is a subordinate factor.

The problem of not having a stomach can thus be reduced to more or less morphological problems, which can be technically solved. The major requirements after total gastrectomy are consequently concerned with the creation of a reservoir and of an anti-reflux mechanism. A number of technical procedures for both have been specified, and their characteristic methods will be contrasted in the following chapter.

Certain trends can be established, although a definitive statement concerning the validity of one method in favor of another is naturally not possible due to the lack of prospective, randomized clinical investigations.

Esophagojejunostomy Following Gastrectomy for Gastric Carcinoma – A Follow-Up Study

M. M. Linder, C. Mennicken, and M. Trede

Introduction

In Mannheim, a staged operative therapy in curable gastric carcinoma is performed. Differentiating factors are: localization, size, and metastasis of the tumor and general aspects such as, age and other preoperative risk factors (Table 1). In small tumors localized in the distal half of the stomach and with probably only perigastric lymph node metastases, a three-fourths gastric resection is thought to be sufficient. Omentectomy is also performed. For large tumors, tumors in the proximal gastric half, and those with probable metastases along the left gastric artery, a gastrectomy is performed (including omentum and spleen). Intestinal continuity is reestablished by jejunal interposition (Longmire). In cases with high risk, old age (70 years of age), and questionable curability, an esophagojejunostomy is done. According to Schlatter, a retrocolic terminolateral esophagojejunostomy is performed and an inframesocolic jejunojejunostomy (Braun) is done in addition.

Material and Methods

From October 1972 until September 1978, 693 patients with gastric carcinoma were operated upon (Table 2). One-fifth of these patients had an exploratory

Table 1. Differentiated operative therapy for gastric carcinoma with the intention of cure

Tumor in the distal half of the stomach, occupation of only perigastric lymph nodes 3/4 Gastric resection	→
Proximal gastric tumor, nodes along the left gastric artery occupied Gastrectomy, reconstruction of continuity: 1) Interposition of jejunum 2) Terminolateral esophagojejunostomy (old age, high risk)	→

Table 2. 693 operations for gastric carcinoma, October 1972 – September 1978

Gastric resection	315	45.4%
Gastrectomy	123	17.8%
Gastroenterostomy	122	17.6%
Exploratory laparotomy	133	19.2%
Total	693	100%

laparotomy only, the tumors were inoperable, but no serious symptoms were present necessitating palliative operations. In 45% of the cases, gastric resection was performed. Gastrectomy was done in 18%.

Intestinal continuity was reconstructed by esophagojejunostomy in 79 (64%) patients, by jejunal interposition in 43 (35%), and esophagoduodenostomy in one (Table 3). Age distribution in esophagojejunostomy showed the preponderance of old patients compared to the jejunal interposition group: one-third of the patients with esophagojejunostomy were over 70 years of age, whereas only one-ninth were over 70 in the group with jejunal interposition.

For the Reisensburg Symposium, the 79 patients with esophagojejunostomy were analyzed. Postoperative complications, hospital mortality, and survival until 1 October 1978 were analyzed. Surviving patients were interrogated by a checklist that included all point of the Ulm catalogue of postoperative criteria for gastric cancer patients. A physical examination and endoscopy with biopsy were planned for each surviving patient.

Results

Ten of 79 (12.7%) patients with esophagojejunostomy died during their hospital stay, four from an anastomotic leakage, three from pulmonary embolism, two from pneumonia, and one from cerebral insufficiency (Table 4). An additional 28 of 79 (35.5%) patients succumbed until October 1978. Contact was lost in three cases. Thirty-eight of 79 (48.1%) patients survived; 33 of 38 (87%) returned the checklist asking for subjective and objective parameters of their postoperative life. There was no sign of recurrence. In 25 of 38 (66%) patients, endoscopy was performed and biopsies taken for histological examination and grading of esophagitis.

Table 3. 123 gastrectomies for gastric carcinoma; reconstruction of intestinal continuity

Esophagojejunostomy	79	64%
Interposition of jejunum	43	35%
Esophagoduodenostomy	1	1%
Total	123	100%

Table 4. 79 esophagojejunostomies (Oct. 1972 – Sept. 1978); follow-up until October 1978

Hospital mortality			10	12.7%
Anastomotic leak	4	5%		
Pulmonary emb.	3	3.8%		
Pneumonia	2	2.6%		
Dead by October, 1978			28	35.5%
Lost contact			3	3.7%
Alive			38	48.1%
Checklist returned	33	87%		
Gastroscopy done	25	66%		
Total			79	100%

History

1) The mean postoperative observation time was only 14.5 months (Table 5).
2) Four-fifths of the followed-up patients were already retired before gastrectomy.
3) Quality of life was rated as good by 27 (82%) patients.
4) Mean frequency of daily food intake was 5.1.
5) Repeated hospitalization was necessary by one patient with ileus. He was successfully treated conservatively.

Symptoms

Six (18%) patients felt deterioration after gastrectomy (Table 6). The poor results were due to reflux in four patients and to burning sensation in one patient. In one patient, no anatomic cause could be found.

Postprandial fullness, abdominal oppression, vomiting, dumping, diarrhea, and heartburn were treated medically.

Body weight was lost in 26 of 33 patients. The mean loss amounted to 15 kg, but the weight was compared to the preoperative state and remains constant today.

Table 5. Follow-up I – history; 33 esophagojejunostomies

1) Mean postoperative observation 14 months	
2) Occupation:	4/5 already retired preop.
3) Quality of life	good: 27
4) Mean food intake/day	5 ×
5) Repeated hospitalization	1 patient (ileus, treated conservatively)

Table 6. Follow-up II – symptoms, 33 esophagojejunostomies.

1) Subjective rating,	better:	18	82% (better + unchanged)
	unchanged:	9	
	deteriorated:	6	18%
2) Postprandial fullness		18	
3) Abdominal oppression		15	
4) Occasional vomiting		7	
5) Dumping		2	
6) Diarrhea		2	
7) Heartburn		14	
8) Body weight vs. preop.			
	gained	4	
	constant	3	
	lost	26	

Table 7. Follow-up III – objective findings; gastroscopy in 25 esophagojejunostomies – histology

Macroscopic appearance:		
Reflux esophagitis	*12*	48%
with symptoms	4	16%
Histological extent of esophagitis:		
Low grade	8	
Extensive	2	25% (Extensive + Ulcerating)
Ulcerating	1	
Dysplasia	1	

Endoscopy and Histology

Macroscopically, 12 of 25 (48%) patients showed signs of reflux esophagitis; there was no stenosis (Table 7). In only 4 of these 12 patients did esophagitis produced symptoms.

Histologically, esophagitis was severe in only 3 of the 12 patients with macroscopic esophagitis. Eight showed low-grade inflammation and one patient demonstrated mucosal dysplasia.

Summary

Patients of the last 6 years (693) with operations for gastric carcinoma are presented. A staged operative therapy was practiced. One hundred and twenty-three gastrectomies were done, intestinal continuity was reestablished in 79 by esophagojejunostomy, and in 43 by jejunal interposition. Old age, poor risk, and uncertain curability represented indications for the time-saving esophagojejunostomy. Three-fourths of the esophagojejunostomy patients were over 60 years of age, one-third over 70. Hospital mortality was 12.7%. No real 5-year survival rates exist as yet. Subjectively, four fifths of the followed-up surviving patients felt equal or better compared to the preoperative period.

Poor results in six (18%) patients were due to reflux in four and heartburn in one. In one case, no anatomic cause could be found. Endoscopically, reflux esophagitis was found in one-half of the patients. But only one-third of these 12 patients had correlating symptoms. Only 3 of 12 patients with macroscopic esophagitis suffered from extensive histological esophagitis.

The results of this follow-up study seem to justify the continued use of esophagojejunostomy, even though it is not so popular. It should be limited, though, to patients of high age, poor risk, and to cases with uncertain curability.

Mortality and Morbidity After Esophagojejunostomy

V. Seeger and F. P. Gall

The value of different methods for reconstruction of the digestive tract after total gastrectomy must be judged according to the incidence of anastomotic leakage, primary mortality, reflux esophagitis, and the patient's postoperative state of nourishment.

In the surgical department of the City Hospital, Fürth, 87 gastrectomies were carried out between 1970 and 1977, 85 were for cancer of the stomach. One-fourth of the patients were over 70 years of age and one-half over 60.

Two different methods of reconstruction were used. In 69 patients, an esophagojejunostomy according to the method described by Graham was performed using a two-layered end-to-side anastomosis. As shown in Fig. 1, the

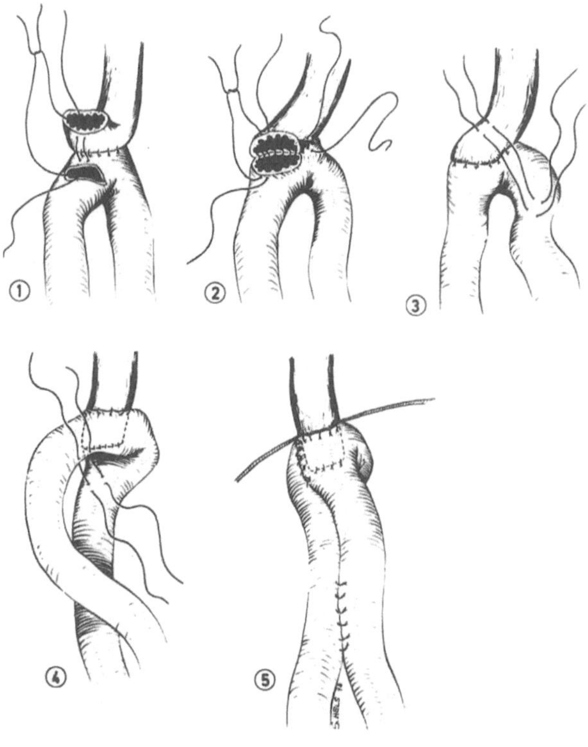

Fig. 1. Technique used in Graham's esophagojejunostomy

Table 1. Types of reconstruction in 87 gastrectomies (1970 – 1977)

Type of reconstruction	n	Primary postop. lethality	Suture insufficiency n	†
Graham's anastomosis	69	3 (4.3%)	2 (2.9%)	1
Roux's anastomosis	18	3 (16.6%)	4 (24.5%)	3
Total	87	6 (6.9%)		

anastomosis is covered by the afferent jejunal loop in a sandwich-like fashion. This results in a jejunal plication similar to that described in Schreiber and Peiper's method. In 18 carcinomas of the gastric stump, reconstruction after gastrectomy was carried out by a Roux-en-Y anastomosis.

Six of 87 patients who underwent total gastrectomy died in the postoperative period; three after the Graham and three after the Roux-en-Y anastomosis. This represents a primary mortality of 6.9%. These operations were performed by eight different surgeons.

The nutritional state of the 58 patients who had follow-up examinations was satisfactory. In 23.2%, the body weight remained stationary; 33.3% of the patients gained an average of 3.3 kg and 42.3% lost an average of 8 kg body weight. No patient suffered from severe reflux esophagitis requiring treatment.

A comparison of the two anastomotic techniques used showed that among 69 patients with a Graham anastomosis, anastomotic leakage occurred in two cases corresponding to 2.9% (Table 1). With a Roux-en-Y anastomosis, on the other hand, 4 of 18 cases (24.5%) showed this complication.

The esophagojejunostomy as described by Graham using a sandwich technique has, in our department, proved to be the most reliable method for reconstruction of the digestive tract after total gastrectomy. It resulted in an incidence of anastomotic leakage of only 2.9%. The Roux-en-Y anastomosis, on the other hand, had an incidence of anastomotic leakage as high as 24.5%. Therefore, in the future, we will use the Graham method exclusively in all total gastrectomies after Billroth-II resections.

Summary

Two different surgical techniques were employed in a total of 87 gastrectomies between 1970 and 1977. In 69 cases, an esophagojejunostomy was constructed using Graham's technique, and in 18 cases, Roux's anastomosis was performed. One-quarter of the patients were over 70 years old and one-half of the patients over 60 years old. The primary lethality of the operation was 6.9%. Suture insufficiency occurred in 2.9% of Graham's anastomoses and in 22.2% of Roux's anastomoses. In follow-up examinations, 58 of the patients were described as satisfactorily nourished. No patient suffered from severe reflux esophagitis.

References

1. Bünte, H., Döring, J.: Erfahruangen mit 200 totalen Gastrektomien beim Magencarcinom: Bruns Beitr. Klin. Chir. *220*, 244–252 (1973)
2. Hegemann, G., Gall, F.: Die Behandlung des Magencarcinoms durch totale Magenentfernung; Dtsch. Med. Wochenschr. *93*, 329–335 (1968)
3. Schreiber, H. W. et al.: Oesophagojejunostomie. Langenbecks Arch. Chir. *338*, 159 (1975)
4. Peiper, H. J., Siewert, R.: Magenersatz. Chirurg *49*, 81–88 (1978)

Jejunal Interposition

R. Pichlmayr, H.-J. Meyer, and G. Tidow

Introduction

If liberal criteria for a gastrectomy are to be used so that it becomes a routine operation – in our case specifically the gastrectomy *"de principe"* – as well as the palliative gastrectomy, it is advisable that the technique used in the subsequent reconstruction be as simple and take as little time as possible [12]. The simplest procedure is said to be the esophagojejunostomy with an anastomosis according to Braun. In previous years, we used this method a total of 65 times; our patients often had severe postoperative reflux complaints despite our using a long jejunal loop and ensuring that the Braun anastomosis was exactly placed and sufficiently deep: thus, it seemed to us that a change in the operative procedure was necessary.

Since 1974, we carry out isoperistaltic jejunal interposition according to Longmire and Beal [8] using a long loop as reported by Gütgemann-Schreiber [4, 13] whereby the modified end-to-side esophagojejunostomy proposed by Seo [16] is performed. A total of 144 patients have been operated using this method, one of whom with a proximal end-to-end anastomosis. In a further 26 gastrectomies, an isoperistaltic segment of small intestine was removed and the anastomosis carried out according to Roux-en-Y-anastomosis.

Procedure

The jejunal loop should be approximately 30 – 35 cm long [4, 8, 13, 18]. In order to obtain a segment of this length and also for reasons of vascular supply, the so-called second jejunal loop is used, that is, that segment beginning approximately 15 – 20 cm distal of the duodenojejunal flexure. Once the blood vessels have been exposed, the proximal mesenteric vessels are cut, whereby the loop to be interposed is supplied asymetrically by the distal mesenteric vessels. Apart from the anastomosis with the duodenum, the distal jejunal segment only has to be mobilized for a short distance. Thus, severance of the distal mesenteric vessels at this stage of the resection is not necessary in most cases, thus providing an additional guarantee of adequate vascular supply [11]. In order that any circulatory disturbances occurring within the jejunal loop as a result of the erroneous cutting of mesenteric vessels are recognized in time, total mobilization of the mesenterium is then carried out as well as the bilateral, i.e., also aboral, severance of the loop of the small intestine *before* commencing the anastomosis. Adequate blood supply and a position of the loop where it is not subject to tension must be guaranteed in order to prevent subsequent necrosis. The loop is retrocolically pulled through a slit in the mesocolon near the duodenojejunal flexure.

The antimesenteric jejunal incision for the proximal anastomosis should be approximately 5 cm long in order to prevent a subsequent stenosis due to scar tissue. We perform an end-to-side esophagojejunostomy. With this procedure, the serosa is adequately covered on all sides, thus providing a form of protection for the anastomosis [11, 15]; furthermore, the weight of the mesenterium pulls on the entire anastomosis and not directly on one point only. The oral end of the segment usually lies under the left subphrenic space; if it is 4–6 cm long, no functional or mechanical disadvantages are to be expected.

The sutures in the proximal anastomosis are placed in a single row; in our procedure, the esophageal mucosa is not penetrated. After the posterior wall of the esophagus has been exposed, only the esophageal musculature is severed and pushed back without cutting the submucosa, so that when the esophageal cuff is removed later, the posterior row of sutures is covered by the proximal, overlapping esophageal mucosa [1]. For the posterior and anterior wall of the anastomosis, seven interrupted sutures in each case seem appropriate, using a non-traumatizing absorbable material (3/0). The jejunoduodenostomy and jejuno-jejunostomy are carried out end-to-end, with our method, in a single row using a non-traumatizing, absorbable material.

To relieve the jejunal loop, the stomach probe is placed in such a position that its perforations lie below the esophagojejunostomy. Abdominal drainage is carried out in the splenic area; if necessary, a second drainage is laid in the subhepatic area.

Both the stomach probe and the drainage are only removed after the possibility of a suture insufficiency has been ruled out by X-ray examination on the fifth postoperative day.

Decisive criteria in judging the results of the substitute stomach after gastrectomy with the isoperistaltic jejunal interposition are the postoperative morbidity and mortality due mainly to suture insufficiency of the esophagojejunostomy [5, 10, 15]. On the other hand, the long-term morbidity is due to the jejuno-esophageal reflux as well as the loss of the stomach in regard to its function as a reservoir [2, 3, 6, 9, 14].

Postoperative Morbidity and Mortality

Anastomotic insufficiency after total gastrectomy can cause a series of different clinical symptoms, depending on the quantity of secretion leaking out, the time at which this occurred, and the adhesions which have thereby developed. Of 235 total gastrectomies, we observed a proximal suture insufficiency 22 times (9.4%); 15 times (10.4%) after jejunal interposition, and 7 times (10.8%) after esophagojejunostomy. As a result of a clear-cut peritonitis, a relaparotomy was performed in three cases, in one case, the insufficiency could be resutured, in two cases external drainage was carried out. Two of the reoperated patients died. In those cases where the symptoms were very protected, the indwelling drainage was still in contact with the insufficiency in 19 patients, thus enabling them to receive conservative treatment, whereby 6 (31.6%) subsequently died.

A proximal anastomotic insufficiency was fatal in eight cases (36.4%); four times (26.7%) after a jejunal interposition, and four times (57.1%) after esophagojejunostomy (Tables 1 and 2). In our opinion, a suture insufficiency, when it occurs at a very early stage (1 – 2 days, postoperatively), should be treated by relaparotomy; one cannot reckon with the spontaneous demarcation of the insufficiency at such an early stage postoperatively – that is, a diffuse peritonitis is likely – and the local tissue conditions at this stage occasionally permit the resuturing of the insufficiency. At a later stage, the procedure taken depends on the patency of the indwelling drainage and on the abdominal findings; if the drainage is still in contact with the insufficiency and/or a severe local or diffuse peritonitis can be ruled out, then a conservative method of treatment is appropriate. Continuous observation of the patient is necessary. In particular, food intake is forbidden, constant aspiration of the secretion from the loop via a transnasal probe, high caloric parenteral nutrition, as well as X-ray

Table 1. Total gastrectomies: rupture of the esophago-enteric anastomosis and postoperative mortality (1 May 1968 – 31 December 1977)

Total gastrectomies		Anastomotic leakage				Postoperative mortality			
		Total		Lethal		Total		Anastomotic leakage	
	n	n	%	n	%	n	%	n	%
Total	235	22	9.4	8	36.4	28	11.9	8	3.4
Esophagojejunostomy	65	7	10.8	4	57.1	14	21.5	4	6.2
Jejunal interposition	144	15	10.4	4	26.7	9	6.3	4	2.8
Roux-en-Y reconstruction	26	0	0	0	0	5	19.2	0	0

Table 2. Total gastrectomies (n = 235). Rupture of the esophago-enteric anastomosis, therapy, and mortality

Anastomotic leakage	Therapy and mortality							
	Conservative				Operative			
n	n	%	n	%	n	%	n	%
Total 22	19	86.4	6	31.6	3	13.6	2	66.7
Esophagojejunostomy 7	5	71.4	3	60	2	28.6	1	50
Jejunal interposition 15	14	93.3	3	21.4	1	6.7	1	100

controls after the 10th day must be carried out. If, however, acute symptoms or signs of peritonitis develop during this treatment, that is, the indwelling drainage does not appear to be effective, then a relaparotomy with copious external drainage, internal aspiration, etc. [17] is necessary. The local resuturing of the anastomosis at this stage is no longer possible (Table 3).

Long-term Morbidity

Our investigations of the number and kind of pathophysiological changes among our patients after gastrectomy are not yet completed. Thus, at present only a preliminary statement can be made. In particular, it should be mentioned that a clinically manifest reflux esophagitis after the isoperistaltic interposition of a long jejunal loop did not occur (Table 4). A duodenojejunoesophageal reflux could not be detected by hepato-biliary sequential scintigraphy [7]. A slight esophageal reflux could be induced during the X-ray examination using the appropriate technique, but this did not appear to be clinically relevant.

We twice observed an additional loss in weight after gastrectomy – admittedly, the group of patients in the follow-up examination was small – whereas the other patients retained their weight or else gained up to 7 kg (Table 5). None of the patients from this group complained of postprandial diarrhea or dumping syndrome.

Table 3. Therapy of proximal suture insufficiency after total gastrectomy

Early insufficiency and diagnosis (1. and 2. day postop.)	*Operative* therapy; if possible resuturing
Late insufficiency and diagnosis (from 3. day postop.)	*Conservative* therapy; absence of acute symptoms or peritonitis *Operative* therapy (drainage); presence of acute symptoms or clear-cut peritonitis

Table 4. Functional results after total gastrectomy and jejunal interposition

Pain of reflux

Postoperative period (months)	Patients (n)	Clinical signs (n)
12	57	0
24	28	0
36	18	0

Table 5. Functional results after total gastrectomy and jejunal interposition

Body weight		
Decrease		2 patients
Steady		11 patients
Increase		12 patients
	total	25 patients
Meals each day		4–10
Postoperative period		4–26 months

Conclusions

1) The jejunal interposition was used a total of 144 times. Between 1974 and 1977, the mortality rate with this method was 6.4%. It is thereby superior to the other procedures used by us.

2) After jejunal interposition, an insufficiency at the esophageal anastomosis occurred in 10.4% which – following conservative therapy in most cases – proved fatal in 26.7%. This is 2.8% of the total mortality rate. The equally high insufficiency rate after the simple esophagojejunostomy according to Graham resulted in a markedly higher mortality even though conservative therapy was applied. This may possibly be due to the fact that the site of the anastomosis was not completely excluded from the passage of the duodenal secretion.

3) The long-term morbidity according to our results is low, that is, reflux complaints did not occur and the nutritive situation was satisfactory.

4) Thus from the functional point of view, the jejunal interposition is suitable for routine use as a substitute stomach following gastrectomy and represents, in our opinion, a satisfactory compromise between simple esophagojejunostomy on the one hand, and complicated operative procedures on the other. The latter, in our opinion, may be used in selected cases. Admittedly, the insufficiency quota in our patients of approximately 10% has not yet been satisfactorily solved. The reasons for the insufficiency, however, may be caused by inadequate surgical technique of the individual surgeon or by a general shortcoming of the method. Perhaps such personal failure – in the last analysis, to a certain extent unavoidable – can be reduced even further, when other kinds of substitute stomachs are used.

References

1. Borst, H. G., Dragojevic, D.: Resektionsbehandlung des Speiseröhrencarcinoms mit Magenüberbrückung. Zentralbl. Chirurgie *99*, 189–190 (1974)
2. Brünner, H., Kempf, P.: Der Dünndarmersatzmagen. Dtsch. Med. Wochenschr. *100*, 1044–1047 (1975)
3. Goebell, H.: Magenersatz, Funktionsausfälle und erforderliche Substitutionstherapie. Chirurg *49*, 89–94 (1978)

4. Gütgemann, A.: Totale Gastrektomie beim Magenkrebs. Chirurg *23*, 474 – 479 (1952)
5. Häring, B., Eckart, J., John, St., de Pena Perez, R., Stallkamp, B., Tung, L. C., Waldschmidt, J.: Die Nahtinsuffizienz der oesophagealen Anastomose nach Gastrektomie und Cardiaresektion. Langenbecks Arch. Chir. *328*, 295 – 310 (1971)
6. Husemann, B., Groitl, H., Zirngibl, H.: Die totale Gastrektomie. Metabolische und chirurgische Aspekte. Munch. Med. Wochenschr. *120*, 561 – 566 (1978)
7. Löhlein, D., Reichelt, H.-G., Hundeshagen, H., Pichlmayr, R.: Die Anwendung einer neuen Methode zur Bestimmung des duodeno- und jejunogastralen Reflux nach Magenoperationen. Chirurg *48*, 588 – 591 (1977)
8. Longmire, W. P., jr., Beal, J. M.: Construction of a substitute gastric reservoir following total gastrectomy. Ann. Surg. *135*, 637 – 645 (1952)
9. Merkle, P., Schlag, P., Krause, F.: Zur Frage der agastrischen Dystrophie nach Gastrektomie. Chirurg *47*, 380 – 383 (1976)
10. Nier, H., Ulrich, B., Jacobs, G., Günther, E., Rumpf, P.: Frühkomplikationen und Spätergebnisse nach totaler Gastrektomie. Langenbecks Arch. Chir. *340*, 263 – 272 (1976)
11. Pichlmayr, R., Grotelüschen, B.: Chirurgische Therapie. Berlin, Heidelberg, New York: Springer 1978
12. Pichlmayr, R., Meyer, H. J., van Alste, H. E.: Die Gastrektomie als Standardoperation beim Magencarcinom. 10th Int. Magensymposium: Magencarcinom – Frühdiagnostik und Therapie. Berlin, 1978. Stuttgart, Thieme, in press
13. Schreiber, H. W.: Radikalität und pathophysiologische Gesichtspunkte bei der Resektion des Magencarcinoms. Langenbecks Arch. Klin. Chir. *314*, 213 – 230 (1966)
14. Schumpelick, V., Begemann, F., Grossner, D., Schwoy, M., Garbrecht, A.: Reflux und Refluxverhütung im operierten Magen. Langenbecks Arch. Chir. (Suppl.) *78*, 7 – 12 (1978)
15. Sanchez, R. E., Gordon, H. E.: Complications of total gastrectomy. Arch. Surg. *100*, 136 – 139 (1970)
16. Seo, T.: Technik der totalen Gastrektomie mit Ersatzmagen: Zitiert nach Tomoda, M. Chirurg *23*, 264 – 268 (1952)
17. White, T. T., Harrison, R. C.: Reoperative gastrointestinal surgery. Boston: Little & Brown 1973
18. Winkler, R.: Der Ersatzmagen. Pathophysiologische und operative Technik. Z. Gastroenterol. *12*, 445 – 452 (1974)

Jejunal Interposition with Plication

R. Winkler, M. Pfeiffer, and H. W. Schreiber

Introduction

Concerning their functional results, the jejunal interposition introduced by Seo-Longmire and modified in the long-loop-type by Gütgemann is well established [1, 2, 9]. The advantages are:
- Orthograde physiological duodenal transit,
- Development of a reservoir capacity,
- Portional emptying,
- Induction of digestion causing a better stimulation and synchronization of duodeno-bilio-pancreatic secretion,
- Prevention of reflux by one-way peristaltics and by occlusion of the esophagus on account of the tension of the filled loop – tension-sphincter-mechanism [8], and
- Function-adapted onset of substitution therapy.

The method is consequent, clear, and comparatively simple. However, the esophagojejunal junction remains a "weak point" regarding operative security as well as postoperative function. Among the factors concerning the high frequency of postoperative leakage in esophageal anastomosis, the most important are:
- Loss of the peritoneal reflection after dissection of the esophagus,
- Longitudinal tension of the organ,
- Absence of well-defined suture layers, and
- Segmental blood supply, forming insufficient arcades.

The blood supply of the distant esophageal margin often seems to be unsatisfactory, because the most important vessels, recurrent from the stomach, have to be cut off. The upper next segmental arteries may attempt to carry out the resection to the mediastinal cavity [3].

If the esophagus is anastomized end-to-end to the isolated jejunal loop, it is connected with another part at risk of necrosis because of worsened blood supply and additional anemia by sutures and esophageal tension. Therefore dehiscence seems unavoidable to some degree and anatomically bound.

Technique

We translocated the anastomosis to the well-supplied proximal third of the interposed jejunum [6, 9, 10]. The anastomosis is done one layer end-to-side, the oral end of the interposed jejunum is closed blindly, and the overlapping part, measuring about 10 – 15 cm is wrapped around the anastomotic region (Figs. 1a – b). Thus, all sutures, at risk of leakage, are invaginated into a peritoneal pouch in analogy to the sandwich-technique. Peritoneal adhesions will form within 8 h, so that necrosis or leakage, developing about the fourth postoperative day, will drain into the jejunal cavity. Additionally, the pouch forms a fundoplication-like closure of the terminal esophagus, thus supporting reflux prevention [6, 7].

The functional length of the interposed loop has to exceed 25 cm so that a total loop of 40 cm has to be isolated and led up behind the transverse colon. The interposed jejunum must form a siphon-like curve. The pouch may also be fixed to the diaphragm.

The remaining anastomosis is done end-to-end. Alternatively, the jejunoduodenostomy may be adapted end-to-side contrapapillary. Thus, duodenojejunal reflux may be reduced and portional emptying of the gastric replacement is supported; on the other hand, duodenal reflux is wanted to some degree in order to improve digestion in the interposed jejunum. Up to now, it has not been decided whether there is any practical advantage of the latter modification.

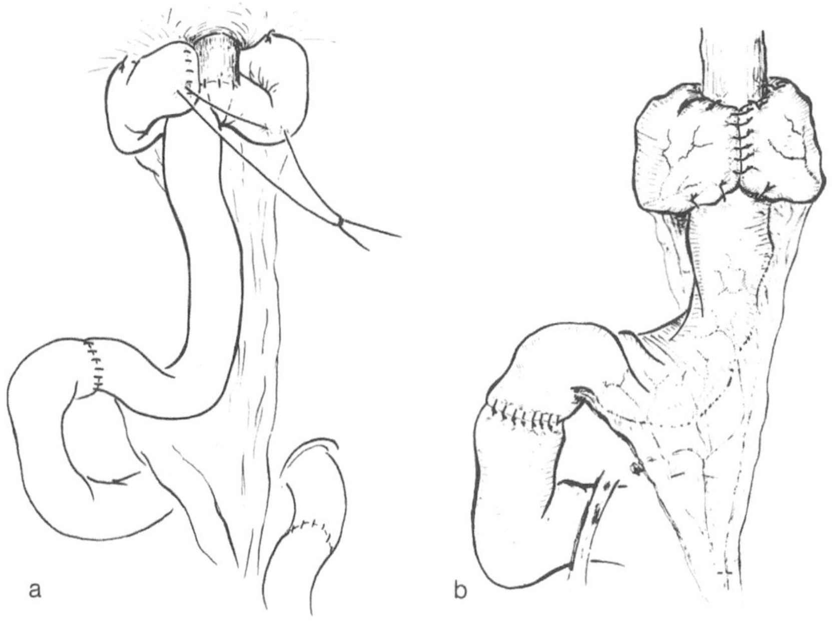

Fig. 1a and b. Scheme of the technique of jejunoplication.
a) The loop is prepared for plication. Note the position of the esophagojejunal junction. Retroesophagically, the pouch is fixed to the diaphragm. b) Completed plication. Note some additional sutures to the esophagus and the interposed jejunum. All suture lines, at risk of leakage, are peritoneally covered

Early Results

Since 1974, the method of jejunal interposition was used in 49 cases of gastric cancer. An amazing initial series of 12 patients with totally uncomplicated outcome was followed by less satisfying results because of enhancement of indications and an increasing number of surgeons performing the operation. In all, we lost six patients (12%). Compared to 1965 – 1973, this means a reduction of postoperative mortality of 13%. (However, this period was characterized by many operative procedures, among which the Graham-Nissen-modification had dominated). The most important reason for this development was the decrease of local complications. While in the former series, 55% of all patients developed local failure, this was now reduced to 33%. The leading complication, anastomotical dehiscence, was reduced from 44% to 22%. Furthermore, these patients had a less dramatic outcome. This may be illustrated by the causes of postoperative death: former, local complications had been the main reason for fatal development in 75%, now it only increased to 50%; in other words, whereas 20% of all patients in the early series died from operation-related complications, this was actually 6% (Tables 1 and 2).

Late Results

Clinical Findings

Naturally the varied technique does not alter the principally obvious fate of gastric cancer patients. As – on account of the high operative risk – indications

Table 1. Postoperative complications: Jejunal interposition with plication 1974 – 1978 (n = 49)

Leakage	apparent	5
	inapparent	6
Abscess (abdominal)		4
Stenosis (transient)		3
Ileus		3
Pancreatitis		1
Pleural exsudation/empyema		8
Cardio-respirat. disturbances		10

Table 2. Postoperative mortality (total number of deaths: 6). Jejunal interposition with plication 1974 – 1978 (n = 49)

Reason	Frequency
Leakage	3
Ileus	1
Pancreatitis	1
Pneumonia, pleural empyema	3
Cardiac infarction	1
Relaparotomy	3

for total gastrectomy are limited, improvement of survival times is not to be expected. Within 2 years after the operation, 41% died from recurrent or metastatic cancer. However, even among these patients – transient – melioration of quality of life was visible. Postoperative loss of body-weight was less severe. Patients free of recurrence regained their operative weight mainly within 6 months, although only a few patients regained their former weight. In the first year, the frequency of meals was reduced from median 8 to 4–5 times; 60% regarded their appetite as being normal. None suffered from deprivation. There were no typical aversions; fatty meals, legumes, and cabbage were most frequently refused. One-third had become annuitant because of their operation. Of the people still at work, one-third didn't feel as potent as before (Compare [2, 3, 5, 9]).

Most of the patients regarded their condition as being satisfactory. Condition and postoperative behavior were well correlated to the degree of information. The well-informed patient, with knowledge of the diagnosis and dubious prognosis, was much more capable of solving his problems, recreated quicker and adapted his personal way of life sooner. Diarrhea was merely obligate in the first postoperative weeks, however, of various intensity and duration. Only few patients spontaneously complained of pain relating to reflux, severe postprandial conditions, or regurgitation. Furthermore, these symptoms were inconstant in the same patient. None had Dumping-syndrome.

Rehospitalization resulted from recurrence [6], benign transient stenosis (3 suture-granuloma-disease), and late inflammatory complications [2].

Serological and Apparative Findings

There were no essential abnormalities among serological examinations at least 6 months after the operation. One-third had a slight normochromic anemia. Serum iron levels were normal in all cases, probably because of a regular substitution therapy. There were no pathological findings in enzyme-reactions, lipid and protein scale, and electrolyte balance. Qualitative analysis of stool showed a deficiency in protein digestion in 60%, in fat digestion in 10%.

Radiologically, the interposed jejunum tends to widen and elongate. This improves the reservoir function as well as the portional emptying. Transit times, therefore, normalized during this time. Filling of the plicating loop could be demonstrated regularly, preventing reflux in all cases (Fig. 2). Sometimes, sliding of the pouch could be observed, however, this did not seem to influence the occluding function.

Endoscopically, however, 30% had a moderate reflux and half of them had mild forms of esophagitis, which were verified histologically. These findings contrast with the radiological ones. In our former series, we had reflux in 80%, esophagitis in 60%, and severe forms in 20%. Biopsy from the interposed jejunum only offered lympho-histio- or plasmocellular infiltration of the submucosal stroma, but no metaplasia. Rigid esophagojejunal anastomosis not due to recurrence was found in five cases, but the anastomotic region could always be passed by the endoscope.

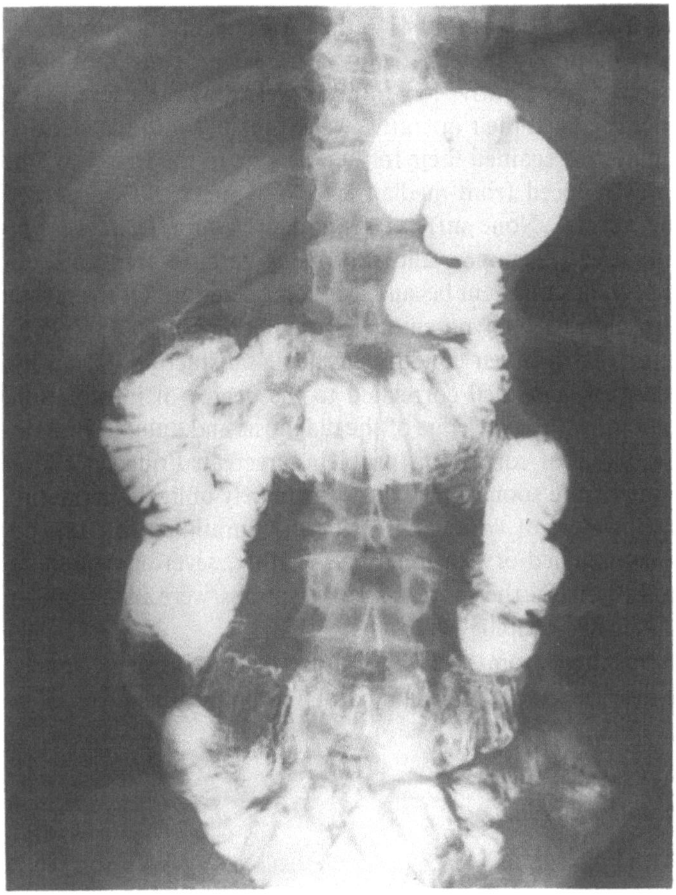

Fig. 2. X-ray of the interposed jejunum. Note the well-filled plicating pouch and the overlength of the interposed jejunum; no reflux to the esophagus

Conclusion

The most important advantages of jejunal interposition with plication concern the improvement of anastomotic healing and reflux prevention. The frequency of complicated or deleterious anastomotic leakage was reduced from 55% to 22%. Death rate due to local complications decreased from 75% to 50%. Whereas formerly the vaste majority of gastrectomized patients had reflux, some of them developing severe ulcerous esophagitis, only one-third of patients with plication suffered from moderate forms of reflux, most of them necessitating no regular therapy. The known advantages of jejunal interposition of Longmire, modified in the long loop type by Gütgemann, are still working. In all, restriction in the quality of life is tolerable, especially if the patient is informed. On account of the greater radicalness in cancer surgery, the results favor a more progressive basis for gastrectomy indications.

References

1. Bernhard, A., Schreiber, H. W., Bartsch, W. M., Braun, O.: Form und Funktion des Ersatzmagens nach totaler Magenresektion. Langenbecks Arch. Klin. Chir. *307*, 261 (1964)
2. Brünner, H., Kempf, P.: Der Dünndarmersatzmagen. Klinik und Ergebnisse nach 51 jejunalen Interpositionen. Dtsch. Med. Wochenschr. *100*, 1044 (1975)
3. Häring, R., Franke, H.: Gastrektomie und Kardiaresektion beim Magenkarzinom. Stuttgart: Thieme 1970
4. Merkle, P., Schlag, P., Krause, F.: Zur Frage der agastrischen Dystrophie nach Gastrektomie. Chirurg *47*, 380 (1976)
5. Schreiber, H. W., Eichfuß, H. P., Farthmann, E., Eckert, P.: Ösophagojejunostomie. Anastomosentechnik. Langenbecks Arch. Chir. *338*, 159 (1975)
6. Siewert, R., Peiper, H. J., Wallat, H.: Erste Erfahrungen mit der Ösophago-Jejunoplikatio. Bruns' Beitr. Klin. Chir. *221*, 343 (1974)
7. Stelzner, F., Lierse, W.: Der angiomuskuläre Dehnverschluß der terminalen Speiseröhre. Langenbecks Arch. Klin. Chir. *321*, 35 (1968)
8. Winkler, R.: Der Ersatzmagen. Pathophysiologie und operative Taktik. Z. Gastroenterol. *12*, 445 (1974)
9. Winkler, R., Wollbrink, W.: Zur Funktion des Ersatzmagens nach Gastrektomie. Med. Welt *29*, 1800 (1978)

Esophagojejunoplication

J. R. Siewert and G. Schattenmann

Since first described in 1973 [3], esophagojejunoplication has become the standard procedure in surgical reconstruction following gastrectomy at the Department of General Surgery of the University of Goettingen. The methodology and results of this procedure are presented in the following context.

Method

Subsequent to total gastrectomy and closure of the duodenum, intestinal continence is restored utilizing the first jejunal loop, which is passed retrocolically into the upper abdomen. A side-to-side enteroanastomosis of about 15 cm in length between ascending and descending limbs of the loop is established approximately 8 cm below the crest of the loop. The blind arch of the loop should effortlessly encompass a distance of about three fingers in diameter. In an area above the ventral suture of the anastomosis, an opening should remain about 3 – 4 cm long, which corresponds with the lumen of the esophagus. The esophageal stump is then sewn into this aperture utilizing an all-layer, one-row suture. The crescent of the jejunal loop is brought behind the esophageal stump when knotting the rear portion of the esophagus. The ventral anastomosis, likewise, entails an all-layer, one-row suture. After completion of the esophagojejunostomy, the lateral segments of the jejunum crescent are pulled forward around the front wall of the esophagus and fastened together with sero-serous singlebutton sutures. The establishment of a tensionless cuff can be guaranteed only if the crescent of the jejunal loop is devised in the above mentioned manner. The cuff tends to embrace the distal esophagus, especially the anastomosis. In order to prevent postoperative complications, it is suggested that the ascending limb be transposed to a position corresponding to the former large curvature. Finally, the jejunal loop is fixed to the edges of the mesocolon opening (Fig. 1).

This operation can also be carried out as an interposition. Accordingly, the jejunal loop must be detached at its base; the descending limb is anastomosed with the duodenum and the ascending limb closed. Small bowel continence is reconstructed by end-to-end anastomosis.

Cases and Indications

Figure 2 shows the underlying diseases that give cause to total gastrectomy in our clinic. When compared to former statistics, it can be concluded that cancer of the

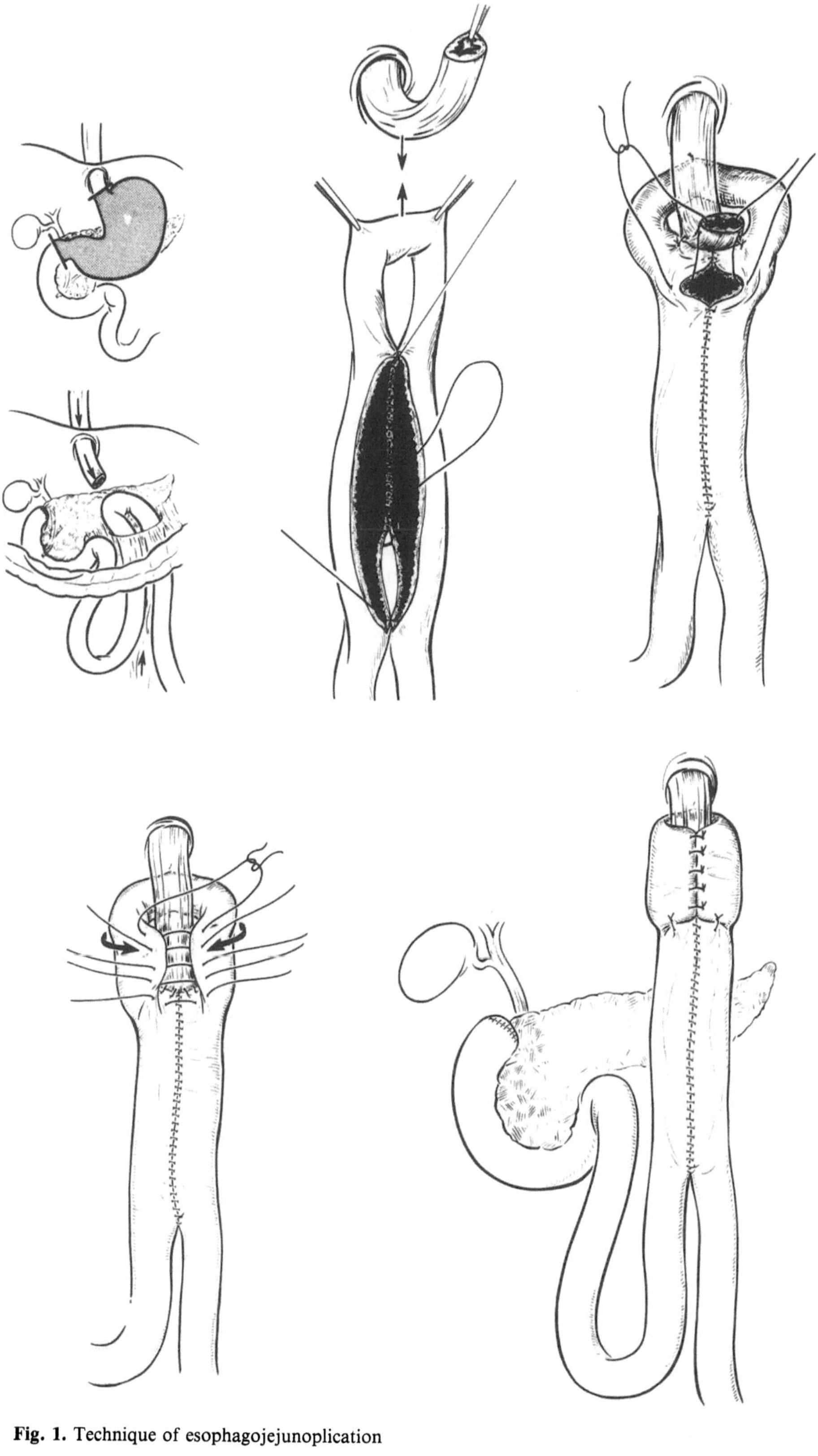

Fig. 1. Technique of esophagojejunoplication

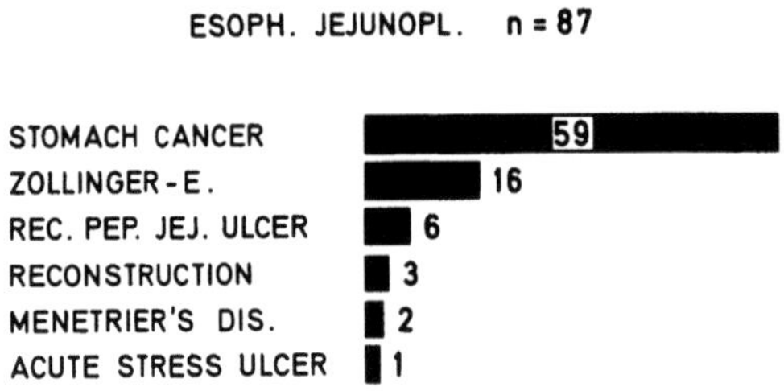

Fig. 2. Underlying disease indications for total gastrectomy

stomach as indicative for total gastrectomy has increased. Until 1974, these malignancies appeared in 51% of cases, increased to 61% in 1976 and now represent 67.5%. On the other hand, the number of cases of Zollinger-Ellison-Syndrome which were gastrectomized has steadily decreased. The possibility of medicamentous treatment for this syndrome has given rise to this trend. At this point, it would be proper to mention a patient who underwent total gastrectomy in a third operation because of recurrent hemorrhaging from acute gastroduodenal lesions. In all, 87 patients were gastrectomized between May 1972 and July 1978 and received esophagojejunoplications. The average age was 59.7 ± 10.5 years. Compared to our studies in 1974 and 1976, there was a noticeable increase in the mean age which, in 1974, was still 51.5 years. The same development can be seen in the increasing number of patients older than 60. In 1974, 24% were above the age of 60, whereas this number increased to 34.5% in 1978. The ratio of males to females was two to one (Fig. 3).

Results

Mortality Rate

Our average mortality rate was 16% (14 of 87 cases). This relatively high rate should perhaps be explained. In the initial phases of clinical studies regarding esophagojejunoplication, operative preference was given to patients with benign diseases, or with malign diseases having a favorable prognosis. Also, the number of operating teams was restricted to two. This series encompassed 28 patients. Of these, one patient died, representing a 3% mortality rate. In view of these good results, our clinic has in recent years continuously expanded the indication for total gastrectomy. This is documented by increasing average ages and by an increasing majority of stomach cancer patients undergoing total gastrectomy. This rate has risen from 51% in 1974 to 67.5% in 1978 (Fig. 4).

Very convincing is the reliability of the operation, which is reflected in the low incidence of esophagojejunal junction incompetence. Our three reported cases of incompetence all occurred during the introduction stage of esophagojejunoplication. All three incompetencies had untroubled outcomes; no patient died of this particular complication. Today, anastomosis incompetence is found in 3.4% of all cases (Fig. 5).

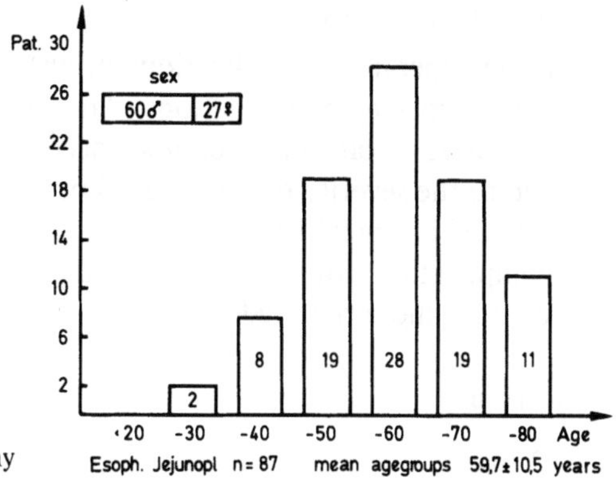

Fig. 3. Age of patients with total gastrectomy

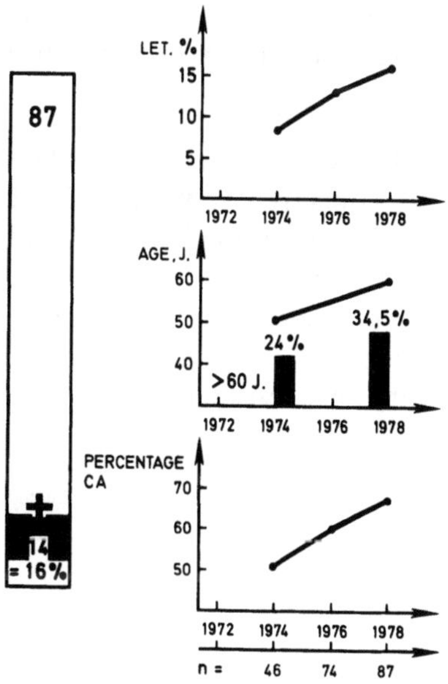

Fig. 4. Mortality rate of total gastrectomy in respect to time, age, and underlying disease

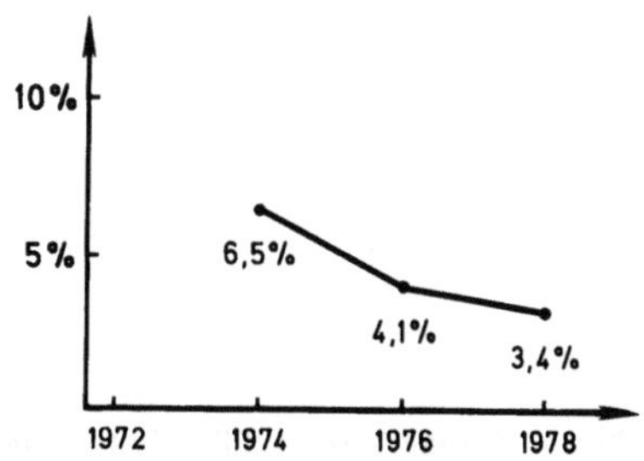

Fig. 5. Anastomosis incompetence in cases with esophagojejunoplication in relation to time

Other Complications

Acute postoperative complications occurred in 35.6% of cases. Figure 6 illustrates the types of complications. The majority of the patients succumbed to postoperative respiratory incompetence due, in all probability, to a high mean age and to the severity of the surgical procedure itself. As before, an ileus of the small bowel is typical following total gastrectomy. Six of our patients developed this complication; four underwent emergency surgery. The mortality rate was relatively low and amounted to 8%.

Follow-up

Of 87 patients who underwent surgery, 14 died in the immediate postoperative period. Seventy-three patients survived gastrectomy and were able to be discharged from the hospital. Of these, 33 patients died from underlying diseases up to 1 July 1978. Four patients could not be located or failed to report for their follow-ups. Consequently, 36 patients were able to participate in the follow-up examinations. The average observation period lasted 28.5 months; patients with benign diseases were observed for 39.6 months, those with malign underlying diseases were observed for 19.5 months (Fig. 7).

Follow-up Mode

Patients were called in for follow-ups after 3, 6 and 12 months, respectively, and subsequently, every 6 months. Intermittently, the findings were classified using the following standardized point system: patients with no complaints were given 0–1 point; those with easily manageable discomfort, 2–3 points; 4–5 points corresponded with low-degree, still treatable symptoms; 6–7 points meant moderate, continuous symptoms despite treatment; patients with continuous symptoms resisting therapy were given 8–10 points. Symptoms occurring during

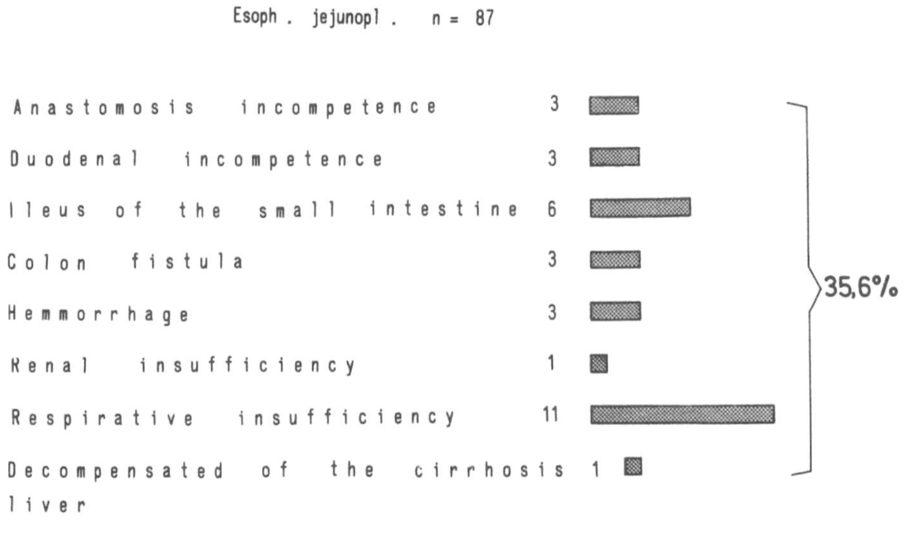

Fig. 6. Postoperative complications in patients with esophagojejunoplication

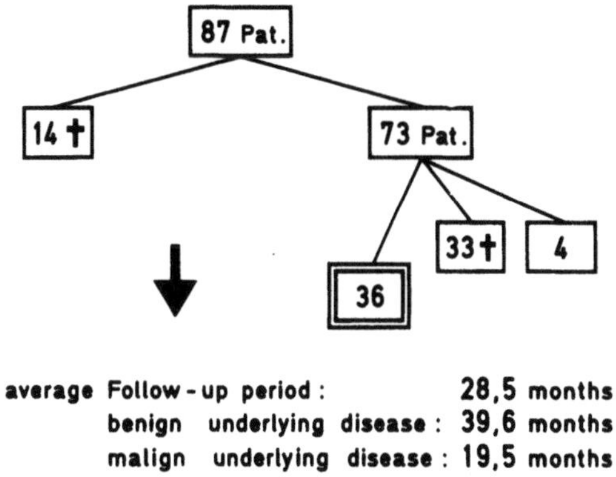

Fig. 7. Follow-up of patients with esophagojejunoplication

a single week were also included in the study. The following symptoms and complaints were acknowledged: heartburn or retrosternal pain, epigastric pain, dumping-like syndromes, diarrhea, and dysphagia.

Each follow-up examination included an upper G. I. series. During the examination, a standardized reflux-provocation procedure was conducted (testing during abdominal compression, with elevated lower extremities, and in a head-down-position). Endoscopy was also carried out. The macroscopic findings of the tubular portion of the esophagus were recorded in the manner set out in the literature, the passage through the anastomosis examined, and finally, the jejunal substitute for the stomach inspected.

Biopsies were taken under visual control from the jejunum and from a point 5 cm above the anastomosis. In order to study the reflux, pH testing was done in accordance with Tuttle and Grossman. For this purpose, 200 ml of 0.1 normal HCl solution with a pH of 1 were fed by tube into the substitute stomach. The tube was then removed and continous pH monitoring 5 cm above the anastomosis initiated. In addition, reflux-provocation through manual or active abdominal compression and elevation of the lower extremities was undertaken. The tests were concluded with manometry, utilizing pentagastrin-stimulation to locate the terminal esophagus muscle tissue.

Clinical Results

The studies which were transformed to a Visick-analog classification, showed excellent or good results in 73% of the cases. Seventeen percent were classified as Visick III, 10% as Visick IV (Fig. 8). The principle signs are illustrated in Fig. 8. There was a surprising congruency between the subjective complaints concerning retrosternal symptoms and the objective findings of the reflux tests. Dumping-like symptoms occurred in 10% of the patients interviewed. This relatively low percentage corresponds well with the findings of other authors. A closer analysis of the postoperative dysphagia in six patients seems necessary. Three of these patients developed immediate postoperative passage obstruction in the anas-

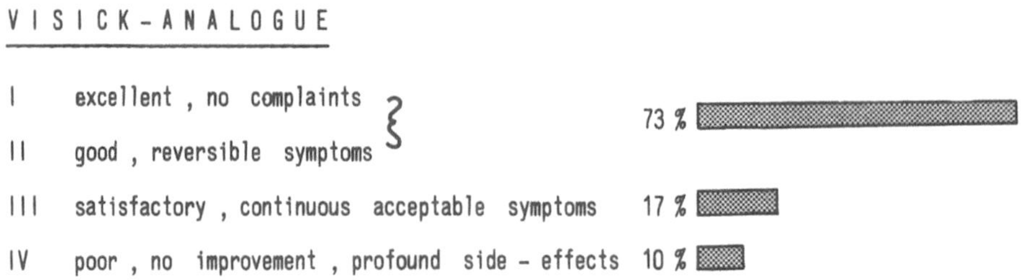

Fig. 8. Subjective results in patients with esophagojejunoplication

tomosis. Bougienage was necessary, which relieved two patients of their symptoms. One patient continued complaining of dysphagia despite normal findings in the upper G. I. series. The remaining three patients complained of dysphagia at a much later date. Here local recurrences of cancer proved to be the cause (Fig. 9).

Table 1 shows additional objective findings with respect to reflux disease, anastomosis status, and body weight variations. Reflux disease was diagnosed when two of the tests used (endoscopy and biopsy, radiology, pH-metry) were positive.

The rate of reflux disease was put at 6.9%. However, it should be mentioned that it was difficult to differentiate between reflux sequelae and surgical sequelae. In 18 cases, severe hyperplasia of the stratified epithelium was found, partly in the form of leukoplakia.

In three patients, stenosis of the anastomosis due to scarring was found and required subsequent bougienage.

With respect to weight variations, most patients showed a positive trend. Compared to the preoperative period, an average weight gain of 4.5 ± 0.4 kg was recorded. However, inspite of this weight gain, the average patient attained only 84.2% ± 14.2% of his ideal body weight.

Radiologically, no patient developed cuff complications, as they are sometimes seen in patients with fundoplication. In all patients, the jejunal substitute stomach dilated increasingly in correlation with the duration of the follow-up study. In part, volumes were reached that easily compare with those of a normal stomach. In this context, it is interesting to note that no patient needed more than four meals a day.

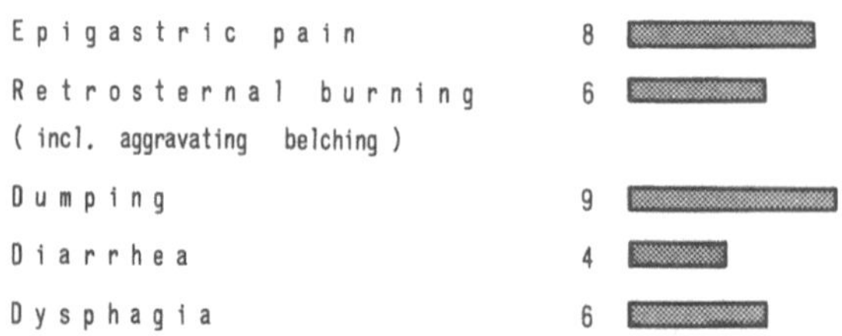

Fig. 9. Subjective complaints in patients with esophagojejunoplication

Table 1. Objective findings in patients with esophagojejunoplication

Objective Findings	
Reflux disease (Endoscopy – Biopsy) Reflux disease (X-ray) Reflux disease (pH-metry)	n = 6 (6.9%)
Anastomosis stenosis	n = 3 (3.4%)
Weight status	+4.5 + 0.4 kg
= ideal body weight	84.2 + 14.23%

Routine lab studies showed normal values in practically all cases. They are presented in Table 2.

Discussion and Conclusion

The ideas that eventually led to the development of esophagojejunoplication were concerned with the frequent postoperative jejunoesophageal reflux following traditional esophagojejunostomy. However, postoperative observations soon proved the fact that jejunal wrapping of the distal esophagus, that is, anastomosis, produced an uncommonly high degree of anastomosis competence. This unique advantage has led to the introduction of esophagojejunoplication as the exclusive standard reconstruction technique following total gastrectomy in our clinic.

This advantage of esophagojejunoplication is well documented here. The rate of anastomosis incompetence was 3.4% of 87 patients. It is important to note that not one patient died because of incompetence. A study of the results of a total of 1444 cases mentioned in the secondary literature indicates the average anastomosis incompetence rate in traditional surgical techniques to be 17.4%. The rate of additional complications (35.6%) compared with rates given by other authors. The total mortality rate of 16% also lay within the framework of published reports (total statistics: 4142 cases with 18.4% mortality). However, the mortality rate has been on the rise in recent years. The main reason for this is the increasingly liberal interpretation of the indication for total gastrectomy. This liberalization is reflected in the continuously rising average age of the patients undergoing surgery and in the high incidence of cancer patients included. It should be mentioned that the indication for total gastrectomy has in recent months been broadened to cover palliative gastrectomies for patients with metastatic stomach cancer. Finally, we would like to point out that total gastrectomy and jejunoplication are at present being performed by every chief resident at the Department for General Surgery in Goettingen. In all, 12 surgeons participated in the surgery of 87 patients.

Our follow-up studies showed that good to excellent clinical results could be attained with this surgical technique in 73% of cases. Laboratory values were all normal. The substantiation of reflux disease can cause great methodological

Table 2. Laboratory values in patients of total gastrectomy and esophagojejunoplication

Laboratory Values		
Total protein	6.8 ± 0.4 g%	(6.2 – 8.0)
Albumin	57.9 ± 6.77%	(57 – 68)
Serum iron	82.5 ± 39.3 µg%	(65 – 175)
Carotin level	46.0 ± 3.2 µg	(100 – 150)

problems. Taking these problems into account, reflux disease could be diagnosed in 6.9% of our patients. In no patient were the symptoms so severe that therapeutic intervention was necessary. The total rate of reflux was markedly below rates given by other authors. A collective statistic showed a reflux rate of 33.6% of 703 cases.

Improved conservative treatment of benign diseases has led to the selective and preferred use of total gastrectomy in the treatment of stomach cancer. The great majority of these patients undergo surgery at a relatively late stage of cancer. Here, an operative approach guaranteeing a high degree of reliability is of great advantage. Pathophysiological considerations, concerning, for example, the necessity of duodenal continence, are of value only to those patients with a prospect of long survival. They are warranted in patients with benign underlying diseases or with cancer to the $T_{1-2}N_0M_0$ stage. All advanced tumors should, in consideration of postoperative reliability, be surgically approached with a technique utilizing jejunoplication.

References

1. Peiper, H. J., Siewert, R.: Magenersatz. Chirurg *49*, 81 – 88 (1978)
2. Siewert, R., Meyer, H., Peiper, H. J.: Technik u. Ergebnisse der Oesophago-Jejunoplicatio. Langenbecks Arch. *343*, 45 – 58 (1976)
3. Siewert, R., Peiper, H. J., Jennewein, H. M., Waldeck, F.: Die Oesophago-Jejunoplicatio. Chirurg *44*, 115 – 120 (1973)

Comparative Analysis of Two Types of Gastric Replacement After Total Gastrectomy

D. Kummer, G. Kieninger, K. Anger, and H. P. Maier

The Surgical Department of the University of Tübingen performed 126 so-called gastric replacements following total gastrectomy between 1959 and 1978. During the first decade, the jejunal interposition of Longmire-Gütgemann [1, 4] was used exclusively, whereas in recent years, the jejunal interposition was done increasingly with an additional anisoperistaltic segment (Fig. 1) developed by Schrader and co-workers [5] in 1971. The latter type of gastric substitute is supposed to provide an increased reservoir function and thus better functional long-term results.

It could be shown that the rate of early postoperative complications and the postoperative mortality of approximately 5% following 83 reconstructions of the Longmire-Gütgemann type and 43 reconstructions of the Schrader type was not higher than following technically simpler methods of reconstruction [2, 3]. This analysis was undertaken to clarify, whether the anisoperistaltic segment really improves the function of the gastric substitute. For this follow-up study, the

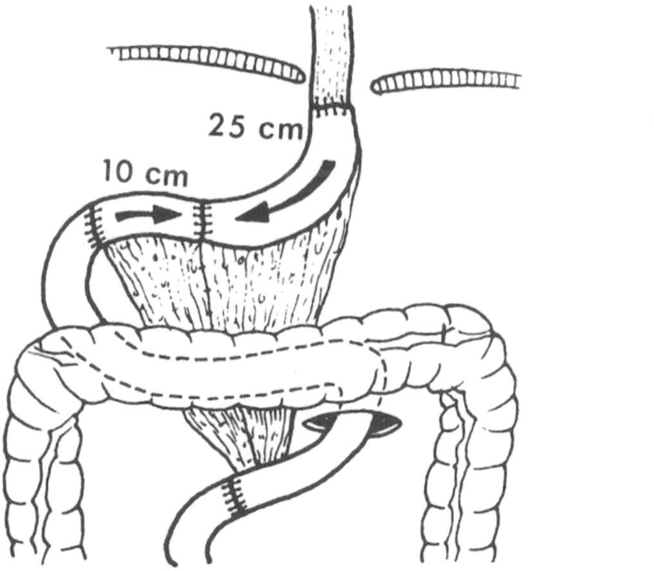

Fig. 1. Gastric substitute by means of iso-anisoperistaltic jejunal interposition

findings of 13 isoperistaltic jejunal interpositions (Longmire-Gütgemann) and of 16 iso-anisoperistaltic jejunal interpositions could be used as a comparison.

This, in relation to the total number of performed operations, only a small number of patients were controlled in periodic intervalls due to the still high rate of gastric cancer operated in an advanced tumor stage and to the rejection of control examinations by patients, who did not understand their necessity. Endoscopic findings could not be included in the analysis, since only one-third of the examined patients agreed to control endoscopy.

The comparison of the anamnestic data (Tables 1 and 2) shows that nearly all patients with a gastric substitute do not feel a considerable impairment to their ability to work. However, with certain reservations, it must be admitted that a good number of the patients have already reached the retirement age, and therefore do not work regularly. Independent of the type of gastric substitute, the patients must have 5 – 7 meals a day. There is no indigestibility of sweet dishes of farinceous products. Only after drinking milk, one-third of the patients reported upper abdominal discomfort. Correspondingly, the great majority of the patients estimated their condition as good and were very satisfied with the result of the operation. Only occasionally did patients complain about weakness, but at the same time still considered their general condition as satisfying (Tables 3 and 4).

Table 1. Anamnestic data following gastric replacement

Isoperistaltic jejunal interposition (*Longmire-Gütgemann*) n = 83
Reexamined n = 13 (6 ♀ /7 ♂)

Mean age (yr)	Time after operation (yr)		Capability		Number of meals (Food intolerance)
	Min.	Max.	Able to work	Reduced	
63	1	13	11/13	2/13	5 – 7 (milk: 3/13)

Table 2. Anamnestic data following gastric replacement

Iso-anisoperistaltic jejunal interposition (*Schrader*) n = 43
Reexamined n = 16 (14 ♀ /2 ♂)

Mean age (yr)	Time after operation (yr)		Capability		Number of meals (Food intolerance)
	Min.	Max.	Able to work	Reduced	
58	1	6	15/16	1/16	5 – 7 (milk: 5/16)

Table 3. Subjective condition and symptoms following gastric replacement

Isoperistaltic jejunal interposition (*Longmire-Gütgemann*) n = 83
Reexamined n = 13

Subjective condition		Feeling of pressure	Eructation	Dumping	Reflux symptoms	Average body weight according to Broca-Index (normal = 1)
Good	Weak					
11/13	2/13	1/13	2/13	2/13	0	0.81

Table 4. Subjective condition and symptoms following gastric replacement

Iso-anisoperistaltic jejunal interposition (*Schrader*) n = 43
Reexamined n = 16

Subjective condition		Feeling of pressure	Eructation	Dumping	Reflux symptoms	Average body weight according to Broca-Index (normal = 1)
Good	Weak					
15/16	1/16	2/16	2/16	5/16	2/16	0.85

Of the patients, 10% – 30% reported postprandial feeling of pressure in the epigastrium, eructation, and dumping complaints. These symptoms were not reduced by the interpolation of a reversed segment. However, specifically, the dumping syndrome was conditioned to a great extent by individual factors, and depended not only on the gastric substitute passage time, as we discovered in follow-up studies after partial gastrectomies.

Whereas 12.5% of the patients with an iso-anisoperistaltic jejunal interposition complained of heartburn, there were no such complaints following isoperistaltic jejunal interposition.

Taking the Broca-Index (ratio of body weight to body height) as a basis, there was on the average, no difference in the weight behavior between the two groups of patients. Likewise, there was no difference in the laboratory results, i. e., in hemoglobin levels and total serum protein (Tables 5 and 6).

The X-ray examination of the gastric substitute, using barium meal mixed with cottage cheese, could prove a reservoir function in 69% of the patients with iso-anisoperistaltic jejunal interposition, but only in 31% of the patients with simple isoperistaltic interposition. It was not astonishing that an esophageal reflux could be demonstrated more frequently within the first group. It remains to be seen, whether a longer isoperistaltic segment (30 – 35 cm) than what we were using recently, can eliminate this complication. Comparing the weight behavior with the radiological findings in both groups, it was clearly demon-

Table 5. Special examinations following gastric replacement

Isoperistaltic jejunal interposition (*Longmire-Gütgemann*)				n = 83		
Reexamined				n = 13		
Laboratory results		Barium meal examination		14-C-Breath-analysis-test		
Mean hemoglobin (g%)	Mean total serum protein (g%)	Reflux	Reservoir function	(Exhalation of activity within 7 hours in % of given activity) n = 9		
				Average	Min.	Max.
13.7	7.2	2/13	4/13	7.9	3.2	11.6

Table 6. Special examinations following gastric replacement

Iso-anisoperistaltic jejunal interposition (*Schrader*)				n = 43		
Reexamined				n = 16		
Laboratory results		Barium meal examination		14-C-Breath-analysis-test		
Mean hemoglobin (g%)	Mean total serum protein (g%)	Reflux	Reservoir function	(Exhalation of activity within 7 hours in % of given activity) n = 10		
				Average	Min.	Max.
12.9	7.3	4/16	11/16	11.5	7.3	16.3

strated that the accidentally or operatively created reservoir function was closely related to the body weight (Table 7). The few patients showing a reservoir function following simple isoperistaltic jejunal interposition have a distinctly higher Broca-Index than those without reservoir function.

Within the group of patients with iso-anisoperistaltic jejunal interposition there is likewise a positive correlation between reservoir function and body weight, except for the patients showing radiologically an esophageal reflux. Two of three considerably underweight patients complained of typical reflux symptoms. This postprandial discomfort evidently restricted food intake so considerably that a drastic decrease in weight resulted, although food utilization was not reduced. This could be proven by measuring fat absorption using the ^{14}C breath-analysis-test. In contrast to preliminary results reported earlier by us [3], in this larger number of patients, a significantly different ($P < 0.01$) fat utilization between the two groups could be demonstrated (Tables 5 and 6). Fat absorption capacity in patients treated with iso-anisoperistaltic jejunal interposition was clearly improved compared with simple isoperistaltic jejunal interposition. In

Table 7. Behavior of body weight in proportion to the reservoir function of the gastric substitute (body weight according to Broca-Index, normal = 1)

Isoperistaltic jejunal interposition (*Longmire-Gütgemann*) n = 13		Iso-anisoperistaltic jejunal interposition (*Schrader*) n = 16	
With reservoir function n = 4 Broca-Index	Without reservoir function n = 9 Broca-Index	With reservoir function n = 11 Broca-Index	Without reservoir function n = 6 Broca-Index
		0.85	0.84
0.9	0.76	without reflux n = 8 Broca-Index 0.9	with reflux n = 3 Broca-Index 0.75

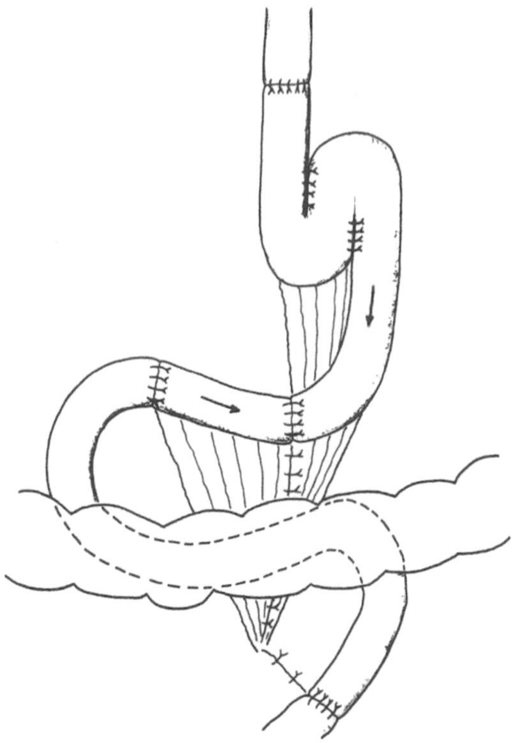

Fig. 2. Gastric substitute by means of iso-anisoperistaltic jejunal interposition and jejunoplication to prevent reflux

some cases of the latter type of gastric substitute, fat absorption was extremely low, whereas maximum fat absorption in the iso-anisoperistaltic jejunal interposition group reached 16.6% of the given amount, which was comparable to the average value of partial gastric resections (n = 4), who were tested as controls. Thus, additional interposition of a reversed jejunal segment in gastric replacement strikingly improved fat absorption capacity.

Based on these data, it was concluded that the gastric substitute consisting of two iso-anisoperistaltic jejunal segments, developed by Schrader [5], provided better long-term results concerning fat absorption than the isoperistaltic jejunal interposition of Longmire and Gütgemann [1, 4]. Therefore, we now use this type of stomach replacement at our clinic routinely in all cases, where a curative total gastrectomy is possible. Since esophageal reflux can neutralize the positive effect of the reversed segment, since it causes a reduced food intake, we have considered using a jejunoplication to prevent reflux into the esophagus (Fig. 2). This modification of our method could be rewarding.

References

1. Gütgemann, A., Schreiber, H. W., Bernhard, A.: Erfahrungen mit der totalen Gastrektomie. Langenbecks Arch. Klin. Chir. *303*, 73–93 (1963)
2. Kummer, D., Buttkereit, K., Koslowski, L.: Frühkomplikationen und Frühletalität verschiedener operativer Methoden bei der Gastrektomie. Langenbecks Arch. Chir. *344*, 195–205 (1977)
3. Kummer, D., Durst, J., Kieninger, G., Anger, K.: Früh- und Spätergebnisse der Ersatzmagenbildung nach Gastrektomie. Vortrag auf dem 10. Internationalen Magensymposium. Berlin: 1978 Stuttgart: Thieme (in press)
4. Longmire, W. P. jr., Beal, J. M.: Construction of a substitute gastric reservoir following total gastrectomy. Am. Surg. *135*, 637–641 (1952)
5. Schrader, C. P., Koslowski, L., Feine, U., Konold, P.: Vergleichende tierexperimentelle Untersuchungen über die Bildung eines Nahrungsreservoirs, seines Entleerungstyps und seiner Auswirkungen auf die Fettresorption. Langenbecks Arch. Klin. Chir. *329*, 242–243 (1971)

The Jejunal Pouch as Stomach Substitute

A. Hollinger, G. Uhlschmid, and F. Largiadèr

After total gastrectomy, reconstruction of the stomach is important for the patient's future well-being. The passage of food has to be unobstructed, free, and at the same time somewhat delayed. Swallowing should be undisturbed. The patient should be able to take normal-sized feeding portions. Bile reflux – a particular unpleasant feeling for the patient – has to be avoided. Reconstruction of the duodenal passage is of minor importance. The interrelationship of gastric-duodenal-biliary and pancreatic secretion is in any event disturbed by the gastrectomy.

Method

After total gastrectomy and closure of the duodenal stump, the jejunum and its mesentery are divided between 8 and 20 cm distal to the ligament of Treitz. The point of division is chosen according to the vascular arcades and to assure sufficient mobility of the distal part, which is blindly closed. The proximal portion is turned in, similar to a walking stick. In this way, a double loop of 15 – 18 cm in length is formed (Fig. 1). The posterior wall is marked by seromuscular

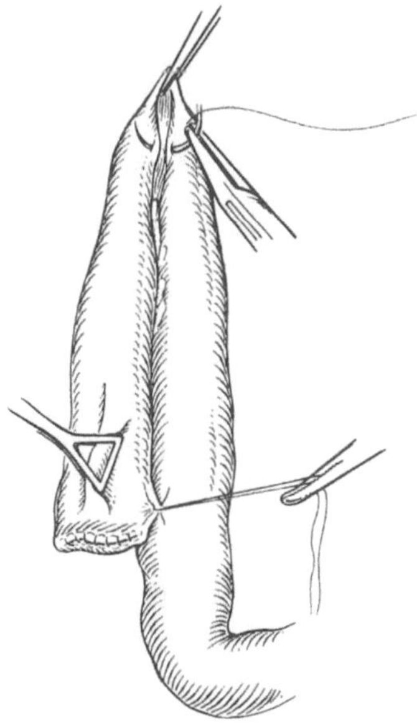

Fig. 1. A jejunal loop of 15 – 18 cm is formed

stitches and is later sewn with a running seromuscular stitch (Fig. 2). The running stitch is interrupted by tying it with the marking stitches. Both lumina are incised close to the suture line at the antimesenteric side (Fig. 3). The often considerable bleeding is controlled by a running, absorbable suture through all layers Finally, the anterior wall, like the posterior wall, is finished by a running seromuscular

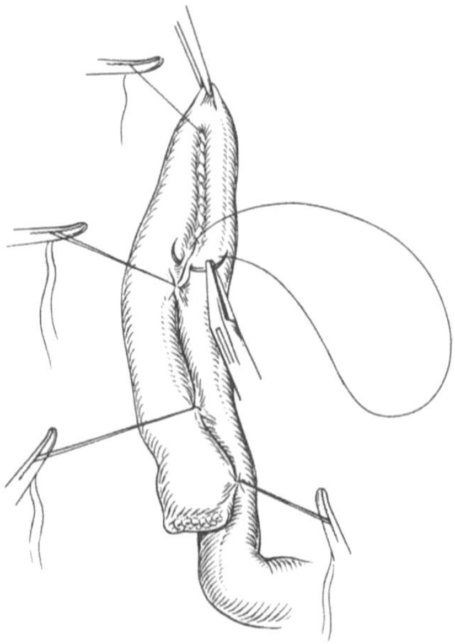

Fig. 2. Suture of the posterior wall of the pouch

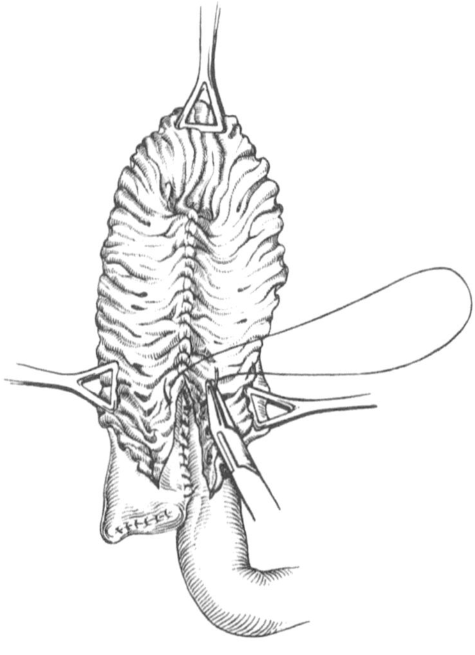

Fig. 3. Both lumina are opened close to the suture line at the antimesenteric side. Running suture through all layers for control of bleeding

stitch (Fig. 4). The gastric substitute is brought into proper position retrocolically and its apex anastomosed to the distal esophagus (Fig. 5). At both sides of the anastomosis we place transfixing stitches lateral-posteriorly and secure the anterior wall at the diaphragmatic peritoneum.

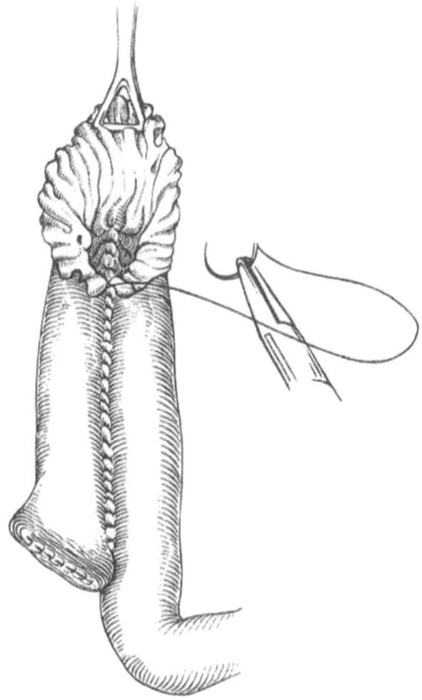

Fig. 4. Closure of the anterior wall of the pouch

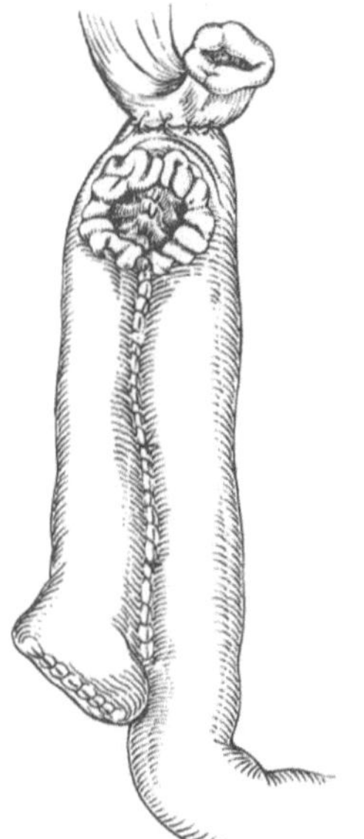

Fig. 5. Anastomosis to the esophagus

Until 5 years ago, all esophageal anastomoses were fashioned this way, and the following cases belong to this group. Today, we add a jejunoplication.

The afferent jejunal loop is anastomosed terminolaterally into the efferent loop of the gastric substitute. Care is taken to have a minimal distance of 30 cm between the distal end of the gastric pouch and the Roux-en-Y anastomosis. This is of particular importance for the prevention of biliary reflux into the esophagus (Fig. 6).

Material

The following are the results of 21 patients with jejunal gastric substitutes after 5 years.

Sixteen patients had cancer, four had a Zollinger-Ellison syndrome and one patient with a strong family history of gastric cancer, had a massive hemorrhage from a gastric ulcer.

Operative Mortality

Within 30 days of surgery, two patients died (9.5%). One patient had a dehiscence of the esophagojejunostomy, the second patient, a bronchopneumonia complicated by sepsis. He also had a second carcinoma in the bronchus.

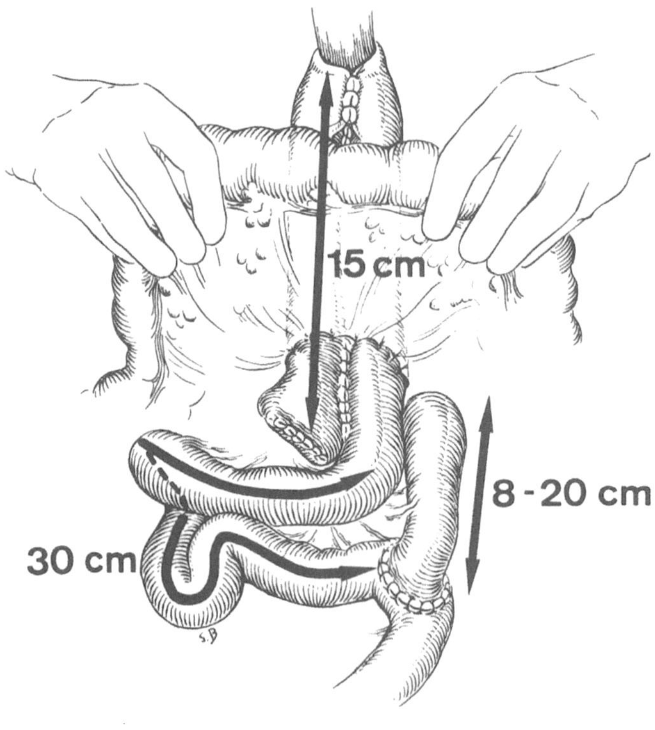

Fig. 6. The completed jejunal pouch

Late Results

The 5-year survival rate was 38%. The cumulative survival rate is presented in Fig. 7. The longest follow-up is 9 years. So far, 15 patients died, ten deaths were due to the cancer and five due to other causes. At the latest follow-up, we were able to examine six patients. One patient complained of occasional dumping symptoms, another patient is able to eat only small portions, but generally feels well and keeps his ideal body weight. A third patient complained of epigastric pain that responded well to a glass of *'schnaps'*. The remaining patients are asymptomatic and consider their operative result as very good.

Discussion

Gastric substitutes by jejunum require a major operation. The esophageal anastomosis is the major source of complications. There were no other operative complications. A small fistula of the esophagojejunostomy doesn't mean disaster under adequate therapy. The operative mortality is comparable with the data of other types of gastric substitutes after total gastrectomy. Late results show half the patients entirely free of symptoms as investigated by direct questioning as well as by inquiries through relatives of patients who died of unrelated causes. In contrast to these results, our late results showed after simple esophago-jejunostomy Dumping syndrome in 77% of cases, bile reflux in 46%, and mild postprandial discomfort in all cases [1].

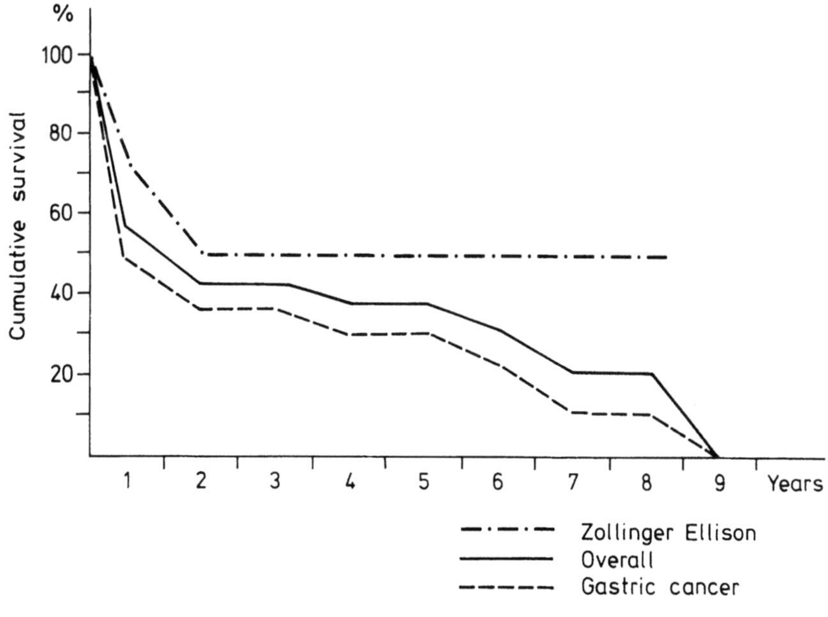

Fig. 7. Actuarial cumulative survival of 21 patients followed for more than 5 years

Possibilities for reconstruction after total gastrectomy are manifold [2, 3]. The stomach substitute, according to Hunt Lawrence-Rodino, is technically not very difficult and should be employed in all cases in which a radical procedure is under consideration and the patient can be expected to tolerate a somewhat longer operation.

References

1. Largiadèr, F., Säuberli, H.: Rekonstruktion nach Gastrektomie, insbesondere mit Jejunumersatzmagen. Helv. Chir. Acta *39*, 883 – 886 (1972)
2. Largiadèr, F., Säuberli, H.: Die totale Gastrektomie. Erster Teil: Möglichkeiten der operativen Rekonstruktion nach Gastrektomie. Bruns. Beitr. Klin. Chir. *7*, 601 – 609 (1972)
3. Säuberli, H., Largiadèr, F.: Die totale Gastrektomie. Zweiter Teil: Resultate von 71 eigenen Fällen. Bruns Beitr. Klin. Chir. *1*, 35 – 44 (1973)

Jejunal Pouch According to Hunt-Lawrence-Rodino with Jejunoplication

Ch. Herfarth, P. Schlag, P. Merkle, and P. Mattes

Technique

In employing the method according to Hunt-Lawrence-Rodino, a reservoir is created by performing a broad enteroanastomosis between the afferent and efferent portion of the jejunal loop used for the esophago-anastomosis subsequent to total gastrectomy. The remaining, disconnected superior jejunal loop is utilized for the esophagojejunostomy, whereby the anastomosis is applied to the descending portion of the loop and the rest of the free superior jejunum is used for the jejunal plication by completely sandwiching the anastomosis. The jejunoplication conforms to the modifications specified by Schreiber [2] and Peiper and Siewert [1]. The determining factor for this method of forming a jejunal pouch is that the afferent loop is disconnected and introduced in form of a Roux-en-Y anastomosis 30 – 35 cm below into the efferent jejunal limb (Figs. 1 and 2).

Surgical Mortality

The listing of surgical mortality after surgery reveals a rate of 19%, which is in accord with the average figure given by the literature (summary Schreiber in [2]).

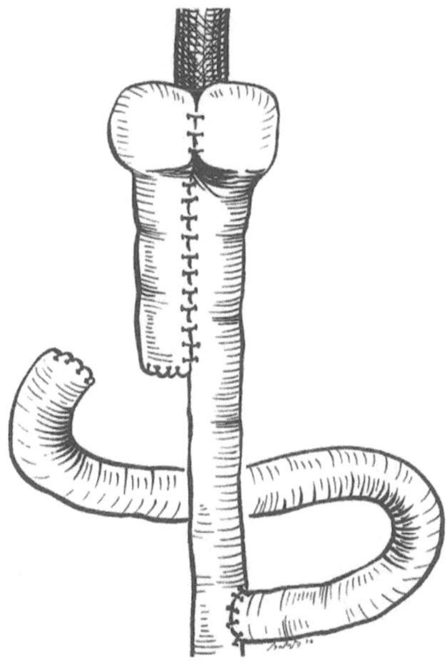

Fig. 1. A jejunal pouch in modification of the Hunt-Lawrence-Rodino method with broad enteroanastomosis of the superior jejunal loop used for the esophagojejunostomy. Introduction of the afferent jejunal loop 30 – 35 cm below the jejunal pouch

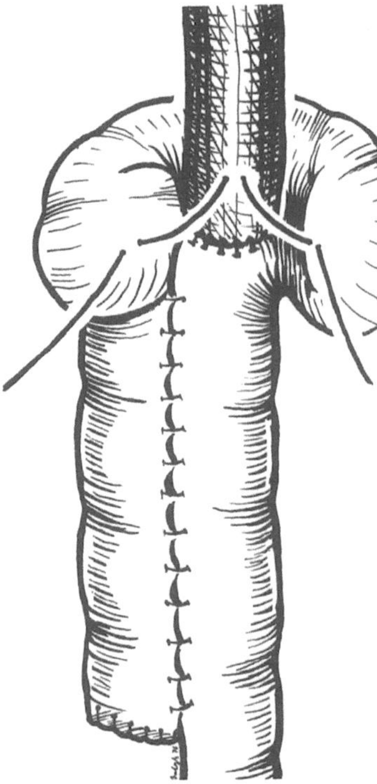

Fig. 2. Jejunoplication done by sandwiching the esophagojejunostomy with the aid of the free cranial jejunal loop above the jejunal pouch

By separating the various groups of our own patients and excluding those patients with extensive cancer (gastrectomy *de nécessité*), considerable differences with an improved mortality rate are found in comparison to those with a gastrectomy indicated by a carcinoma localized in the antrum or the inferior corpus. If in analyzing the surgical mortality only the gastrectomies for early cancers (n = 12) are taken into consideration, a mortality of 0% is determined. This analysis of mortality after surgery exposes a problem of postoperative collective statistics, which are prone to considerable variation in dependence on the selection of the patient pool. The literature contains a not insignificant number of noncancerous stomach lesions with subsequent gastrectomy included in the calculations (Peiper, 1978).

Reexamination

In order to test the effects of one certain type of gastrectomy as a surgical procedure, a number of postulates must be fulfilled, which are summarized in the following:

a) The surgical procedure must be standardized.

b) A sufficient interval must have elapsed between operation and reexamination (1 year).

c) The surgery performed on the patient must have been "curative".

d) The patient must appear clinically and diagnostically free of cancer.

e) The patient must be willing to undergo the various diagnostic procedures.

When adhering to these strict criteria, the number of cases for evaluation becomes drastically reduced. In our own hospital, 311 cases of gastric cancer were surgically treated from July 1974 through November 1977. Of these patients, 189 were operable and 82 were subjected to a total gastrectomy. On 52 patients alone, the typical procedure explained above was performed as representing a curative therapy from the surgical point of view. Of these patients, 25 were available for reexamination at least 1 year after the date of the operation and were subjected to a general clinical examination. Only a fraction was willing to undergo more intensive diagnostic procedures (Fig. 3)[1].

The following factors were considered for the reexaminations after total gastrectomy with jejunal pouch and jejunoplication:

a) Subjective criteria, such as appetite, sense of fullness, contentment, productivity – criteria, the value of which should not be underestimated, as they after all determine the quality of life of patients with a low average survival rate.

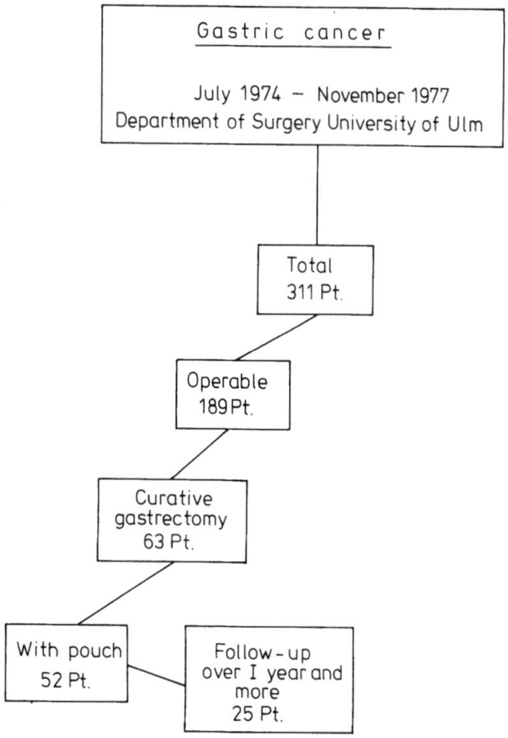

Fig. 3. Patients with gastric cancer (July 1974 through November 1977), General Surgery Clinic, University of Ulm. In 63 of 189 operable cases of a total of 311 patients, a curative gastrectomy was possible. On 52 of these, a jejunal pouch was applied in modification of the Hunt-Lawrence-Rodino method. On 25 patients, follow-up was maintained over more than a year.

[1] This striking reduction in the number of a group of patients selected for reexamination demonstrates the kind of problems a single center has to solve, if strict clinical criteria for reexamination are to be applied. It supports the desire for multicenter coordination in the pursuit of such examinations, which would still leave the difficulty of defining uniform criteria.

b) Clinical and diagnostic criteria, such as weight, X-ray examinations, endoscopy with biopsy, manometry, gastric clearance time, and examination of fat absorption.

c) Laboratory parameters: Hemoglobin, protein, vitamin A, iron, calcium, phosphat.

Results

Subjective Criteria

State of Health

In answer to the question of whether they felt very good, good, fair, or poorly, almost 4/5 of the patients considered their state of health to be very good or good. Four patients designated their general condition as only fair, and two felt definitely poor. It should be mentioned of these last two patients, that they were already in poor general condition preoperatively (Fig. 4).

Complaints

Considering the patients complaints, there were quite a number of these described by half of the patients despite their claims of well-being, with reflux

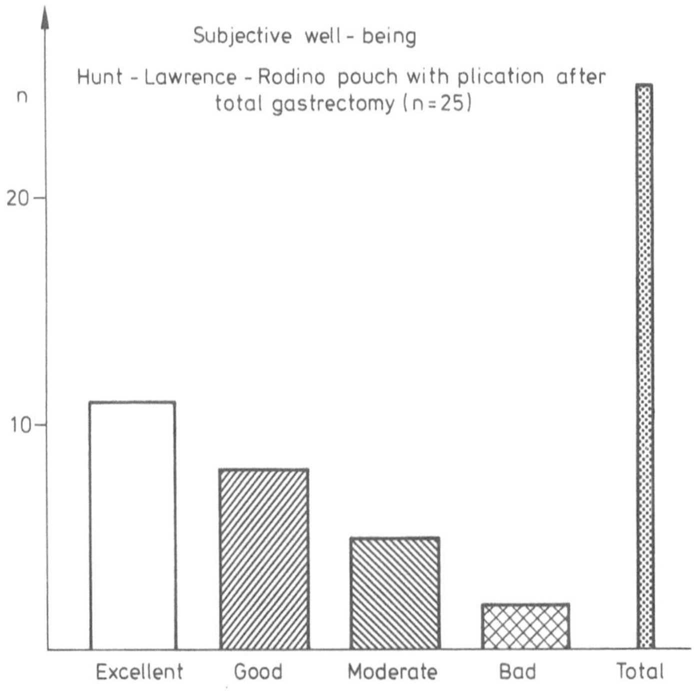

Fig. 4. Follow-up examination after gastrectomy: Subjective well-being

and diarrhea being the most frequent, followed by dysphagia and dumping symptoms. Remarkably, lack of appetite was no great factor among the complaints (Fig. 5).

Food Incompatibility

Upon closer questioning, only ten of the reexamined patients had no food incompatibility, whereas the rest complained of more or less intolerance towards milk or sugar or meat and fat (Fig. 6).

Capacity for Work or Productivity

Of the 25 patients reexamined, 19 demonstrated complete capacity for work or, if they were beyond the age of pension, full productivity. Two patients were sent into pension before their time, although no reduction in their productivity was in evidence. Four patients showed a postoperative reduction of productivity (Fig.7).

Clinical Diagnostic Criteria

Weight

The ideal weight was chosen to be the major parameter for determining weight fluctuation. Whereas all patients were slightly overweight preoperatively, an almost ideal weight could be recorded postoperatively. In no case could undue weight reduction be determined (Fig. 8).

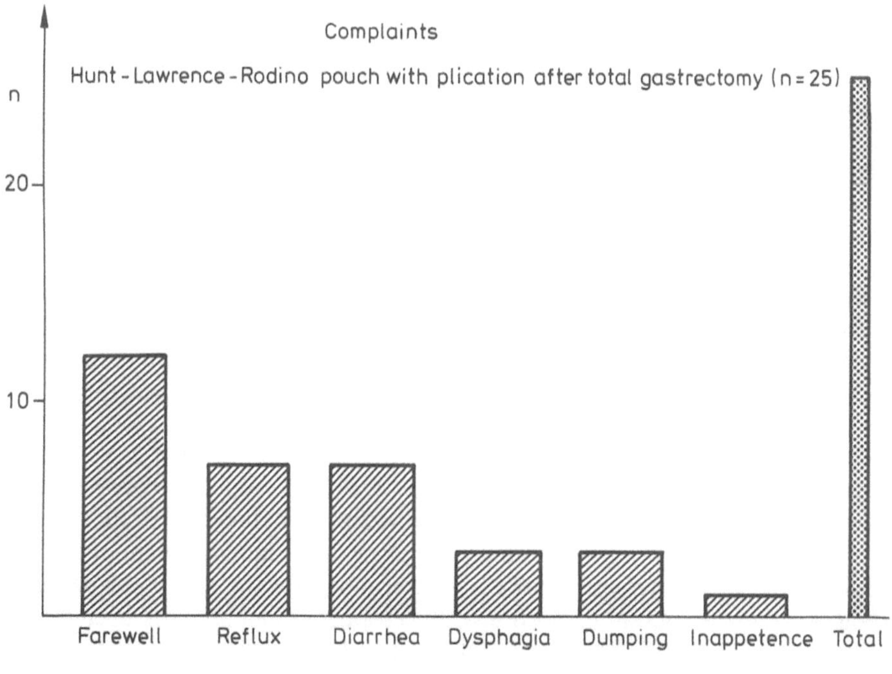

Fig. 5. Follow-up examination after gastrectomy: Complaints

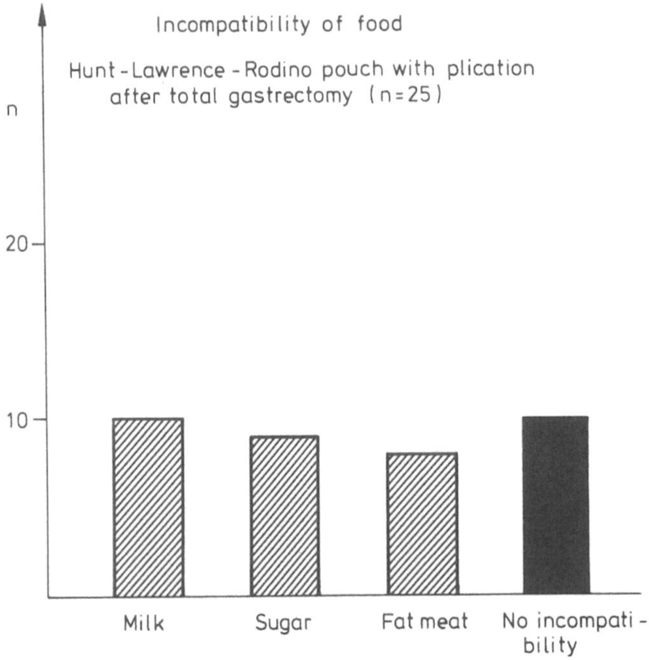

Fig. 6. Follow-up examination after gastrectomy: Food incompatibility

X-ray Examination

Barium enemia revealed the typical picture of a gastriform outpouching of the small intestine in gastrectomized patients with jejunal pouch. Whereas the postoperative control revealed a relatively slight stomach reservoir, reexamination 1/2 – 1 year later showed a reservoir with a capacitative volume of 400 – 600 ml (Fig. 9). The jejunoplication was easily displayed radiologically. Essential for radiological examination was the fact that only a small percentage of cases exhibited reflux upon provocation during the examination (Fig. 10).

Endoscopic Examination

There was no endoscopic evidence of severe esophagitis found in any of the cases examined, and only one patient exhibited a bioptically proven slight esophagitis. There were no more severe morphological changes of the esophagus (Fig. 11).

Esophageal Manometry

Manometry of the esophagus produced a positive lower esophageal pressure profile in a third of the cases. In these patients, the abdominal portion of the esophagus was not removed during gastrectomy because of the modest extent of the carcinoma. A negative pressure profile was determined for the rest of the patients. In these cases, the abdominal portion of the esophagus had been removed as well (Fig. 12). It was not possible to correlate the esophago-manometric findings with the clinical complaints of the patients, with a possible radiological determination of reflux, or with the histological proof of esophagitis.

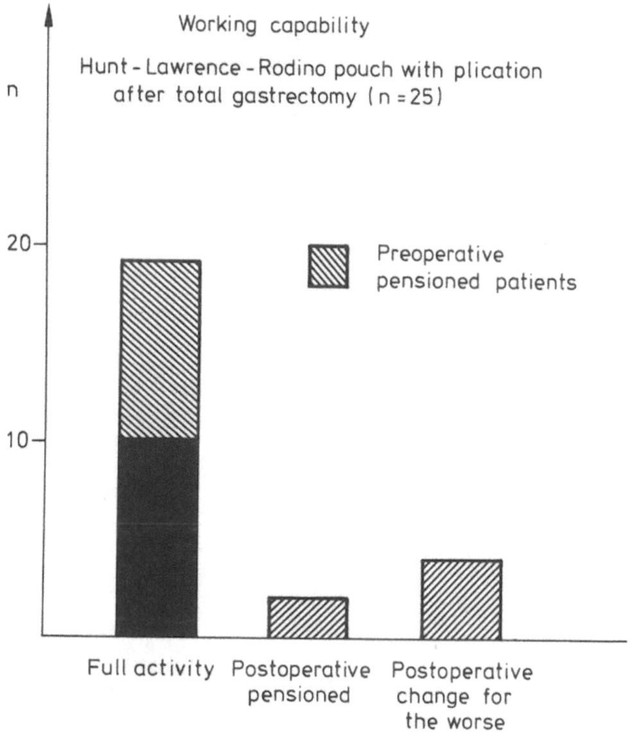

Fig. 7. Follow-up examination after gastrectomy: Capacity for work and productivity

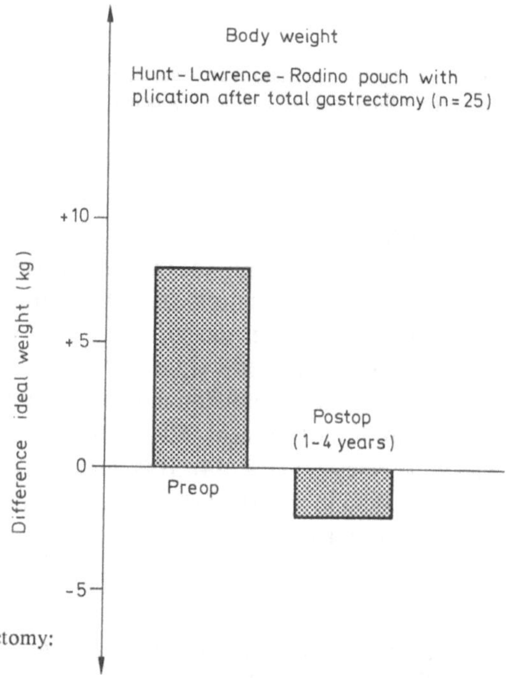

Fig. 8. Follow-up examination after gastrectomy: Weight maintenance

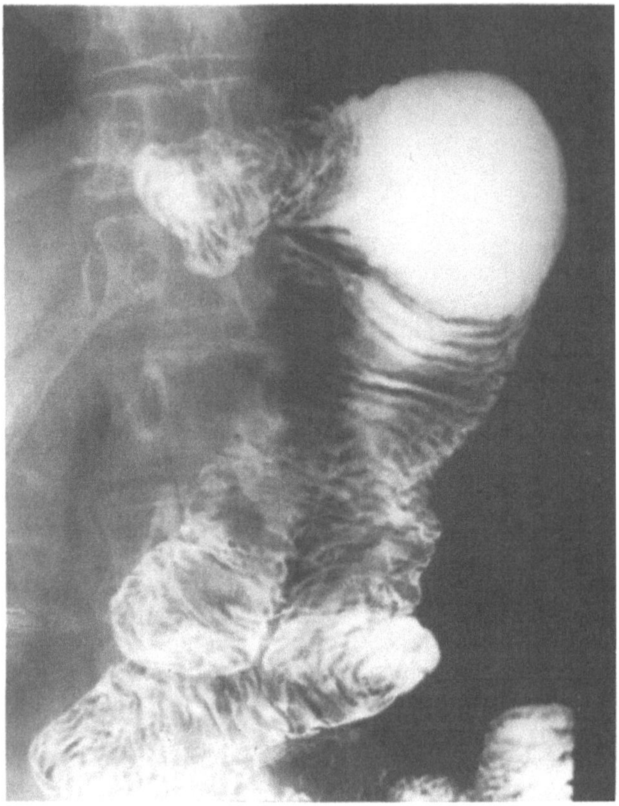

Fig. 9. Follow-up examination after gastrectomy: Passage of barium contrast medium through a jejunal pouch 1 year after gastrectomy

Gastric Clearance[2]

The sequence scintigraph was the most advantageous aid in determining the question of reservoir formation and of the portioned evacuation from the jejunal pouch. Oat meal gruel mixed with ^{99}Tc-S colloid was given and the substitute stomach was divided into separate "regions of interest" (Fig. 13). The declining activity curves in the individual gastric regions demonstrate the vacillation or the evacuation of the test meal. The examined cases show 10 of 13 as having developed a good reservoir (Fig. 14). It is interesting to note that the evacuation proceeded slower than in a normal stomach, i.e., the clearance from the jejunal pouch is distinctly decreased.

---

[2] We thank for these investigations and the figures Priv. Doz. Dr. A. Sonntag, Department of Radiology III, of University Ulm.

Fig. 10a

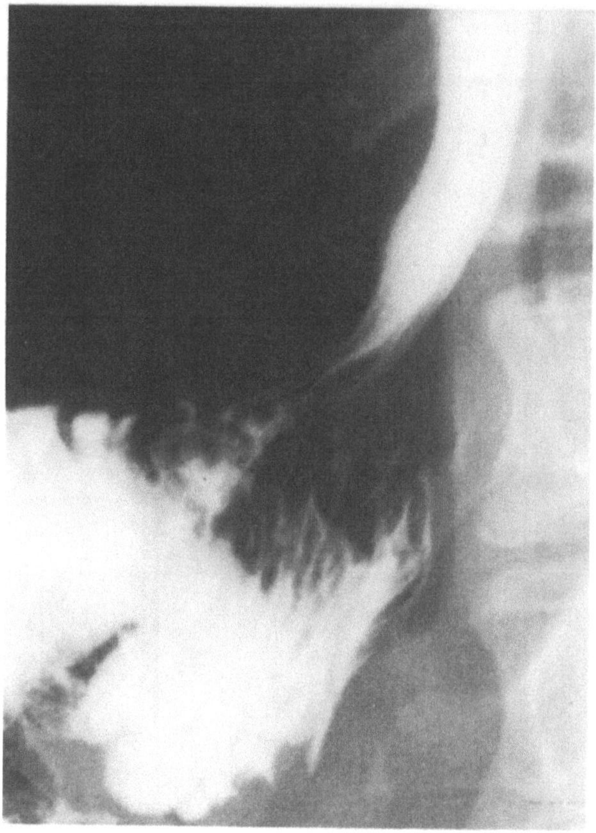

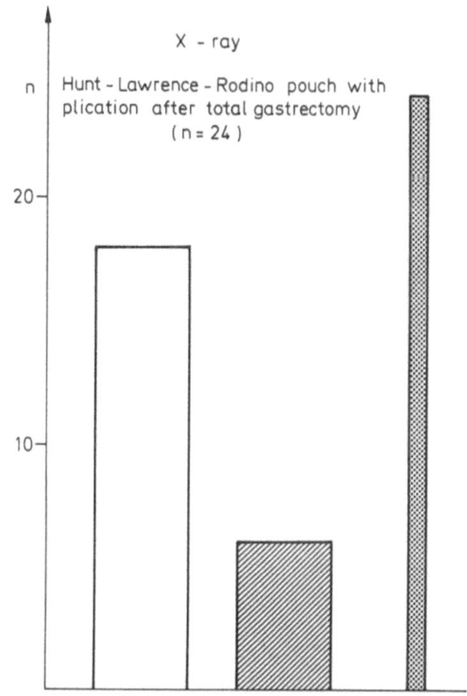

Fig. 10b

Fig. 10a and b. Follow-up examination after gastrectomy: Preservation of reflux by the jejunoplication (X-ray-method)

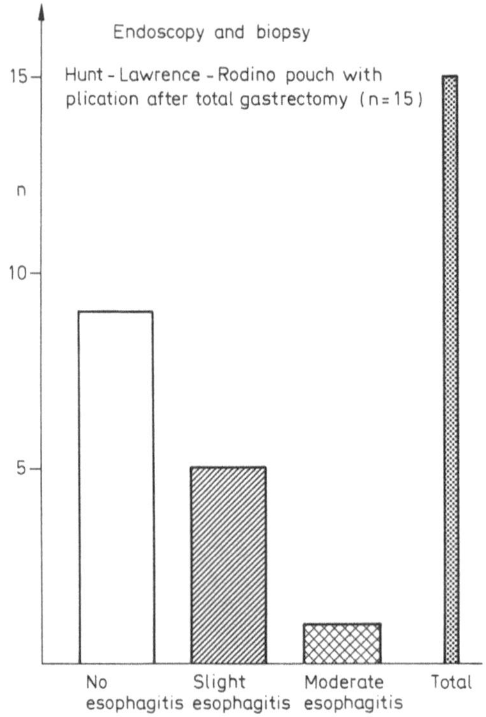

Fig. 11. Follow-up examination after gastrectomy: Endoscopy and biopsy of the terminal esophagus. Esophagitis was diagnosed histologically but not endoscopically

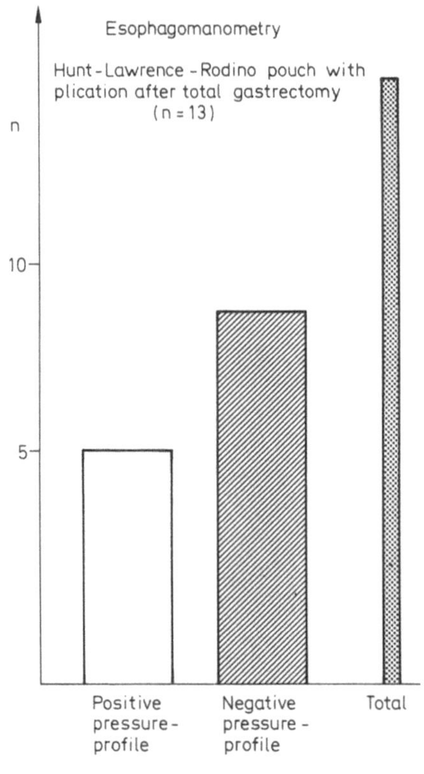

Fig. 12. Follow-up examination after gastrectomy: Esophageal manometry. Positive pressure profile with remaining terminal esophagus

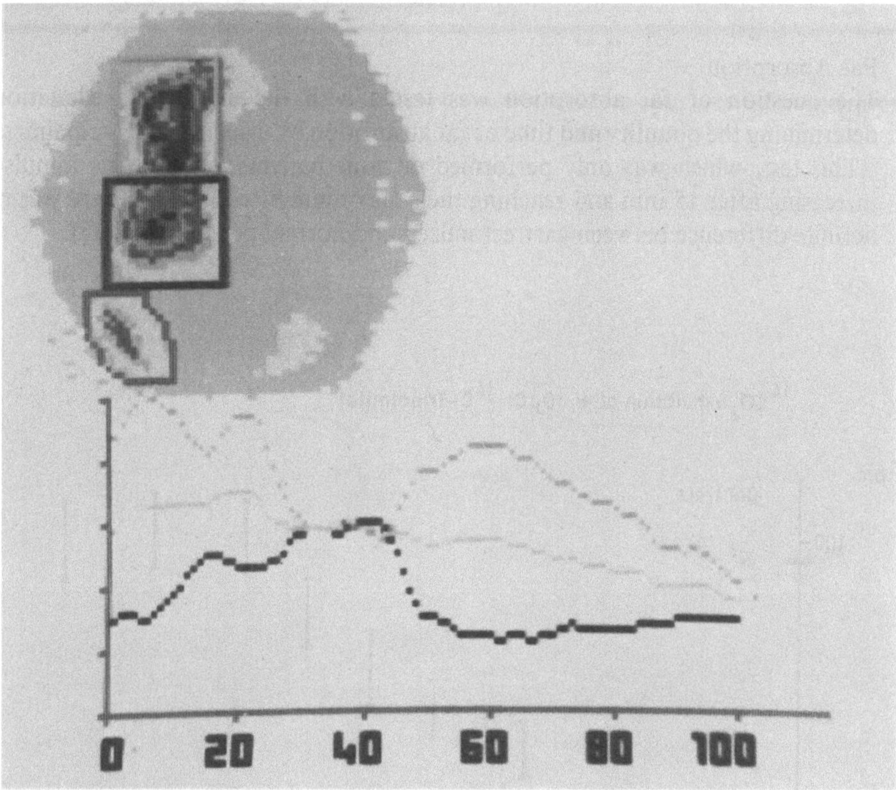

Fig. 13. Follow-up examination after gastrectomy: Sequence scintigraphy using ^{99}Tc-S-colloid added to oat meal gruel as a test meal. Demarcation of the substitute stomach with subdivisions of separate "regions of interest"

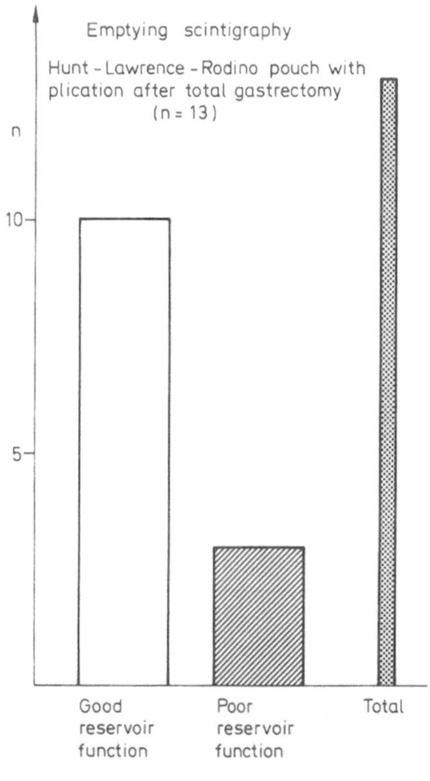

Fig. 14. Follow-up examination after gastrectomy: Clearance scintigraphy of the jejunal pouch

Fat Absorption
The question of fat absorption was tested with the aid of ^{14}C-exhalation, determining the quantity and time of fat absorption by dispensing ^{14}C-tripalmetat

This test, which was only performed on four patients, showed the impulses increasing after 15 min and reaching their maximum after 3 – 4 h. There was no definite difference between gastrectomized and normal persons (Fig. 15).

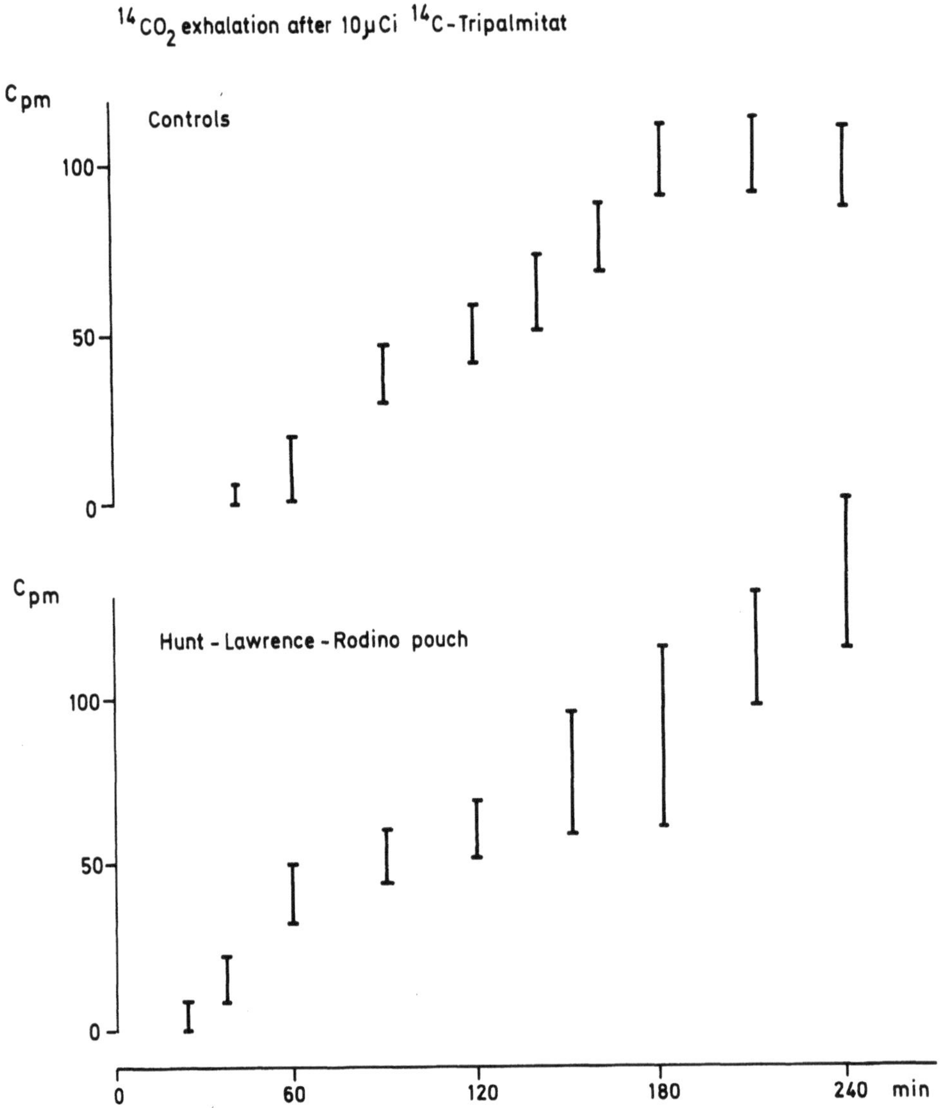

Fig. 15. Follow-up examination after gastrectomy: The ^{14}C exhalation after gastrectomy shows no differences in comparison with normal persons

Laboratory Parameters

With the exception of a reduction of vitamin A, none of the laboratory criteria showed anything remarkable (Fig. 16).

Summary

The following facts arising from the series of reexaminations with jejunal pouch formation and jejunoplication according to a modification of Hunt-Lawrence-Rodino should be particularly noted:

The number of reexaminations is scant, because strict postulates had to be maintained. According to the self-evaluations regarding well-being, there is a remarkably large number of contented patients, although definite complaints could be recorded for half of the patients upon direct questioning. The fact that there was no anorexia is also remarkable. The high rate of intact productivity is in accord with the favorable results obtained for the other criteria. The constant weight maintenance indicates good adaptation to the lack of a stomach. Reflux complaints were voiced by some patients, though no reflux or evidence of severe reflux esophagitis was demonstrable. Reservoir formation within the jejunal pouch was proven by the X-ray examination. The clearance of a test meal yields

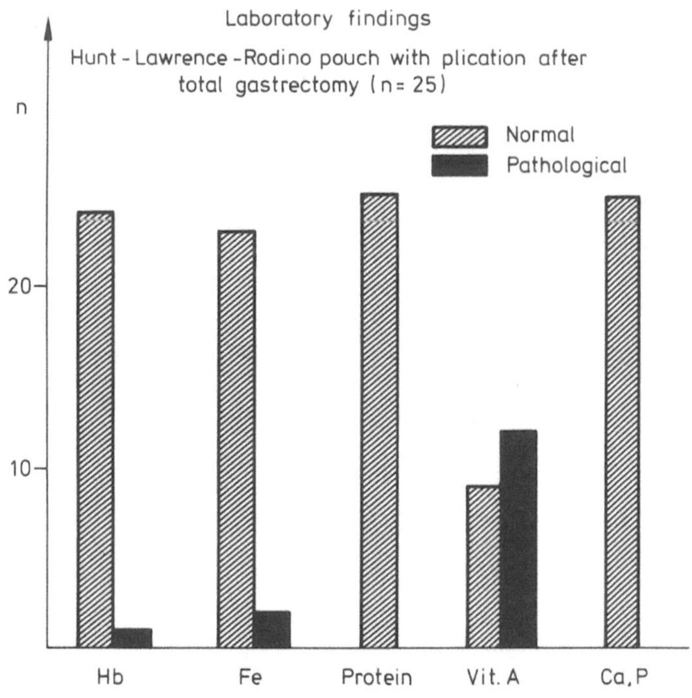

Fig. 16. Follow-up examinations after gastrectomy: Laboratory findings

distinctly delayed evacuation figures, a fact which could possibly explain the low number of patients exhibiting early and late postalimentary syndrome. The absorption of fat does not seem to be inhibited, although the reduction of the vitamin A level determined could be an indication for a delayed adaptation of fat absorption.

Conclusion

If by the concept of stomach substitute, the prevention of reflux, sufficient reservoir capacity, and an adequately portioned evacuation is meant, then the described method of jejunal pouch with jejunoplication in modification of the procedure of Hunt-Lawrence-Rodino can be chosen as its closest approximation. This stomach substitute is of course no substitute in the sense of a replacement of physiological functions, such as nutrient breakdown and working humoral and neural kinetics. In this sense, the concept of a substitute stomach remains something of a euphemism.

References

1. Peiper, H. J., Siewert, R.: Magenersatz. Chirurg *49*, 81 – 88 (1978)
2. Schreiber, H. W., Eichfuss, H. P., Schumpelick, V.: Magenersatz. Chirurg *49*, 72 – 80 (1978)

Jejunal Pouch After Total Gastrectomy: A Study of Different Substitutes for the Stomach

H. G. Beger and R. Bittner

The prognosis of patients with gastric cancer is determined by their biological age [3], the extent of diffusion of the tumor, and the histological type of the cancer [7]. In addition, the operative therapeutic influences encumbers the prognosis because of the frequency and difficulties of postoperative complications.

When considering the individual reconstruction techniques after a gastrectomy, two questions present themselves:

1) Of what significance is the duodenum for the alimentary passage?

2) Which substitute stomach ensures an adequate reservoir for uninterrupted assimilation of nutriments as well as an evacuative function?

Recent studies show the duodenum passage to be of great value for the assimilation of nutriments and glucose homeostasis [1, 2]. However, studies are still necessary when considering the reservoir and evacuative function of a substitute stomach. An evaluation of individual reconstruction techniques after gastrectomy can therefore, with today's knowledge, be obtained only with the provision of a long-term postoperative and tumor-free course of progress.

In the following, operative techniques with and without a jejunal interposition will be compared with the aid of examination results of patients who, on the average, had a gastrectomy more than 12 months beforehand.

Patients

Twenty-two patients were involved in the study and were examined on the average, 13.8, 15.3, and 22.3 months after gastrectomy. Sex differences, age, as well as the occurrence of postoperative examinations are indicated in Table 1.

Table 1. Clinical data of the patients included in the study. Groups I and II: patients after total gastrectomy following cancer of the stomach

Substitute stomach	Pat. (n)	Sex (m/f)	Age (Yrs) $\bar{x} \pm SD$	Postop. (Months) $\bar{x} \pm SD$
Hunt-Rodino pouch[a]	6	3/3	61.0 ± 5.0	13.8 ± 5.6
Interposition C[a]	8	5/3	48.4 ± 13.8	15.3 ± 9.2
Interposition Z[b]	8	6/2	45.8 ± 8.3	22.3 ± 13.1

[a] Gastric cancer.

[b] Zollinger-Ellison Syndrome.

Fourteen patients had gastric cancer with the following tumor stages: one patient had multicentered early cancer. Of 13 patients having advanced cancer, five patients represented Borrman I; seven patients, Borrman II, and one patient, Borrman III. Eight patients had a gastrectomy due to a Zollinger-Ellison syndrome. In the course of aftercare, all patients were regularly treated and received a controlled substitution of vitamin B_{12} and iron.

Operative Techniques

Using macroscopic criteria with the inclusion of the intraoperative frozen section diagnosis, a so-called radical operation was possible in all the patients with gastric cancer. In principle, those patients with a gastrectomy following gastric cancer, an esophageal cuff (2 cm) as well as a narrow ring (1 cm) of the post-pyloric duodenum was included in the resection.

For six patients, a reconstruction was made using the Hunt-Rodino technique [5, 6]. The Roux-en-Y anastomosis lay 20 cm aboral to the jejunal substitute stomach. In 16 patients, the jejunal loop was interposed, using the Longmire-Gütgemann-Schreiber technique [9] between the esophagus (end-to-side) and the duodenum (end-to-side/end-to-side). The restoration of the jejunal continuity was followed with an end-to-end anastomosis.

Reexamination Results

Subjective Judgment Criteria

By direct questioning of the patients, frequency of pain, epigastric fullness, pressure in the upper abdomen, vomiting, frequent outbreak of perspiration with

Table 2. Frequency of abdominal complaints after total gastrectomy

	Hunt-Rodino pouch	Interposition (Longmire-Gütgemann)	
		Gastric cancer	Zollinger-Ellison
	6 Pat.	8 Pat.	8 Pat.
Pain[a]	1	2	0
Epig. fulness	1	2	0
Pressure	2	1	2
Vomiting	1	1	1
Dumping	2	1	1
Diarrhea	1	1	2
	22%	16%	12%

[a] Dependent upon nutrition.

dizzy feelings, and tachycardia related to nutrition (Dumping syndrome) as well as diarrhea, were found to exist. As indicated by Table 2, the preceding symptoms were considerably more rare in patients with a jejunal interposition, than in patients with a Hunt-Rodino pouch.

A statistical assessment of the differences was not possible due to unlike conditions, i.e., average age of the groups of patients and variability of the illness. With regard to the ability to work and normal living (Table 3), the number of those again fully fit was only 1 of 6 patients with a Hunt-Rodino pouch, but 12 of 16 patients with a jejunal interposition. Although patients with a Hunt-Rodino pouch were, on the average, 10 years older than those with a jejunal interposition, a balance in favor of the jejunal interposition as the reconstruction technique of choice after gastrectomy, resulted from this difference.

Objective Judgment Criteria

In the objective assessment of patients after gastrectomy, weight, hemoglobin, blood sugar, serum protein and serum-iron concentration were examined (Table 4). In particular, with regard to the relationship of the postoperative body weight, a clear difference was to be seen between patients with a Hunt-Rodino pouch and patients with a jejunal interposition: an increase in weight occurred in only 1 of 6 patients with a Hunt-Rodino pouch, but it occurred in 11 of 16 patients with a jejunal interposition. The patients who had a Hunt-Rodino pouch, in regard to blood glucose concentration and serum-iron concentration, had pathological average values; in regard to the hemoglobin concentration and total protein, they had the lowest mean values.

Considering histological criteria, a reflux esophagitis was on the whole, in all patients, a rare discovery: histological signs of esophagitis were found in 2 of 5

Table 3. Frequency of disability to work and limitations in the way of life in patients after total gastrectomy

	Hunt-Rodino pouch	Interposition (Longmire-Gütgemann)	
		Gastric cancer	Zollinger-Ellison
	6 Pat.	8 Pat.	8 Pat.
Ability to work			
not capable	5	4	–
limited	1	1	2
fully capable		3	6
Way of life			
limited	2	5	1
unchanged	4	3	7

Table 4. Body weight, hemoglobin, blood glucose, serum protein, and blood-iron concentration in patients after total gastrectomy

		Hunt-Rodino pouch	Interposition (Longmire-Gütgemann)	
		6 Pat.	Gastric Cancer 8 Pat.	Zollinger-Ellison 8 Pat.
Weight	+/−/±/Pat.	1/1/4	4/1/3	7/0/1
Hemoglobin	g%	11.1 ± 1.3	12.9 ± 1.5	13.6 ± 0.6
Blood glucose	mg%	102 ± 17	86.3 ± 14.4	72.8 ± 9.1
Protein	g%	6.1 ± 0.3	6.6 ± 0.5[a]	7.1 ± 0.2[a]
Iron	μmol/liter	11.1 ± 5.0	16.3 ± 8.2[a]	21.8 ± 6.3[a]

[a] 7 Pat.

Table 5. Frequency of esophagitis after total gastrectomy

	Hunt-Rodino pouch	Interposition (Longmire-Gütgemann)	
	6 Pat.	Gastric cancer 8 Pat.	Zollinger-Ellison 8 Pat.
Esophagitis macrosc.	5/6	4/8	1/8
Esophagitis histolog.	2/5	1/8	1/8
Reflux esophagitis (X-ray)	3/6	2/8	1/8

patients with a Hunt-Rodino pouch and in 2 of 16 patients with a jejunal interposition (Table 5). Those patients with pains related to nutrition also had simultaneously, signs of a reflux esophagitis.

Summary

Twenty-two patients were examined after gastrectomy, on the average, longer than 1 year postoperatively, with regard to criteria of morbidity.

Patients with a Hunt-Rodino pouch showed a difference of 22% in frequency of upper abdominal pains in comparison to patients with a Longmire-Gütgemann-Schreiber jejunal interposition. A clear difference in favor of those patients with a jejunal interposition existed in particular, in regard to the reintegration to "normal" life.

Patients, who because of a Zollinger-Ellison syndrome had a gastrectomy, had the most favorable examination results in comparison to patients who were operated upon because of gastric cancer.

References

1. Adams, J. F.: The clinical and metabolic consequences of total gastrectomy. Scand. J. Gastroenterol. *2*, 137–146 (1967)
2. Bittner, R., Beger, H. G.: Die Glucosehomöostase nach Gastrektomie. In: Magenkarzinom: Frühdiagnostik und Therapie. Beger, H. G., Oshima, H., Bergemann, W. (eds.). Stuttgart: Thieme 1979 (in press)

3. Bittner, R., Beger, H. G., Kraas, E., Gögler, H.: Magencarcinomchirurgie auch bei über 70-jährigen? Langenbecks Arch. Chir. *344*, 293 – 307 (1978)
4. Gütgemann, A., Schreiber, H. W., Bernhard, A.: Erfahrungen mit der totalen Gastrektomie. Langenbecks Arch. Klin. Chir. *303*, 73 – 93 (1963)
5. Hunt, C. J.: Construction of food pouch from segment of jejunum as substitute for stomach in total gastrectomy. Arch. Surg. *64*, 601 – 608 (1952)
6. Largiadèr, F., Säuberli, H.: Die totale Gastrektomie – Möglichkeiten der operativen Rekonstruktion nach Gastrektomie. Bruns' Beitr. Klin. Chir. *219*, 601 – 609 (1972)
7. Laurén, P.: The two histological main types of gastric carcinoma: Diffuse and so-called intestinaltyp carcinoma. Acta Pathol. Microbiol. Scand. *64*, 31 – 49 (1965)
8. Peiper, H. J., Siewert, R.: Magenersatz. Chirurg *49*, 81 – 88 (1978)
9. Schreiber, H. W., Eichfuß, H. P., Schumpelick, V.: Magenersatz. Chirurg *49*, 72 – 80 (1978)

Quality of Life and Stomach Replacement

H. Troidl, K.-H. Menge, W. Lorenz, K.-H. Vestweber, H. Barth, and H. Hamelmann

Aim of the Study

In our opinion, the following four criteria determine chiefly the *quality of life* after total gastrectomy:

1) Physical fitness.
2) Capability to work and to resume the preillness occupation.
3) Absence or only insignificant, easily tolerable existence of alimentary complaints and dysfunctions.
4) Overcoming the psychological trauma of the disease.

The aim of this study was therefore to investigate, these parameters after two often used reconstructive methods following total gastrectomy: Longmire-Gütgemann interposition versus Hunt-Lawrence-Rodino pouch.

Patients and Methods

The study consisted of five men and one woman (with gastric cancer which underwent total gastrectomy (Table 1).

The reconstruction of the gut was accomplished after randomization of the patients either with Longmire-Gütgemann interposition or with Hunt-Lawrence Rodino pouch.

Table 1. Peculiarities of the patients and early results

Features	Longmire-Gütgemann (n = 3)	Hunt-Lawrence-Rodino (n = 3)
Age (years)	62 – 68	47 – 70
Sex (m/f)	2/1	3/0
Weight (preop., kg)	57 – 79	60 – 60
Tumor stage (AIC, 1972)	$T_3N_1M_0$, $T_3N_2M_0$, $T_3N_1M_0$	$T_2N_1M_0$, $T_3N_0M_0$, $T_3N_1M_0$
Time duration of surgery	4.6	4.6
Complication, surgical	1/3 (Ileus)	1/3 (biliocutaneous fistula)
medical	1/3 (Pneumonia)	0/3
Duration of hospitalization (days)	28 – 52	18 – 143
Tumor recurrence, local	1/3	0/3
distant	0/3	0/3

The treatment and the course of the examinations of the patients were standardized within our systematic follow-up clinic as described earlier [2, 3]:

1) Diagnostic findings and additional information through patient questionnaire (outpatient).
2) Preoperative preparation (at least 4 days hospital stay); hyperalimentation (at least 3 500 kcal).
3) Operation with standardized indication and technique – only 2 surgeons and pathologist.
4) Postoperative treatment: hyperalimentation.
5) Monthly follow-up examination with questionnaire.
6) Systematic follow-up examination (6 months after operation). Outpatient in the surgical department. Hospital admission in the medical department.
7) Nutritional history with diary.

Results

1) The characteristic complaints over digestion, one of the four criteria for the definition of quality of life, are shown in Table 2. It is conspicuous that the patients are disturbed by belching, especially those with Hunt-Lawrence-Rodino gastric substitute. This complaint was also evident in the self-assessment of the patient and in the assessment of the panel. Dysphagia was found in two of the three patients with Longmire-Gütgemann interposition, whereby the statement of the patient concurs with the panel. Notable were the patients with the Longmire-Gütgemann stomach, who lost their feeling for hunger 6 months after the operation. On the other hand, light dumping in all patients with a Hunt-Lawrence-Rodino stomach was diagnosed. A self-assessment of this characteristic from the patient was, of course, not possible. There were almost no differences or significant results in the symptoms: heartburn, inappetence, fullness,

Table 2. Quality of life 6 months after operation

	Longmire-Gütgemann (n = 3)		Hunt-Lawrence-Rodino (n = 3)	
Criterion	Physician	Patient	Physician	Patient
Belching	1/3	0/3	3/3	3/3
Heartburn	1/3	1/3	0/3	0/3
Dysphagia	2/3	2/3	0/3	0/3
Lack of hunger	3/3	3/3	0/3	1/3
Lack of appetite	1/3	1/3	0/3	0/3
Fullness	1/3	2/3	2/3	1/3
Diarrhea	1/3	1/3	0/3	0/3
Dumping	1/3	2/3	0/3	0/3

and diarrhea, whereby heartburn was especially interesting with regards to a possible reflux.

2) The characteristic physical ability, as criterion for the assessment of the quality of life, is shown in Table 3. It is clear from this table that these criteria, i. e., ability to leave the hospital and non-confinement to bed were shown by the three patients with Longmire-Gütgemann. In one of the three patients which Hunt-Lawrence-Rodino, a biliocutaneous fistula after gallbladder necrosis occurred. This patient could not leave the hospital and was confined to be until exact diagnosis and reoperation (cholecystectomy) could be performed.

3) In the assessment of the quality of life, on the basis of the principal ability *to overcome the psychological trauma*, an interesting result was obtained. At the time of systematic follow-up between the sixth and the eighty month, none of the patients worked in his former profession, and although physically fit, could not work in their utmost capacity as before the operation. More important was the knowledge that all the patients without any differences in this factor were afraid of a recurrence of the disease, which was described as producing quite an influence on the quality of life.

4) Our assessment of the general clinical condition in stomach cancer patients (Table 4) analogous to Visick's staging for peptic ulcer patient, has shown its usefulness. None of the six patients was classified into group 1, 6 months after the operation. Patients G. P. and W. W. achieved the grade 3, whereas patient W. W. was given grade 3 by the physician; the patient judged himself with a better grade. This was more distinct by Mrs. K. E.; the physician placed her into grade 5 because of local recurrence, while the patient assessed herself satisfactorily with grade 3. The patients with Hunt-Lawrence-Rodino assessed themselves one grade better and the judgement of the panel in the estimation of their general condition, namely, grade 2, was unanimous. However, J. J., the patient with the biliocutaneous fistula, who was reoperated, was classified into grade 5, whereas the patient judged himself one grade better. The patients with Hunt-Lawrence-Rodino obtained for themselves as well as from the physician, a better total judgement. On the other hand, it was also evident that the patient estimated his judgement on his general health condition a nuance better than the attending physicians.

Table 3. Quality of life 6 months after operation: physical ability

	Longmire-Gütgemann (n = 3)		Hunt-Lawrence-Rodino (n = 3)	
Criterion	Physician	Patient	Physician	Patient
Not dormant	3/3	3/3	2/3	1/3
Dormant, but not confined to bed	0/3	0/3	0/3	1/3
Confined to bed	0/3	0/3	1/3	1/3

Table 4. Grading of the overall clinical condition after total gastrectomy. This includes three of the main factors for quality of life: physical fitness, capability to work and to resume pre-illness occupation, and absence of existence of alimentary complaints and dysfunctions

Stage	Definiton	Attributes
1	Very good	Physical fitness corresponding to age. Capability to work, especially in the pre-illness occupation. No alimentary complaints or dysfunctions.
2	Good	Physical fitness corresponding to age. Capability to work, not necessarily in the pre-illness occupation. Mild alimentary complaints or dysfunctions (only moderate hunger or appetite, epigastric fullness, dumping, etc.), which only insignificantly disturb the patient's general well-being if he is properly adapted (e. g., by diet). Medical treatment is only occasionally necessary.
3	Satisfactory	Physical fitness diminished, but the patient can leave the house. Incapability to work, but the patient is occupied with activities in the family or elsewhere. Moderate alimentary complaints or dysfunctions which can be influenced only by continuous medical treatment.
4	Unsatisfactory	Physical fitness considerably diminished, the patient generally cannot leave the house. Incapability to work, only insignificant activities in the family. Severe alimentary complaints or dysfunctions which cannot sufficiently be influenced by continuous medical treatment. Considerable difficulties in stabilizing body weight. Hospitalization sometimes necessary.
5	Failure	Recurrence of tumor, metastasis, or reoperations. No physical fitness, the patient generally cannot leave bed and is without any drive. Body weight cannot be stabilized, hospitalization is repeatedly necessary.

5) Weight behavior, a parameter which certainly contributes to the quality of life with regards to physical fitness, is shown in Table 5. All patients, without exception lost 6 kg mean weight despite hyperalimentation in the postoperative phase. From the time of discharge from the hospital to the time of follow-up, a trend could be recognized: the patients with a Hunt-Lawrence-Rodino estimated the weight loss more positive.

6) A interesting result was the calculation of the daily caloric intake on the basis of the records from the dairy over 14 days prior to the systematic follow-up (Table 6). Because of loss of hunger and appetite, especially in the patients with Longmire-Gütgemann interposition, a daily caloric deficit resulted. On the other hand, the patients with the Hunt-Lawrence-Rodino pouch had a positive balance of calories with the exception of the patient J. J., who had a biliodigestive fistula at the time of calculation.

7) The tests, which were indicators for an eventual prevailing disturbance of absorption, vitamin B_{12} absorption, carbohydrate intake, and iron resorption, and the chymotrypsin test, as the last possible indication for an exocrine pancreas function, showed no difference between the two employed methods for stomach reconstruction (Table 7). Despite the presence of duodenal passage in the patients with Hunt-Lawrence-Rodino interposition, the three patients had no better fat absorption. It was almost in all cases elevated above the normal value. The xylose test, as an indicator for carbohydrate intake, was unchanged and showed no

Table 5. Weight changes (kg) in gastric cancer patients after 2 types of stomach substitutes. ("Ideal weight" recommended by Statist. Ball. Metrop. Life Insurance Co. 40, Nov. – Dec. 1959)

Surgical technique	Longmire-Gütgemann				Hunt-Lawrence-Rodino			
Patient	K. E.	G. P.	W. W.	x̄	Z. K.	Q. K.	J. J.[a]	x̄
In hospital	−6	−6	−7	−6.3	−5	−8	−11	−8.0
6 months postop.	−3	−7	−3	−4.3	−3	+2	− 2	−1.0
% of the ideal weight	96	103	93	97.3	95	90	77	87.3

[a] Biliocutaneous fistula.

Table 6. Nutritional parameter in gastric cancer patients after 2 types of stomach substitutes

Surgical technique	Longmire-Gütgemann			Hunt-Lawrence-Rodino		
Patient	K. E.	G. P.	W. W.	Z. K.	Q. K.	J. J.[a]
Caloric intake as:						
Protein (g)	15	60	55	65	110	60
Fat (g)	25	95	75	120	175	40
Carbohydrate (g)	50	155	200	215	455	125
Intake (kcal)	516	1765	1765	2260	4165	1200
Requirement (kcal)	1600	2250	2440	2000	3500	2000
Deficit	−1084	− 485	− 675	+ 260	+ 665	− 800

[a] Biliocutaneous fistula.

Table 7. Metabolic functional tests in gastric cancer patients after 2 types of stomach substitutes. ↑ = pathologically increased; ↓ = pathologically decreased; ↔ = no change

Functional test[a]	Changes	Longmire-Gütgemann (n = 3)	Hunt-Lawrence-Rodino (n = 3)
Fat excretion/day	↑	2/3	2/3
Vitamin A test	↓	0/3	1/3
Xylose test	↔	3/3	3/3
Schilling test			
without intrinsic F.	↓	3/3	3/3
with intrinsic F.	↓	3/3	3/3
Chymotrypsin in faeces	↓	1/3	1/3
Iron absorption	↔	3/3	3/3

[a] Accomplishment and estimation according to the synopsis from Menge et al. [1].

difference for both methods. The Schilling test showed, without exception, a reduced vitamin B_{12} absorption for both methods with and without an intrinsic factor. The chymotrypsin test, as indicator for exogenous pancreas function, was in one case, namely in J. J., surely in pathological range, while otherwise it was scarcely within the so-called low, normal range. Despite removal of all the acid-producing cells, the iron absorption in all six patients was unchanged.

8) All the laboratory investigations of the blood and the serum electrolytes were in normal range in all patients.

9) In the patients' history on nutrition, the patients reported incompatibility of dairy products and fatty foods; in addition salads, cucumber, and coffee. Differences and/or trend toward a difference between both methods were not found.

10) Two patients (G. P. and W. W.) reported aversion to particular foods as well as fatty foods, acidic cucumber, and potato salad. All the patients kept to diet despite contrary instruction, in contrast to patients with Hunt-Lawrence-Rodino.

Conclusions

The study showed that the factor quality of life in the selected definition was an important and comprehensible feature, whereby the study clearly showed that the fourth criterion of quality of life, namely, the overcoming of the psychological trauma, was recognized as the most important one. A similar, important result was the fact that the patient, after total gastrectomy, could have a daily caloric intake deficit up to 1 000 cal because of poor food intake. The causes for this are, however, not malabsorption, but rather the loss of hunger and appetite.

The usual, employed metabolic tests as indicators for fat and carbohydrate absorption, etc. after total gastrectomy are, like parameters for discrimination of reconstruction procedures after total gastrectomy, of little importance. Differences between the two applied procedures after total gastrectomy, i.e., Hunt-Lawrence-Rodino pouch and Longmire-Gütgemann interposition, were not found due to the small number of patients.

References

1. Menge, K. H., Rieken, O. E.: Dünndarmfunktionsdiagnostik. Z. Gastroenterol. *16*, 198–205 (1978)
2. Rohde, H., Troidl, H., Lorenz, W.: Systematic follow-up: A concept for evaluation of operative results in duodenal ulcer patients. Klin. Wochenschr. *55*, 925–932 (1977)
3. Troidl, H.: Einrichtungen einer systematischen Kontrolluntersuchungsklinik. Langenbecks Arch. Chir. *347*, 467–480 (1978)

Summary: Experiences With Various Types of Reconstructive Procedures After Gastrectomy

Long- and short-term results after gastrectomy are determined by the type of reconstruction of the alimentary tract. The goal of all reconstructive procedures must be:

1) Prevention of reflux esophagitis.
2) Prevention of Dumping syndrome.
3) The lowest possible failure rate obtained with a technically uncomplicated procedure.

Maldigestion and duodenal passage are of clinically subordinate significance, since the maintenance of an orthograde duodenal passage could not be proven to yield physiologically more advantageous results. There is a general consensus that reflux esophagitis can be prevented most effectively by jejunal interposition with a sufficiently long loop or jejunal pouch formation with a deep Roux-en-Y anastomosis. The function of an additional jejunal plication lies not so much in the creation of an antireflux mechanism, but rather in its capacity as a safeguard against rupture of the anastomotic seam. If the intraabdominal esophagus is preserved, the lower esophageal sphincter can remain functional. Adequate circulation is indispensible for this. The extent of the influence of a radicular ligature of the arteria gastrica sinistra on the circulation is uncertain.

No definitive statement concerning the best reconstructive procedure after gastrectomy is possible to date. Any comparative critique of individual methods fails for lack of uniform protocols of reexamination. If a scrupulous follow-up program is adhered to, many more long range complications are registered. Figures over dumping after jejunal interposition, for instance, fluctuate between almost never and one-third of the cases.

As a prerequisite for the evaluation of the surgical procedures, an investigation including not only the surgical result, but also a painstaking survey of long range results and, above all, data concerning the general psychological situation of the patient is much in demand. In order to compile sufficient case material and to be able to compare the different procedures, such a study can only be made in cooperation with various medical centers. A uniform catalogue of criteria, however, is indispensible in this effort.

10 Adjuvant Therapeutic Measures

A Tentative Synopsis of the Nutritional Problems Encountered in Patients Afflicted with Malignant Neoplasia

K. Schultis, W. Fekl, and O. Brand

Hypotheses on the Development of Malignant Cachexia

Unaccountable weight loss is frequently an early symptom of malignant neoplasia. Since it can be assumed that the exogenous food supply is generally not lacking in nutrients, this change in weight, which can range from simple weight loss to deleterious marasmus, must occur for other, mostly endogenous reasons. The main hypotheses under discussion are an increased consumption due to the tumor, alterations of the gastrointestinal tract, anorexia of unknown origin, and alterations of the intermediary metabolism.

1) Increased Consumption due to the Tumor

The possibility that tumor metabolism specifically differs from the norm has been under consideration for some time. The increasing evidence that the difference in the metabolism of tumor and host is quantitative rather than qualitative does not, however, negate the possibility of an increased consumption of individual nutrients. If, for example, a metabolic pathway, whose integrity depends on the presence of a specific vitamin or amino acid, becomes significantly overactive in a tumor, the corresponding partner of the reaction pattern may thus be insufficiently available to the intermediary metabolism of the host.

2) Alterations of the Gastrointestinal Tract

The reasons for nutritional disturbances due to changes in the gastrointestinal tract can be manifold. They range from mechanical obstructions by the primary tumor or its metastases to gastroenteric malassimilation as a complication of the basic ailment or its therapy, and include severe disturbances of homeostasis as produced by enteral fistulae. A known percentage of patients with malignant neoplasms exhibits symptoms of hunger dystrophy due to malassimilation.

3) Consuming Diseases

Marasmus, as an empirical concomitant to the so-called consuming diseases, is in its definition still highly hypothetical. Although cachexiae developed in the course of malignant neoplasms reveal certain uniform features, the exact nature and location of the disturbances evidenced by increased consumption remain obscure. Forced synthesis of specific proteins of the immunological system such as C-reactive proteins, immunoglobulin, or other globulins, and increased leukopoesis can conceivably play a part in this.

4) Anorexia of Unknown Origin

Anorexia is an additional factor in the development of malignant cachexia, and of the utmost concern to cancer patients, their families, and the nursing staff. Hardly of psychogenic or even psychosomatic origin in patients with malignant neoplasia, its cause remains unknown. The hypothesis that the lack of appetite may be caused by an excess of some metabolites remains to be proven [2, 22].

5) Alterations of Intermediate Metabolism

Although quantitative variations from the physiological norm have been affirmed in tumor metabolism, no qualitative deviations have as yet been verified.

The literature contains contradictory reports on the changes in the intermediary metabolism of the organism. On the one hand, hyperglycemia is manifest as a disturbance of glucose tolerance [4], for instance, whereas, on the other hand, there are reports of hypoglycemia as a result of high glucose turnover in the tumor [1]. There is an intricate functional relationship of malignant tumor and host organism [21]. It seems reasonable to assume that metabolic characteristics of the tumor interact with those of the host as to constitute specific syndromes (Table 1).

Calman [6] compiled a list of these specific abnormalities (Table 2). In an earlier paper, the same author describes a reduction in co-enzyme A activity. It is as yet uncertain, whether this is due to a deficit of pantothenic acid, or whether this central co-enzyme is lacking in other components, such as cystine [7].

Other syndromes frequently observed concomitant to malignant neoplasia are diabetic metabolism, protein catabolism, delayed or absent immune response [8], and hemorrhagic diathesis. They all contribute to the constellation of nutritional problems confronting the cancer patient and the practitioner.

Table 1. Neoplasia as functional interaction of tumor and host organism. The active components of the tumor evoke the specific reaction syndromes in the host which make up the total clinical picture of neoplasia (According to Straeuli)

Tumor	Host
Increase of cells	Mechanical/functional disturbances
Penetration/Formation of metastases	Danger to life
Metabolism	Syndromes
Antigenicity	Immune reactions

Table 2. Decreased concentrations for patients with malignant neoplasia (according to Calman)

Anemia
Hypoalbuminemia
Deficiency of:
Vitamin A
Carotene
Thiamine
Leukocytic ascorbic acid
Folic acid
Vitamin B_{12}

Specific Nutritional Problems in Gastric Cancer

A reduced nutritional status was determined for the majority of patients with malignant neoplasia by means of the so-called anthropometric methods, which provide parameters (Table 3) for the assessment of nutritional status. The indication for therapeutic supplementary nutrition derived therefrom requires a closer look at the specific nutritional problems encountered with gastric cancer.

The decline of gastric cancer morbidity in recent years and the considerable difference of occurrence in various countries are obvious indications for the pathogenic significance of exogenous factors. Eating habits, such as the consumption of animal fats, smoked meats, and soy products significantly influence the etiology of stomach cancer.

Significant observations can be made when studying case histories of gastric cancer patients under nutritional auspices. There is frequently an aversion to meats. Except for the case of cardiac carcinoma, nutritional disturbance due to the obstruction of stomach passage by a primary malignant tumor is uncommon, whereas complications are often caused by obstructive metastases. These can lead to choledochal and/or Wirsung's duct stenosis and result in maldigestion particularly of fats, but also of proteins and carbohydrates. Hemorrhage, occult or macroscopically evident, is not uncommon for gastric cancer, and constitutes

Table 3. Parameters to assess nutritional status

Standard parameters	
Weight/height	Albumin
Triceps skinfold	Creatinine index[a]
Mid-upper arm circumference	Lymphocyte count
Mid-upper arm muscle circumference	Iron-binding capacity/Transferrin
	Prealbumin
	Cellular immune response (skin test)

[a] Calculation $\frac{\text{Measured creatinine}}{\text{Ideal creatinine}^{b}} \times 100.$

[b] The ideal creatinine in ng can be determined by the ideal weight:
Ideal weight for men × 22
Ideal weight for women × 17

Table 4. Survey of results obtained with parenteral nutrition in cancer patients

Author	No. of patients	Duration of parenteral nutrition	Type of treatment	Results
Schwartz (71)	10	17 – 84 days	Chemotherapy	↑ Appetite ↑ Weight ↑ Chemotherapeutics
Heller (72)	30	42 days	Radiotherapy Chemotherapy	↑ Chemotherapeutics ↑ Tolerance
de Matteis (73)	23	12 days	Operation	↑ Weight ↑ Albumin ↑ Wound healing
Lanzotti (75)	38	9 – 41 days	Chemotherapy	↑ Immune response
Bozetti (76)	44	1 – 16 weeks	Chemotherapy Radiotherapy	↑ Weight ↑ Lymphocyte transformation ↑ Albumin
Copeland (77)	406	∅ 23 days	Chemotherapy Radiotherapy	↑ Immune response ↑ Albumin ↑ Chemotherapeutics >50% Decrease in tumor size (↑) Survival time
Eriksson (77)	50	5 – 109 days ∅ 26	Operation Chemotherapy Radiotherapy	↑ Lymphocytes ↑ T-cells ↑ B-cells ↑ Transferrin
Gulajev (77)	31	During radiotherapy	Radiotherapy	↑ Tolerance of radiotherapy Full treatment possible in contrast to control group
Holter (77)	30	10 days postoperative	Operation	↑ Albumin Weight gain
Moghissi (77)	10	5 – 7 days preoperative 6 – 7 days postoperative	Operation	Positive *N*-balance uncomplicated postoperative course
Solassol (78)	1350	1 – 4 months	Operation Chemotherapy Radiotherapy	Restoration of the nutritional status Well being
Kohlschütter (78)	7	7 – 30 days	Chemotherapy	↑ Tolerance ↑ Quality of life

an additional, significant factor for the development of preoperative cachexia, since it enhances the malnutritional status.

Fasting in the course of perioperative diagnostic treatment and postoperative care, quite apart from the postaggression metabolism after the operation itself, contributes to the nutritional deficit. Nutritional problems in the acute postoperative phase, barring complications, are usually checked after 4 – 6 days. The previously emaciated patient, of course, is much more severely affected by the consequences of the catabolism associated with postaggression metabolism than the patient without prior metabolic impairment [17].

The gastric cancer patient's situation is postoperatively defined by the type of operation he has undergone, by the impact of the side effects of adjunct oncotherapeutic measures on his nutritional intake and his intermediary metabolism, and by the course of the affliction itself.

Aspects of Nutritional Therapy

The implications of the nutritional situation of cancer patients are so grave, that a physician should be very circumspect in this regard, particularly pertaining to the prescription of fasting periods even for diagnostic purposes.

Therapeutic nutritional restrictions with the aim of inhibiting or perhaps reversing tumor growth are certainly not indicated in view of the cancer patient's precarious condition. It can conversely be argued, that an optimum supply of nutrients would result in a maximum rate of mitosis, which again would provide the necessary prerequisite for schematic therapy based on mitotic synchronization.

A partial survey of recent results obtained with parenteral nutrition in cancer patients shows positive influences on a number of vital variables (Table 4).

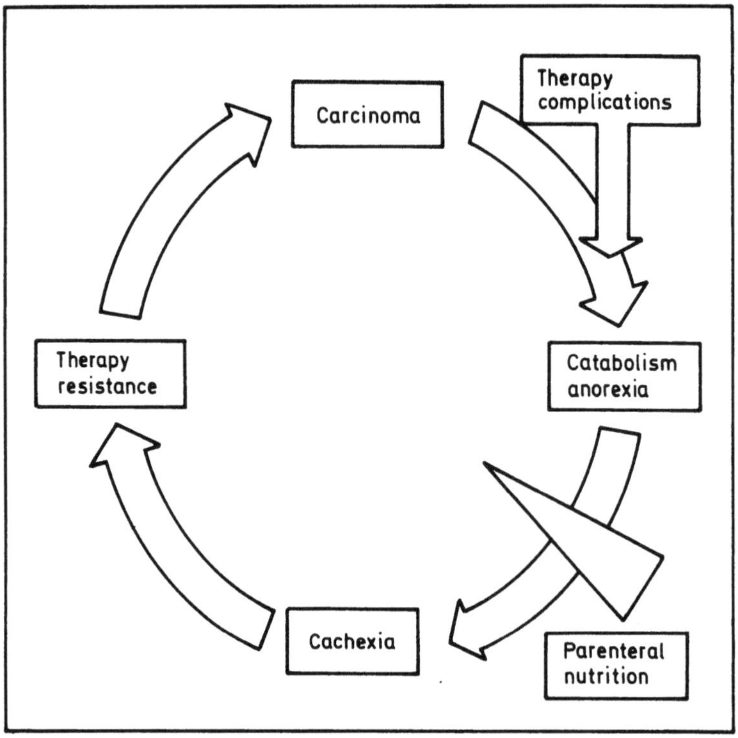

Fig. 1. Vicious circle in carcinoma

Conclusion

The mechanical and metabolic interaction of a tumor with the host organism especially affects the nutritional status of the patient, and therefore the possibility and the success of surgical intervention as well as the postoperative prognosis and quality of life. A malignant and untreatable cancer condition with anorexia, catabolism, and cachexia constitutes a vicious circle activated by noxae, which in turn affect the patient (Fig. 1). Consistent parenteral nutrition provides the only means of breaking this vicious circle.

References

1. Ardenne, von, M.: Die Stimulierung des Stoffwechsels der Zellen als Waffe gegen Krankheiten und Krisenzustände. Phys. Med. Reh. *14*, 321–332 (1973)
2. Batz, K., Truog, P., Nagel, G. A.: Unterstützende allgemeinmedizinische Maßnahmen in der Tumortherapie. In: Internistische Krebstherapie. Brunner, K. W., Nagel, G. A. (eds.), Berlin, Heidelberg, New York: Springer 1976
3. Blackburn, G. L., Bistrian, B. R., Maini, B. S., Schlamm, H. T., Smith, M. F.: Nutritional and metabolic assessment of the hospitalized patient. J. Parent. Ent. Nutr. *1*, 11–22 (1977)
4. Bodansky, O.: Biochemistry of human cancer. 1. general metabolic characteristics in cancer. New York: Academic Press 1975
5. Bozetti, F., Terno, G., Pupa, A., Uccellini, M., Rota, G., Emanuelli, H.: Iperalimentazione parenterale nei pazienti con neoplasia avanzata. Tumori *62*, 623–644 (1976)
6. Calman, K. C.: Nutrition and cancer. In: Nutritional aspects of care in the critically Ill. Richards, J. R., Kinney, J. M. (eds.), Edinburgh: Churchill Livingstone 1977
7. Calman, K. C.: Nutritional support in malignant disease. Proc. Nutr. Soc. *37*, 87–93 (1978)
8. Copeland, E. M., Daly, J. M., Dudrick, S. J.: Nutrition as an adjunct to cancer treatment in the adult. Cancer Res. *37*, 2451–2456 (1977)
9. Eriksson, B., Douglass, H. O., Homan, P., Milliron, S., Fitzpatrick, J., Nava, H.: Hyperalimentation as an adjunct to the treatment of cancer of the upper gastrointestinal tract. IPEN *1*, Nr. 4 (1977)
10. Heller, K. L.: The Effect of fat on complete parenteral nutrition on the nitrogen balance. 9th International Congress of Nutrition, Mexiko 1972
11. Holter, A. R., Fischer, J. E.: The effects of perioperative hyperalimentation on complications in patients with carcinoma and weight loss. J. Surg. Res. *23*, 31–34 (1977)
12. Kohlschütter, B., Jehn, U.: Die parenterale Ernährung bei aggressiver Chemotherapie verschiedener Neoplasien. Onkologie *1*, 31–34 (1978)
13. Lanzotti, V. J., Copeland, E. M., George, S. L., Dudrick, S. J., Samuels, M. L.: Cancer chemotherapeutic response and intravenous hyperalimentation. Cancer Chemother. Rep. *59*, 437–439 (1975)
14. DeMatteis, R., Hermann, R. E.: Supplementary parenteral nutrition in patients with malignant disease. Cleve. Clin. Q. *40*, 139–145 (1973)
15. Moghissi, K., Hornshaw, J., Teasdale, P. R., Dawes, E. A.: Parenteral nutrition in carcinoma of the oesophagus treated by surgery: Nitrogen balance and clinical studies. Br. J. Surg. *64*, 125–128 (1977)
16. Schultis, K.: Postaggressionsstoffwechsel als Adaptation und als Krankheit. In: Postaggressionsstoffwechsel – Grundlagen, Klinik, Therapie. Heberer, G., Schultis, K., Hoffmann, K. (eds.), Stuttgart: Schattauer 1976
17. Schultis, K.: Pathobiochemische Grundlagen des Postaggressionsstoffwechsels. Langenbecks Arch. Chir. (in press)
18. Schwartz, G. F., Green, H. L., Bendon, M. L., Graham, W. P., Blakemore, W. S.: Combined parenteral hyperalimentation and chemotherapy in the treatment of disseminated solid tumors. Am. J. Surg. *121*, 169–173 (1971)
19. Solassol, C., Joyeux, H.: Künstlicher Gastrointestinaltrakt bei Magen-Darm-Krebs. Onkologie (in press)

20. Souchon, E. A., Copeland, E. M., Watson, P., Dudrick, S. J.: Intravenous hyperalimentation as an adjunct to cancer chemotherapy with 5-Fluorouracil. J. Surg. Res. *18*, 451 – 454 (1975)
21. Sträuli, P.: Neoplasien. In: Klinische Pathophysiologie. W. Siegenthaler (ed.), 3rd ed. Stuttgart: Thieme 1976
22. Theologides, A.: Why cancer patients have anorexia? Geriatrics *31*, 69 – 71 (1976)
23. Wirths, W.: Ermittlung des Ernährungszustandes. In: Ernährungslehre und Diätetik, Bd. III. Angewandte Ernährungslehre. Cremer, H. D., Hötzel, D. (eds.), Stuttgart: Thieme 1974

Total Parenteral Nutrition in Regional Surgery for Gastric Cancer

H. Joyeux, Cl. Solassol, J. B. Dubois, and H. Pujol

The prognosis for patients with cancer of the stomach is still very poor; the 5-year survival rate of approximately 13% for those patients whose cancer was diagnosed between 1955 and 1959 has not improved to any degree since that time [2]. Gastric cancer tends to metastasize to regional lymph nodes and to exhibit a diffuse lymphatic spread in the gastric wall. It also shows a tendency to vascular invasion, which may have no relationship with the involvement of the lymph nodes or the lymphatic system. Lymphatic spread may extend across the pylorus into the duodenum and may involve the esophagus. The greatest prognostic factor after surgical resection is the presence or absence of lymph node involvement. Today, thanks to extemporaneous histopathological studies of regional lymph nodes following frozen section, additional extensive tissue resection can be performed upon demand when positive lymph node involvement is detected during the surgical procedure. Malnutrition is a common occurrence during the course of gastric cancer; the imbalance may be severe and artificial nutrition, primarily parenteral, may be the only effective means of restoring and maintaining a proper nutritional status in these patients. From 1972 to 1977, 227 cases of gastric cancer were treated at the Montpellier Cancer Institute and total gastrectomy of necessity was performed in 48 cases using the specific guidelines for regional surgery of gastric cancer. In all cases, parenteral nutrition was incorporated into the therapeutic program [14].

Malnutrition in Gastric Cancer

In general, cancer as a disease can cause malnutrition under three different circumstances which can be associated: nutritional intake inferior to basic daily requirements, digestive malabsorption, and enhanced metabolic requirements. Complete anorexia, or anorexia relative to specific foods, is often one of the revealing symptoms of the tumor. Pain and anxiety are not always the cause of this reduction in food intake. Anorexic agents produced by the tumor cells might be shown to play some part in this process. Compression of the digestive tract by a tumor situated within the lumen, or altering the lumen from without, will cause dysphagia and/or gastric intolerance. The 227 gastric cancer patients who were seen at the Montpellier Cancer Institute, including 48 patients who underwent total gastrectomy out of necessity, were studied in order to determine the specific contributing factors of this malnutrition syndrome.

Malnutrition Preceding the Start of Cancer Therapy (Tables 1 and 2)

A quantitative reduction in nutritional intake is often noted with a global 10% – 70% decrease in the daily energy and protein ration. No specific deficiencies were revealed by various investigations into the individual patients' dietary habits. Dysphagia and epigastric discomfort are the most frequent causes of the reduction in food intake. Loss of weight is commonly encountered (84%); its importance correlates well with the size of the tumor (5% – 30% decline from the normal weights of the patients). Anorexia is not a constant finding, but it is observed in 30% of the cases.

A protein-losing gastropathy may be seen alone [2], or with atrophic or hypertrophic gastritis and steatorrhea; the major resulting disturbances are low serum albumin and globulin levels.

Thus, a majority of patients with cancer of the stomach present with a negative nitrogen balance before the start of antineoplastic therapy (Table 6).

Malnutrition as a Result of Cancer Treatment

Even though the combined use of radiotherapy and surgery in gastric cancer is still not a universally acknowledged method of therapy, it seems probable that

Table 1. Malnutrition in gastric cancer; 1972 – 1977: 227 patients

Reduction of food intake	Dysphagia-pain	20%
	Weight loss	84%
	Anorexia	30%
Protein-losing-gastropathy	Hypoalbuminemia	73%
	Hypoglobulinemia	69%
	Steatorrhea	12%
	Atrophic or hyperthrophic gastritis	41%

Table 2. Malnutrition in gastric cancer: Nitrogen losses

	Nitrogen losses and requirements
1. Frequent occurrence during the preoperative period Negative nitrogen balance	10 – 20 gN/24 h
2. Regional surgery 4 – 8 h Visceral resection Lymphadenectomy Multiple anastomoses	50 – 100 gN/24 h
3. Constant occurrence during the postoperative period – Loss of plasma and lymph fluid (protein – rich drainage)	5 – 10 gN/24 h
– Basal requirements, paralytic ileus	10 – 15 gN/24 h

this combination, in the form of pre- or postoperative radiotherapy, will become the treatment of choice in cases where the tumor is extensive and the lymph node involvement positive [1]. It has been our policy to submit all those patients whose tumors are not excisable to this form of palliative treatment; this mode of therapy was found to be all the more tolerable and acceptable to the patient when partial or total parenteral nutrition was added as an artificial means of nutritional support.

As it were, irradiation of the upper abdomen has a strong catabolic effect on the underlying tissues in that it causes radiation injuries in previously afflicted portions of the esophagus, stomach and duodenum, as well as parts of the pancreas and colon [4].

The total gastrectomy procedure is not routine; it is only indicated in cases where total excision becomes necessary because of the extent of the lesions, as in 48 of our patients. In each case, the principles of regional surgery were applied [13]. Lasting between 5 and 10 hours, this extensive type of procedure is associated with an important intraoperative loss of protein, lipids, and electrolytes which must be strictly compensated for (whole blood, plasma, albumin, and electrolyte solutions). This replenishment must be continued throughout the postoperative phase because of renewed losses due to the repeated drainage of the peritoneal cavity as a safeguard against infection and peritonitis due to anastomotic leakage. A lipid-protein-ion losing drainage has been individualized along with a corresponding biological syndrome (Table 3). In addition to the losses described above, there is a reduction in the energy and protein intake (basal requirements); the oral route is barred from use for periods ranging from

Table 3. "Lipid-protein-ion-losing drainage." Biological syndrome in regional digestive surgery

	Intraoperative hemorrhage	Intraoperative and postoperative plasma losses	Intraoperative and postoperative lymph fluid losses
Proteins g/liter	160	51	62–91
Fibrinogen g/liter	3–7	3–7	3–7
Lipids g/liter	3.5–8	3.5–8	10–42
Cholesterol g/liter	1.5–2.7	1.5–2.7	1.5–2.7
Electrolytes mEq/liter			
Na^+	117–141	117–141	117–141
K^+	3.3–5.6	3.3–5.6	3.3–5.6
Cl^-	89–102	89–102	89–102
HCO_3^-	9–20	9–20	9–20
Ca^{++}	2.1–5.1	2.1–5.1	2.1–5.1
PO_4^{--}	3.2–6.5	3.2–6.5	3.2–6.5
Mg^{++}	1–1.4	1–1.4	1–1.4

3 to 4 weeks because of a prolonged state of paralytic ileus caused by the injury of perivascular nerve fibers during lymph node biopsies.

Metabolic Disorders Following Regional Gastrectomy

The disturbances are easily recognized in that every major nutrient is usually altered (Table 4). The imbalance is observed as soon as oral alimentation is reinstated, most often around the beginning of the third postoperative week. The altered anatomical and physiological conditions account for a prolonged period of adaptation of the organism lasting between 2 and 4 weeks following the start of oral alimentation. Correctly adapted nutritional support is used in order to maintain a metabolic setting in which the first course of chemotherapy can be safety initiated (5-FU, mitomycin C, BCNU, and adriamycin according to a planned regimen). It is a well-known fact that the 80% failure rate for curative surgery is related to the presence of established metastatic foci outside the operative field rather than to dislodged tumor cells. Thus, it would seem imperative to administer intensive and protracted chemotherapy in an attempt to eliminate metastatic disease.

Total Parenteral Nutrition System

Our system essentially comprises: a mode of venous access allowing for total or partial parenteral nutrition, which is left in place during the entire period of nutritional support; a U-shaped rubber bag specifically designed for artificial nutrition, and able to contain a daily ration of nutritive mixture, and two types of infusion pumps, a portable one for ambulatory use and one for bedside use.

The Nutritive Tube

The hyperosmolarity of the nutritive solutions and the comfort of the patient make it necessary to use a deep venous trunk as a vascular access route. The Teflon-Scurasil cannula which is used has an internal diameter of 2.7 mm and an external diameter of 4.5 mm. It is inserted end-to-side into the superior or inferior vena cava through one of their tributaries [11].

Table 4. Metabolic disorders following regional gastrectomy

Maldigestion of carbohydrates 30%	Positive D-xylose test Lactase deficit
Maldigestion of lipids 20% – 40%	Triglycerids and fatty acids Steatorrhea
Protein deficit	Reduction of caloric-nitrogen intake Hypoalbuminemia
Iron, Vit. B_{12}, folic acid, and Vit. D malabsorptions	

The principles of the technique used since 1971 are shown in Fig. 1. The access route is chosen so as not to restrict limb movement. Cannulation is performed under surgical conditions using local anesthesia. The Teflon-tipped silicone rubber cannula is secured within the collateral of a large-diameter deep venous trunk. The proper placement of the Teflon tip is verified in all cases by the free back-flow of blood into an aspirating syringe. Hypertonic infusate will be delivered at a uniform rate ensuring rapid dilution of the infusate in an area of high blood flow and precluding the introduction of a foreign body into the mainstream of blood flow; thus, it minimizes the risks of phlebitis and thrombosis. The Scurasil tubing runs along a subcutaneous tunnel over 15 – 20 cm and its exit is located either in the paramamillary or paraumbilical area (Fig. 2). Providing that these cannulas are placed under circumstances of strict surgical asepsis, they can be left in place without difficulty for more than one year's time.

This mode of vascular access is used for parenteral nutrition lasting more than a month. For average term nutritional support (2 – 8 weeks), we use indwelling radio-opaque silicone catheters. These are placed in the superior or inferior vena cava under local anesthesia and strict surgical conditions: they must be replaced every 8 weeks in order to prevent deep vein thrombosis, but there have been a few instances in which catheters were left in place without any incidents for up to 12 month's time in patients who were undergoing sequential chemotherapy.

The Silicone Rubber Bag

We have developed a portable container which can hold the daily ration of nutrients. This container is a one-piece silicone rubber (Scurasil) bag. Its char-

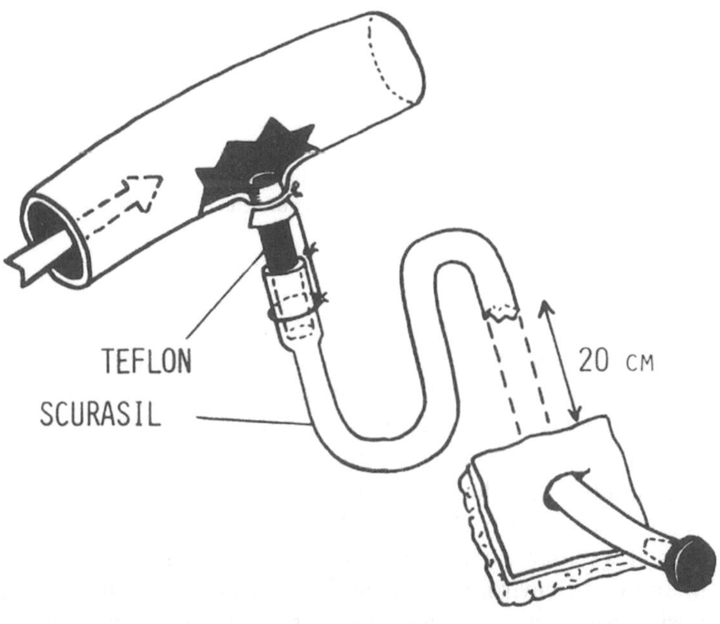

Fig. 1. Cannulated collateral of a deep venous trunk. The end of the Teflon tip is placed at the junction of the collateral with the deep venous trunk. The distal end of the Scurasil cannula runs along a subcutaneous tunnel to its exit site

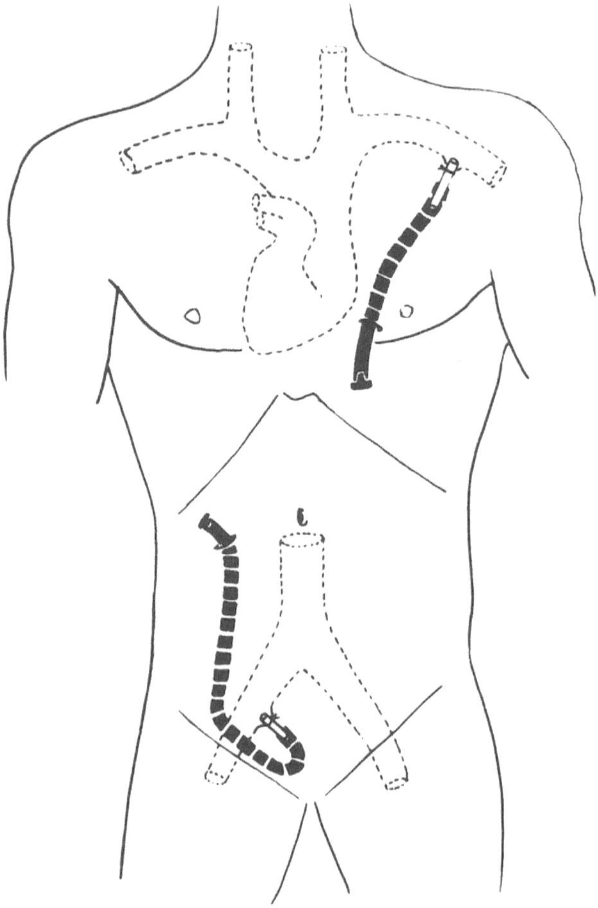

Fig. 2. The implantation of the cannula is made end-to-side to a fixed part of a deep vessel either on the superior vena cava or the inferior vena cava

acteristics are as follows: U-shape, weight 350 g three opening [two lateral openings for washing, one central opening for filling and infusion (Fig. 3)]. The two lateral openings can be closed with Teflon plugs, strongly adhering to the silicone. The central opening is at the lowest point of the bag; the feedline starts here in continuity with the bag. Holes for suspension are provided at each end. This Scurasil container is flexible, collapsible, and washable. It can be sterilized and thus, it is reusable: sterilization is done in a vacuum pan and filling is performed in an aseptic environment under laminar air flow. The plugged bags are placed upside down on a special stand after having been completely emptied; with the force of gravity, ten bags can be filled in 30 min. The full bags are then stored in a room at 4 °C.

The Nutritive Mixtures

All the nutrient constituents of the daily parenteral diet are mixed together in the same flask for simultaneous infusion (Fig. 4). Studies of bacteriological, physicochemical, and biological preservation performed on the complete mixture (stored at 4 °C) gave excellent results, the mixture having first been tested in dogs. The composition of the nutrient mixture is tailored to the patient's present needs, while also taking into account his weight prior to the disease. Adequate caloric and nitrogen intake is provided in order to obtain an improvement in the patient's general condition, as well as a gain in weight and a positive nitrogen balance. An optimal calorie-to-nitrogen ratio of 150–200 kcal/g of nitrogen is maintained. Thus, we have determined different formulas for normonutrition and hypernutrition. The average diet used for parenteral nutrition is shown in Table 5. A miniaturized battery-driven portable pump with dimensions specially calculated for ambulatory and bedside use has now been developed (Fig. 4). Its total weight, including batteries is 470 g. The pump can run for 30 h and is capable of maintaining a constant flow against pressures of up to 200 mmHg. The flow can be set at three different speeds; permitting a gradual increase in flow speed at the beginning of the perfusion and a gradual decrease at the end, thus allowing progressive variations in the osmolar load. This pump is incorporated into the perfusion line and is attached to a specially designed vest for use in ambulatory artificial nutrition.

Table 5. Nutritive mixtures for normo-(N_1, N_2, N_3) and hyper-(H_1, H_2) parenteral nutrition

	Normonutrition			Hypernutrition	
	N_1	N_2	N_3	H_1	H_2
Water ml	2500	2500	3000	3000	3000
Dextrose g	160	150	250	375	375
Lipids cal	0	1000	1000	1000	1500
Nitrogen g	6.25	6.25	10–12.5	12.5–15	15–25
Total Calories	640	1600	2000	2500	3000
Na mEq	50	50	50	121	121
K mEq	48	48	48	80	80
Cl mEq	84	84	84	117	117
Mg mEq	4	4	4	28	28
Ca mEq	8	8	8	16	16
Acetate mEq	10	10	10	42	42
Sulfate mEq	4	4	4	5	5
Lactate mEq	4	4	4	40	40
Phosphate mEq	8	8	8	40	40
Fe mg	1	1	1	1	1
Cu mg	0.84	0.84	0.84	0.84	0.84
Mn mg	1.48	1.48	1.48	1.48	1.48
Co µg	1.47	1.47	1.47	1.47	1.47
F mg	1.45	1.45	1.45	1.45	1.45
I µg	1.52	1.52	1.52	1.52	1.52

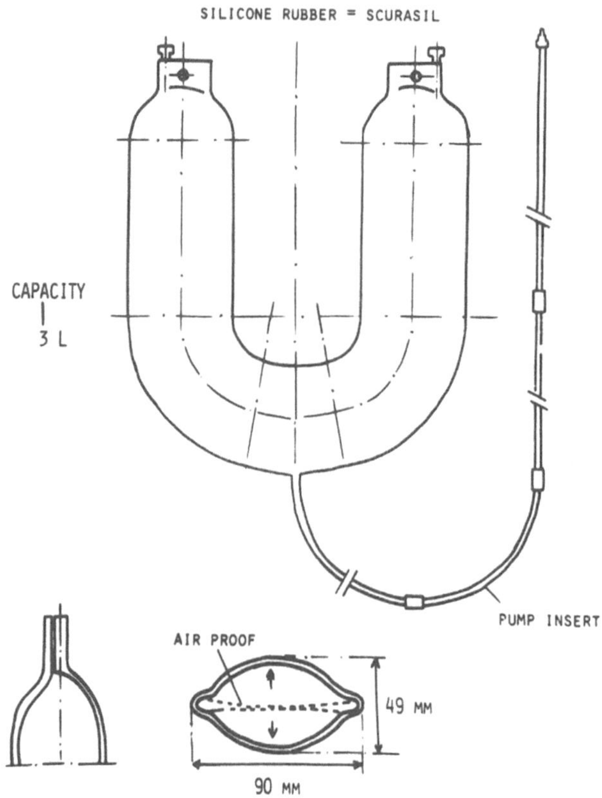

Fig. 3. Bag with the lowest outlet leading into the perfusion tube which is in continuity with the main reservoir

Administration of Solutions

Carbohydrates are provided in the form of anhydrous glucose solutions of 10%, 15%, 20%, 30%, and 50% starting with the 10% solution and increasing to each succeeding level after adjustment periods of 4 – 5 days. Tolerance is evaluated by clinical impressions and fractional urinary sugars, with insulin being used conservatively when required. Fat is provided as a soybean base emulsion (Intralipid 20%) and protein as a crystalline amino acid solution, containing 20 – 30 g of nitrogen/liter. Electrolytes are provided in different amounts for normonutrition and hypernutrition. Micronutrients are added to the nutritive solution each day (Table 5). Simultaneous infusion of the nutrients has several advantages. First, repeated manipulation of the feedline and its attendant risks are avoided. Second, the daily infusion period is reduced to 8, 12, or 18 h instead of the 22 h which would be required if each nutrient subunit were infused separately. The limiting factor in the infusion time is the 50% glucose solution, a liter of which cannot be infused in less than 12 h, and we prefer 24 h in order to be on the safe side.

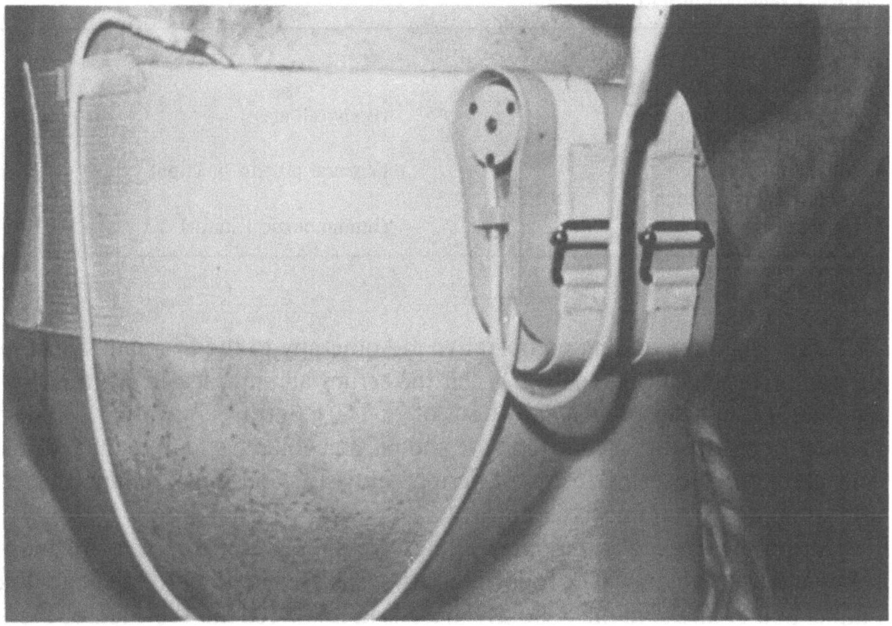

Fig. 4. Miniaturized infusion pump attached to special waistband

Both daytime and nocturnal infusion periods are determined. Between infusion periods, the cannula is disconnected from the feedline, filled with a solution of heparin and capped in order to prevent backflow and thrombosis. Strict aseptic and antiseptic measures must be taken in the preparation and administration of the mixtures and in the day-to-day care of the infusion cannula in order to ensure safe long-term intravenous feeding. A reduction in the number of infectious complications associated with this system is related to the fact that there is only one connection between the nutritive tube and the feedline which is in continuity with the rubber bag.

Our Experience with 48 Patients

The Nutritional Regimen for Extensive Gastric Cancer

This regimen can be divided into three phases:

During the *preoperative phase*, a vascular access is taken (most often a silicone catheter for average-term parenteral nutrition is used) and nutritional support is provided as soon as the patient returns from the operating room. The normonutrition mixture which is first administered provided between 640 and 1600 calories depending on the water and electrolyte requirements. This period varies from 4 to 15 days in length (average: 9 days), according to the nutritional status of the patient as judged by the standard criteria (Table 6). Since January

Table 6. Evaluation of nutritional status

1. Loss of weight	
2. Triceps skinfold (fat reserve)	
3. Arm muscle circumference Creatinine/height ratio	(Body cell mass)
4. Albumin, transferrin Total lymphocyte count	(Visceral protein function)
5. Hypersensitivity skin tests	(Immunological status)

1978, we have been adding preoperative radiotherapy to the program whenever the tumor is clinically palpable. When the serum albumin levels are very low, albumin is administered on a daily basis of 25 – 50 g (intravenous) for 5 – 15 days in order to restore the oncotic pressure and plasma volume and to reduce edema. This allows for better perfusion of peripheral tissues and thus, a more efficient utilization of the administered nutrients.

During the *surgical procedure*, solutes are supplied on the basis of blood losses and urine volume. The following formula is used in order to calculate fluid intake: hourly intake in ml = hourly diuresis in ml + 100 ml + evaluated blood losses in ml. The replacement of the extracellular volume deficit is accomplished with the use of balanced electrolyte solutions (approximately 500 ml per hour). The protein deficit is evaluated at 30 g during a total gastrectomy procedure, but losses may reach 187 g if surgery lasts longer than 6 h and multivisceral resection is performed.

In the *postoperative phase,* parenteral nutrition is initiated immediately upon the patient's return from the operating room with a normonutrition mixture containing the basic requirements for electrolytes, carbohydrates, lipids, and nitrogen in the form of crystallized amino acids. Electrolytes, energy, nitrogen, and minerals are channelled through the central veins (via the silicone catheter), whereas adjustments of the plasma volume of electrolyte levels are made through the superficial veins. In general, a superficial vein is taken during the first 4 – 6 days; from then on all the nutritional requirements are met using the central veins and specially adapted mixtures ($N_3 - N_4$). Oral food intake is allowed after the eighth or the fifteenth day, but its nutritional value is nil until at least the twenty-first day. As a result, parenteral nutrition must be maintained until the latter date. Afterwards, and depending on the patients' nutritional autonomy, parenteral nutrition can be used on a partial or intermittent basis (every second or third day) (Table 7).

Depending on the lymph node involvement and the nutritional status of the patient, the first course of chemotherapy can be initiated before the patient's release on the 45th day or later.

Oncologic Treatment of 48 Patients with Gastric Cancer

Radiotherapy. – The therapeutic association of radiotherapy and surgery is carried out whenever the tumor is clinically palpable and whenever the esophagogastric

Table 7. Total parenteral nutrition in gastric cancer

Preoperative period	
Normonutrition 1200 – 2000 calories/24 h 8 – 15 gN	4 – 12 days
Postoperative period	
Normo ± Hypernutrition 1500 – 3000 calories/24 h 10 – 18 gN	10 – 21 days

region is involved in the tumor process. The objective of this association, as in the treatment of rectal and esophageal cancer, is to obtain a reduction in tumor mass during the preoperative phase, as well as a possible eradication of tumor islets in the adjoining lymph nodes and surrounding soft tissues. The program calls for a total of 2200 rad in ten fractions over 11 days.

Regional surgery. The block of tissue resected includes the entire stomach, gastrocolic ligament, and greater omentum. The decision to extend the resection toward the splenic hilus is based upon the results of extemporaneous lymph nodes biopsies: if one or more lymph nodes are positive, the spleen, and possibly the tail or body of the pancreas are resected. Complete hepatic pedicle and celiac axis lymphadenectomy is performed whenever any one or more of these nodes are positive. The same applies for lymph nodes situated around the gastroduodenal artery and at the origin of the mesenteric vessels. In 17 of 48 cases, all the lymph nodes were negative; in 31 cases, the resection was extended to include the hepatic and splenic pedicles. In seven cases, the tail or body of the pancreas was also resected; in three cases, transverse colectomy was performed as well as inferior third esophagectomy in three other cases.

Chemotherapy. The first course of chemotherapy is initiated at the onset of the third postoperative week if the bone marrow smear and blood cell count are satisfactory (Vincristine, 5-FU, and BCNU).

Preliminary Results

The overall operative mortality rate (first month) for the 48 patients was 12.5%, which is identical to that of the historical group of 93 patients [8].

The percentage of operable patients has been constantly increasing since 1972. In 1972, only 3% of the patients with gastric cancer were deemed capable of undergoing regional gastrectomy; the percentage reached 15% in 1974, 28% in 1976, and 34% in 1978 so far.

Survival rates: the 1-year survival rate for patients who underwent surgery between 1972 and 1976 was 52%. The 2-year survival rate for patients who underwent surgery between 1972 and 1975 was 28%. The 3-year survival rate for patients who underwent surgery between 1972 and 1974 was 19%. The 5-year survival rate for patients who underwent surgery between 1972 and 1973 is very poor; 5%, all of whom had been found to be lymph node negative. In general, death was attributed to metastatic disease; pulmonary (10%), hepatic (25%), cutaneous (8%), bone (6%), and peritoneal with regional disease (51%).

Conclusion

From 1970 to 1977, an artificial gut system was used in 1350 patients suffering from gastrointestinal cancer. This type of prolonged intestinal assistance was recognized to be an important adjuvant in anticancer therapy with indications prior to, during, and following the traditional course of treatment.

In gastric cancer, total parenteral nutrition allows for extensive regional resection of tumor masses with a minimum of surgical risk. Thanks to total nutrition, we can implement the most efficient association of current therapeutic modalities. The 1–4 year survival rates, which are currently being reported, offer no great hope for an early increase in the size of the 5-year disease-free population. A comfortable and prolonged survival time are the only results which we can currently guarantee. In addition to the progress which is still to be made in the field of local tumor reduction, a more effective control of the general metastatic disease must necessarily be sought out. The same problems apply to all types of cancer [6].

References

1. Asakawa, H., Takeda, T.: High energy x-ray therapy of gastric carcinoma. J. Jap. Soc. Cancer Ther. *8*, 362–371 (1973)
2. Carter, S. K., Comis, R. L.: Gastric cancer: Current status of treatment. J. Nat. Cancer Inst. *58*, 567–578 (1977)
3. Copeland, E. M.: Intravenous hyperalimentation as an adjunct to cancer patient managements. Cancer Bull. *30*, 102–107 (1978)
4. Dubois, J. B., Joyeux, H., Yakoun, M., Pourquier, H., Solassol, Cl.: Total abdominal irradiation and parenteral nutrition: An experimental study in the dog. Biomedicine *25*, 123–125 (1976)
5. Dudrick, S. J., Ruberg, R. L.: Principles and practice of parenteral nutrition. Gastroenterol. *61*, 901–910 (1971)
6. Haagensen, C. D.: Disease of the breast. 2nd. ed., pp. 455–458. Philadelphia: Sander 1971
7. Joyeux, H., Astruc, B., Solassol, Cl.: Guide of artificial nutrition. (in press)
8. Pujol, H.: La chimiothérapie complémentaire de la chirurgie dans les épithéliomas digestifs. Nouv. Presse Med. (1978) (in press)
9. Shils, M. E.: Nutrition in neoplastic diseases. In: Modern nutrition in health and disease. Goodhart, R. S., Shils, M. E. (eds.), 5th ed. Philadelphia: Lea & Febiger 1973
10. Solassol, Cl., Joyeux, H.: Artificial gut in gastro-intestinal cancer. In front. Gastroenterol. Res. *5* (1978)
11. Solassol, Cl., Joyeux, H., Etco, L., Pujol, H., Romieu, Cl.: New techniques for long term intravenous feeding. An artificial gut in 75 patients. Ann. Surg. *4*, 179 (1974)
12. Solassol, Cl., Joyeux, H., Romieu, Cl.: Long term total parenteral nutrition. An artificial gut. Proceedings of the International Congress on Parenteral Nutrition. Montpellier (1976)
13. Solassol, Cl., Joyeux, H., Solassol, Ch., Pujol, H., Romieu, Cl.: Chirurgie régionale des cancers du pancréas. Chirurgie *104*, 131–140 (1978)
14. Solassol, Cl., Joyeux, H., Dubois, J. B.: Total parenteral nutrition (TPN) with complete nutritive mixtures: An artificial gut in cancer patients. Nutr. Cancer (1978). (in press)
15. Wretlind, A.: Complete Intravenous feeding. Theoretical and experimental background. Nutr. Metab. *1*, 14 (1972)

Immunological Changes During a Perioperative Parenteral Hyperalimentation in Gastrointestinal Cancer

M. Betzler, M. Gollwitzer, H. D. Flad, and Ch. Herfarth

It is known that parenteral nutrition plays a major role in patients with neoplasia in the alimentary tract before and after surgery until intestinal function has recovered to permit oral feeding. It is supposed by the group of Copeland [2] that cell-mediated immunity may be restored by proper nutritional replenishment.

In a pilot study, the distribution of lymphocyte subpopulations in the peripheral blood and skin tests with recall antigens have been examined in cancer patients for getting further information about immunological changes during the pre- and postoperative period under parenteral nutrition.

Material and Methods

Forty-two patients with gastric and colorectal cancer comprised the study (Table 1) and were treated with two different solution regimens (Table 2) concerning the calories and the concentrations of amino acids and carbohydrates, starting from the sixth preoperative day. The evaluation of the operative procedure is shown in Table 3.

Table 1. Localization of the gastrointestinal tumors

Localization of the tumor	Group 1	Group 2
Stomach (n)	19	8
Colon/Rectum (n)	3	12
Total (n)	22	20

Table 2. Pre- and postoperative intravenous hyperalimentation solutions

Solutions (ml)	Group 1 1500 Aminofusin L 600 1500 Triofusin E 1000	Group 2 2000 Triofusin E 1000 1000 Tutofusin OP S
Amino acids (g)	75	0
Carbohydrate (g)	520	550
Calories (kcal)	2400	2200

Table 3. Number (n) of patients and evaluation of operation

	Group 1 (n)	Group 2 (n)
Operable	9	14
Curative	5	8
Curative?	9	6
Inoperable	13	6
Palliative	2	1
No resection of the tumor	11	5

Table 4. List and timing of immunological tests

1. Lymphatic subpopulations (6th and 1st day pre-, 1st and 10th day postoperatively).
1.1. Lymphocyte count.
1.2. Relative distribution and absolute number of T and B lymphocytes in the peripheral blood (rosette techniques).
2. Skin tests (6th day pre-, 10th day postoperatively).
2.1. Tuberculin (5 I.U.).
2.2. Varidase (1250 I.U./0.1 ml).
2.3. Candida albicans (0.5%).

The lymphocyte count, the absolute number of T and B lymphocytes and their relative distribution in the peripheral blood were tested six and one day before and one and ten days after the operation. The T and B lymphocytes were determined by modified rosette techniques [1, 3]. As recall antigens for skin testing at the sixth day pre- and the tenth day postoperatively, we used Tuberculin, Varidase, and Candida albicans (Table 4).

Results

The absolute number of T and B lymphocytes shows for both groups the same increase between the first and fourth control as the lymphocyte count (Tables 5, 6, and 7).

The relative distribution of these lymphocyte subpopulations did not really change during the observed period (Table 6 and 7).

A remarkable increase was noted for the absolute number of T lymphocytes of inoperable patients who received the amino-acids-containing solution (Table 5).

In some patients, a normalization of T and B cell numbers could be observed during the parenteral nutrition without any significant difference between the two groups. The operative procedure did not provoke any different changes between the two regimens.

Table 5. Absolute number of Lymphocytes/μl ($\bar{x} \pm S_x$) in the peripheral blood

Patients		Preoperative		Postoperative	
		I	II	III	IV
Group 1	(n = 22)	1629 ± 618	1731 ± 649	2282 ± 851	2347 ± 860
Operable	(n = 9)	1282 ± 519	1566 ± 748	2525 ± 1127	2502 ± 1144
Inoperable	(n = 13)	1870 ± 579	1845 ± 575	2093 ± 538	2239 ± 624
Group 2	(n = 20)	1651 ± 710	1651 ± 570.1	2272 ± 858.3	2279 ± 806
Operable	(n = 14)	1731 ± 749	1685 ± 471	2462 ± 758	2544 ± 626
Inoperable	(n = 6)	1464 ± 630	1572 ± 805	1831 ± 987	1660 ± 889

Only one patient, who had initially a negative skin test had a positive skin test during the period of 16 days of parenteral nutrition. In the other patients, we could not observe a conversion of the preoperative skin test. All three skin tests in five patients (3 patients, group 1; 2 patients, group 2) and two of the three skin tests in 12 patients (6 patients, group 1; 6 patients, group 2) remained negative during the course.

No difference was seen between the two solution groups concerning weight gain, which was not significant during the 16 days, the number of postoperative complications, and the time of hospitalization.

Conclusion

The lymphocyte subpopulations, especially the absolute numbers, show during a perioperative parenteral nutrition with 2400 and 2200 kcal, respectively, an increase corresponding to the lymphocyte count, without any marked difference between the two groups. Both of the solutions are qualified to counterbalance the preoperative catabolic situation, which is reflected in a preoperative lymphopenia. This form of parenteral nutrition did not influence a preexisting cellular immunity, but on the other hand, it has to be considered that the nutritional status of the patients examined was not reduced to such an extent that changes of the immune status could occur.

From these results, it is concluded that patients should be supported during their perioperative period by parenteral nutrition with hypercaloric regimens and simultaneously monitored by sensitive immunological tests, e. g., delayed hypersensitivity to DNCB and lymphocyte proliferation in vitro.

Table 6. Absolute and relative number of T lymphocytes ($\bar{x} \pm S_x$)

Patients	Preoperative				Postoperative			
	I		II		III		IV	
	Absol. (/µl)	Rel. (%)	Absol. (/µl)	Rel. (%)	Absol. (/µl)	Rel. (%)	Absol. (/µl)	Rel. (%)
Group 1 (n = 22)	1239 ± 62	73.5 ± 10.2	1346 ± 92	74.0 ± 10.0	1793 ± 71	68.7 ± 13.9	1745 ± 86	71.8 ± 10.5
Operable (n = 9)	1351 ± 52	78.3 ± 9.1	1434 ± 61	73.8 ± 11.4	1652 ± 104	61.3 ± 13.9	1826 ± 103	70.2 ± 9.1
Inoperable (n = 13)	1034 ± 60	70.0 ± 10.8	1136 ± 31	74.1 ± 9.4	1596 ± 63	74.3 ± 11.3	1663 ± 68	72.3 ± 10.6
Group 2 (n = 20)	1294 ± 68	75.8 ± 9.0	1299 ± 64	75.8 ± 12.5	1694 ± 87	71.7 ± 11.4	1679 ± 77	71.7 ± 8.4
Operable (n = 14)	1278 ± 60	75.9 ± 9.3	1354 ± 47	79.3 ± 5.7	1848 ± 73	73.6 ± 7.1	1413 ± 93	72.7 ± 8.0
Inoperable (n = 6)	1141 ± 61	74.9 ± 9.2	1172 ± 86	67.7 ± 20.0	1352 ± 99	67.4 ± 17.9	1262 ± 70	69.4 ± 9.8

Table 7. Absolute and relative number of B lymphocytes ($\bar{x} \pm S_x$)

Patients	Preoperative				Postoperative			
	I		II		III		IV	
	Absol. (/µl)	Rel. (%)	Absol. (/µl)	Rel. (%)	Absol. (/µl)	Rel. (%)	Absol. (/µl)	Rel. (%)
Group 1	352 ± 20	20.4 ± 4.9	339 ± 20	18.3 ± 5.2	447 ± 29	18.1 ± 5.9	446 ± 29	17.5 ± 6.2
Operable	289 ± 18	21.1 ± 5.5	309 ± 22	17.8 ± 6.0	496 ± 35	17.9 ± 5.8	496 ± 38	17.7 ± 7.0
Inoperable	390 ± 20	19.9 ± 4.5	353 ± 19	17.8 ± 5.4	409 ± 18	18.9 ± 3.8	420 ± 27	17.4 ± 7.3
Group 2	339 ± 22	18.9 ± 5.6	311 ± 17	17.8 ± 4.5	450 ± 26	18.7 ± 4.4	430 ± 25	17.8 ± 4.6
Operable	352 ± 24	18.6 ± 6.0	314 ± 17	17.3 ± 4.9	484 ± 25	18.7 ± 4.7	503 ± 23	18.4 ± 4.9
Inoperable	308 ± 19	19.6 ± 5.1	322 ± 21	19.3 ± 3.6	369 ± 25	18.7 ± 4.0	292 ± 20	16.2 ± 3.8

References

1. Betzler, M., Flad, H. D., Schlag, P., Herfarth, Ch.: Untersuchungen zum zellulären Immunstatus bei Normalpersonen, Nichtmalignom- und Malignompatienten. Onkologie *1*, 133 – 136 (1978)
2. Copeland, E. M., McFadyen, B. V., Lanzotti, V. J., Dudrick, S. J.: Intravenous hyperalimentation as an adjunct to cancer chemotherapy. Am. J. Surg. *129*, 167 (1975)
3. Kaplan, M. E., Clark, C.: An improved rosetting assay for detection of human T lymphocytes. J. Immunol. Methods *5*, 131 (1974)

Results of Surgery for Gastric Cancer and Effect of Adjuvant Chemotherapy

Hiroaki Nakazato and Hajime Imanaga

Introduction

Although surgery and chemotherapy have progressed by technical improvements of diagnostic methods for gastric cancer during the past decade, the goal of complete cure is far from obtained except in the early stage of gastric cancer. The purpose of this study is to report results of curability of patients suffering from gastric cancer with surgical treatment and combined adjuvant chemotherapy.

Methods

We recognize that the curability of a patient depends on the stage of the disease at the time of initial treatment. The stage depends on many factors, such as demographic factors, history of the illness, current state of the disease, histology, and physical condition. Some of these factors especially tumor invasion, extension of metastases, and host factors may have a close relationship with the prognosis of the patient. On the other hand, the stage also seems to correspond with the types of surgical procedures which are performed.

Our study involved 1628 patients who underwent surgery for gastric cancer at our hospital between 1964 and 1973. These cases were divided into three groups according to surgical procedures. A curative resection was performed on 995, 283 had a noncurative resection, and 305 had a nonresection that consisted of exploratory laparotomy, gastrojejunostomy, gastrostomy, or jejunostomy.

The definition of curative and noncurative resection is shown in Table 1. The classification is based on "The General Rules for the Gastric Cancer Study in Surgery and Pathology in Japan" [4] and the rules of the WHO International Reference Center [18]. According to these rules, curative resection is defined as follows: no peritoneal dissemination, no hepatic metastasis, complete dissection of the regional nodes, and negative cancer infiltration to the cut margin of stomach.

Postoperative survival rates were computed by the actuarial method [13] without correction for age; patients who died within 30 days after operation were excluded from the calculations. There were 45 operative deaths for an operative mortality of 2.8%. Patients who died of causes clearly unrelated to the gastric cancer or its treatment were also excluded from the calculations. Such patients made up 4.7% of the curative resection group and a small percentage of the other

Table 1. Definition of curative and noncurative resections

Factors	Curative	Noncurative
Peritoneal dissemination	Po	$P_1P_2P_3$
Hepatic metastases	Ho	$H_1H_2H_3$
Relation to n(+)-number and R-number	$n \leq R^a$	$n > R$
Cancer infiltration to the cut margin of stomach	ow(−) aw(−)	ow(+) aw(+)

[a] R-number means type of gastric resection based on the degree of lymph node removal.

groups. Thus, survival statistics were based on approximately 93% of the pool of 1628 patients.

The effect of adjuvant chemotherapy with mitomycin C (MMC) was determined by a cooperative study involving 19 hospitals under the auspices of the Japanese Ministry of Health and Welfare. Adjuvant chemotherapy was given by random allocation to patients who underwent curative resection for gastric cancer. A total of 2636 patients were involved in these studies. Effectiveness was determined by calculation of the actuarial method with correction of age. The specific chemotherapy protocols will be described in relationship to the results.

Survival After Different Operative Procedures

Figure 1 shows the survival curves of patients who underwent curative and noncurative gastrectomy and nonresection. As seen by the lowest curve, most of the patients who did not have resection of the gastric cancer died within 1 year and all patients died within 2.5 years. The patients who underwent noncurative resection had a better survival rate than those with nonresection. Although most of the patients died within 3 years of operation, there was a 12.2% survival rate for 5 years and a 9.7% survival rate for 8 years. It was not possible to explain with any certainty the long-term survival of 9.7% of the patients who underwent noncurative resection. It could have been due to an error, or to rare, spontaneous regression of the tumor that was left behind [1]. Of the 995 patients who underwent curative resection, in which all macroscopic cancer was removed, 63.7% survived for 5 years and 58.3% survived 8 years.

Limitation of Surgical Procedure

When the cancers were classified according to the staging system of the Japanese Research Society for Gastric Cancer (Table 2), it was found that survivals were directly related to the stage of gastric cancer at the time of operation. The survival rates in the ninth postoperative year were 80% for patients who had had

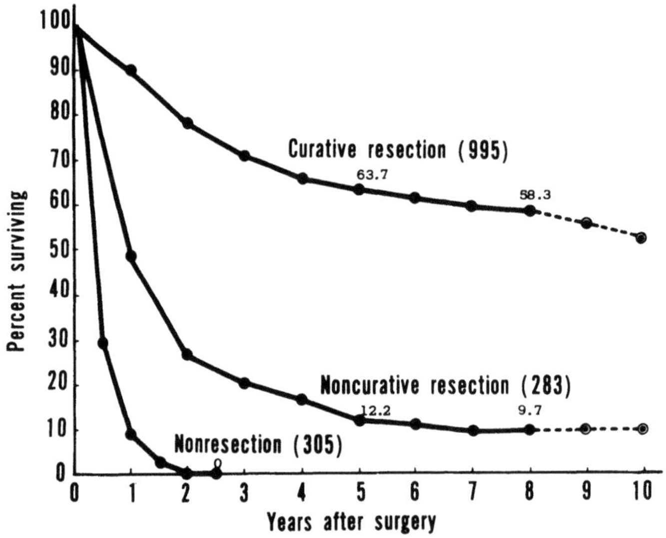

Fig. 1. Postoperative survival curves of gastric cancer patients – classified by curability based on surgical procedure. Cumulated from Dec. 1964 to Dec. 1973; calculated in Jan. 1975. Dead cases (n = 45) within 30 days postoperatively were excluded. Number of patients in parentheses

stage I cancer, 48% for patients who had had stage II cancer, and 19% for patients who had had stage III cancer. By definition, no patients with stage IV cancer underwent curative resection.

In patients subjected to curative resection, it would be of value to determine the degree to which serosal invasion and regional lymph node metastases influence prognosis.

With regards to the influence of serosal invasion, Fig. 2 shows the survival rates of patients with and without extension of the cancer to the gastric serosa in the previously mentioned curative series. Sixteen operative deaths within 30 days postoperatively and 48 deaths from cases unrelated to gastric cancer were excluded in the curves. The 8-year survival rate was 86.8% in the 461 patients

Table 2. Classification of gastric cancer by staging system of Japanese Research Society for Gastric Cancer and 9-year survival

Stage	Peritoneal dissemination	Hepatic metastases	Regional lymph node metastases	Serosal invasion	9-year survival
I	P_0	H_0	n_0	s_0	80%
II	P_0	H_0	n_1, n_2	s_1	48%
III	P_0	H_0	n_3	s_2	19%
IV	P_1, P_2, P_3	H_1, H_2, H_3	n_4	s_3	–[a]

[a] No patients with stage IV underwent curative resection.

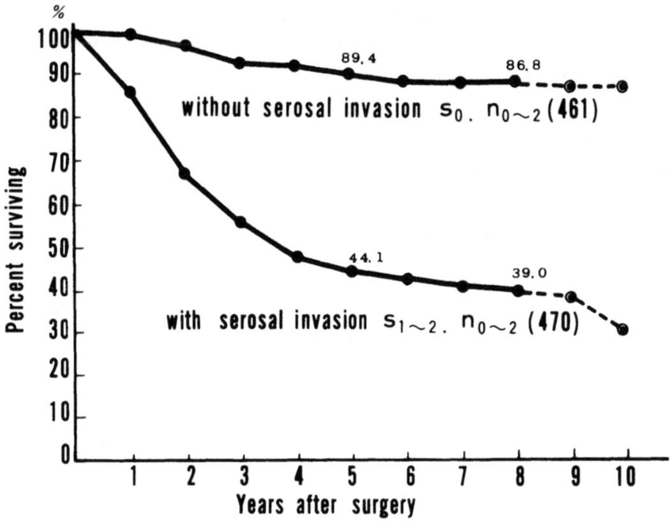

Fig. 2. Postoperative survival curves in curatively resected patients classified by serosal invasion. Cumulated from Dec. 1964 to Dec. 1973; calculated in Jan. 1975. Dead cases (n = 16) within 30 days and noncancerous deaths (n = 48) were excluded. Number of cases in parentheses

with cancers that did not invade the serosa. In contrast, only 39% of 470 patients who had serosal invasion survived for 8 years. The former group, to be called s-negative group, consisted of m, sm, pm, and ss cases in the histopathological category, respectively.

When the carcinoma involved the mucosa or submucosa, but did not reach the muscularis propria, the type of lesion is termed "early gastric cancer", and the 5-year survival rates were 94.3% in m cases, and 93.1% in sm cases [7]. Therefore, it may suggest that while the cancer invasion remains within sm, we can almost cure the patients. Then, in the study, excluding both m and sm cases from the s-negative group, we evaluated prognosis for 148 patients with postmucosal cancers [9].

There were 33 deaths within 7 years of operation. Fourteen deaths were excluded from the calculations; 12 were unrelated to the gastric cancer and two were of unknown causes, giving a survival rate of 85.8%. The types of recurrence in the 19 patients who died of cancer are shown in Table 3. The most common type of recurrence was hematogenous metastasis, usually to the liver. Local recurrence and recurrence from lymphogenous metastases were uncommon. On the other hand, as shown in Table 4, lymph node metastases n_1 and n_2 were found at the time of operation in 59, or 39.9% of the pm patients. So, approximately 40% of the patients had cancer in the regional lymph nodes in the resected specimen. These findings indicate that it was possible to surgically eradicate all local disease, including cancer in lymph nodes, and that recurrence was due mainly to cancer cells in the blood vessels or bloodstream.

Therefore, our conception may be extended as follows: when the cancer remained in the s-negative stage, most of the patients could be cured with

Table 3. Type of recurrence in postmucosal (pm) gastric cancer patients[a]

Hematogenous metastases	Hepatic	9	10
	Other	1	
Lymphogenous metastases			3
Peritoneal dissemination			2
Recurrence of the cut margin			2
Nondifferentiated recurrence			2
Total of recurrent death			19

Rate of total recurrences 19/134 (14.2%)
Rate of hematogenous metastases 10/19 (52.6%)

[a] Excluded 12 cases of noncancerous death and 2 cases of unknown causes of death.

Table 4. Lymph node metastases in 148 pm patients

	n(−)	$n_1(+)$	$n_2(+)$
Number of cases	89	34	25

curative resection, with the exception of hematogenous metastases. In contrast, as mentioned before, only 39% or 470 patients who had serosal invasion survived for 8 years. The types of recurrence were studied in 97 of the patients by Yamada [20]. Local recurrence in the peritoneal cavity, such as peritoneal dissemination was about 64%. This is much more common in patients with serosal invasion than in those without it.

Table 5 shows the relationship of both serosal invasion and lymph node metastases to 5-year survival in patients who underwent curative resections. Although both factors had a deleterious influence on survival, the negative effect of serosal invasion was greater. In fact, in the absence of serosal invasion, the prognosis of patients with lymph node metastases was still quite good. The 5-year survival rate was 74.8%.

The relationship of the histology of the gastric cancers to the presence or absence of serosal invasion was also examined in the current series. Overall, the

Table 5. Five-year survival rates related to lymph node metastases and serosal invasion in 931 patients who had curative resections of gastric cancer

No. of patients	Lymph node metastases	Serosal invasion	5-year survival (%)
368	−	−	92.0
93	+	−	74.8
145	−	+	61.1
325	+	+	36.9

ratio of poorly differentiated to well-differentiated adenocarcinomas of the stomach was 4 to 1. In the cases without serosal invasion, the ratio was 2 to 1, whereas in the cases with serosal invasion, the ratio was 23 to 1 (Table 6).

Survival curves of well-, moderately, and poorly differentiated adenocarcinomas (Fig. 3) were classified by the presence or absence of serosal invasion. It is interesting that in the absence of serosal invasion, survival rate was fairly high even in the poorly differentiated type, and a high survival rate in the presence of serosal invasion was only observed in the few cases of the well-differentiated type. As might be expected, although poorly differentiated cancers were more rapidly and extensively invasive, a good prognosis was obtained in the cases without serosal invasion.

Effect of Adjuvant Chemotherapy and Curative Resection on Survival

For some years, it has been hoped that the combination of chemotherapy and radical gastric resection would improve the curability of gastric cancer. Studies in the United States with triethylenethiophosphoramide (thiotepa) as an adjuvant to gastric surgery demonstrated no effect on survival of patients with carcinoma of the stomach [10, 13, 19]. Studies in Vienna by Karrer and co-workers [6] showed that long-term, intermittent use of cyclophosphamide (CPA) was less effective in gastric cancer than in lung cancer. In Japan, a number of studies on surgical adjuvant chemotherapy have been undertaken; the results have been unclear [2, 3, 5, 8, 12, 14, 15, 17]. Currently, in the hope of improving the survival rate obtained by curative resection of gastric cancer, investigations in 19 cooperating hospitals have conducted four separate studies on surgical adjuvant chemotherapy with MMC.

The protocols of the four phase III-type studies are summarized in Table 7. All of them are controlled therapeutic trials with random allocation. In study I and study II, all patients were followed-up for more than 10 years. Data analysis has been almost completed at present, but it is still going on in studies III and IV. Therefore, studies I and II should be mentioned here.

As seen in Table 7, in study I, MMC was given intravenously in a dose of 0.08 mg/kg twice a week for 5 weeks, starting on the day of surgery. In study I, high-dose MMC was used for only 2 days. The drug was given intravenously in a dose of 0.4 mg/kg on the day of surgery and 0.2 mg/kg on the following day. Each of

Table 6. Histological relationship of gastric cancer to presence or absence of serosal invasion

	Well-diff. adenoca.	Moderately diff. adenoca.	Poorly diff. adenoca.	Other types
s(−)	36	70	76	36
s(+)	4	47	92	17
Total	40	117	168	53

Curatively resected cases in A.C.C. (1973 ~ 1976)

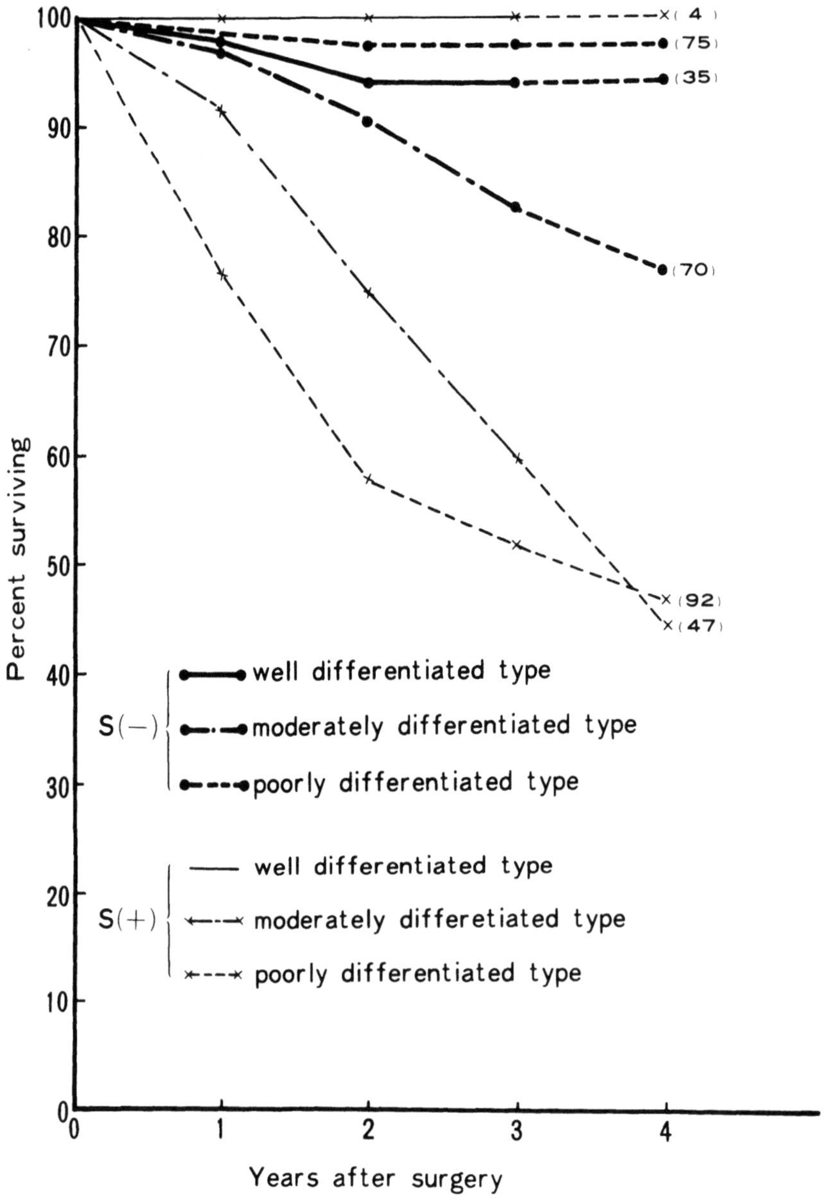

Fig. 3. Survival curves classified by histological type and serosal invasion (1973 ~ 1976)

the studies consisted of the cases of curative resection only as a control group. The results of study I, in which moderate-dose MMC was given for 5 weeks, are shown in Fig. 4. The difference in survival rate between 236 treated cases and 267 controls stands at 14.1% after 5 years postoperatively. The difference is statistically significant. Moreover, distributions of some background factors, such as age, sex, stage, s, and n factors are also statistically identical in both groups.

Table 7. Schedule for adjuvant chemotherapy

Study method		Dose schedule	Inclusion of patients	Cumulative cases *
I	systemic intermittent middle-dose	curative resection; 5 (weeks); MMC 0.08 mg kg twice week	Jan. 1965 ~ June 1966	714
II	systemic short-term high-dose	MMC 0.4 mg kg on the day of surgery; MMC 0.2 mg kg on the day following surgery	July 1966 ~ Oct. 1968	669
III-A	arterial one-shot high-dose longterm	8 – 15 – 6 (weeks); CPA daily 100 mg for 40 days; MMC hepatic 13 mg, splenic 7 mg, peritoneal 6 mg	Mar. 1969 ~ Dec. 1970	567
III-B	arterial one-shot high-dose	MMC hepatic 13 mg, splenic 7 mg, peritoneal 6 mg		
IV-A		The same as the method of I-study	Jan. 1971 ~ Dec. 1973	686
IV-B	systemic intermittent middle dose	MMC 0.04 mg kg; 5FU 5 mg kg twice week; CA 0.4 mg kg		

MMC: Mitomycin C; CPA: Cyclophosphamide; 5FU: 5-fluorouracil;

CA: Cytosine arabinoside.

* Include control group

Figure 5 shows the survival curves of the treated and control groups according to the stage of cancer, as defined by the previously mentioned staging system. The difference between the control and treated groups in patients with stage II cancer was large and highly significant during every year after surgery, but it was not significant in stage III cancer.

The 83 patients who died of recurrences in study 1 were analyzed further with regard to the presence of serosal invasion and lymph node metastases in the resected specimen and the subsequent incidence and mode of cancer recurrence. The results of this analysis are shown in Fig. 6. Patients who did not have serosal invasion and were treated with MMC did not develop liver metastases, in contrast to the controls. Patients who had serosal invasion developed hepatic metastases with almost the same frequency in the treated and control groups. With regard to recurrence in the form of peritoneal dissemination, the differences between the treated and control groups were not significant, whether or not the resected specimen showed serosal invasion or involved lymph nodes. Thus

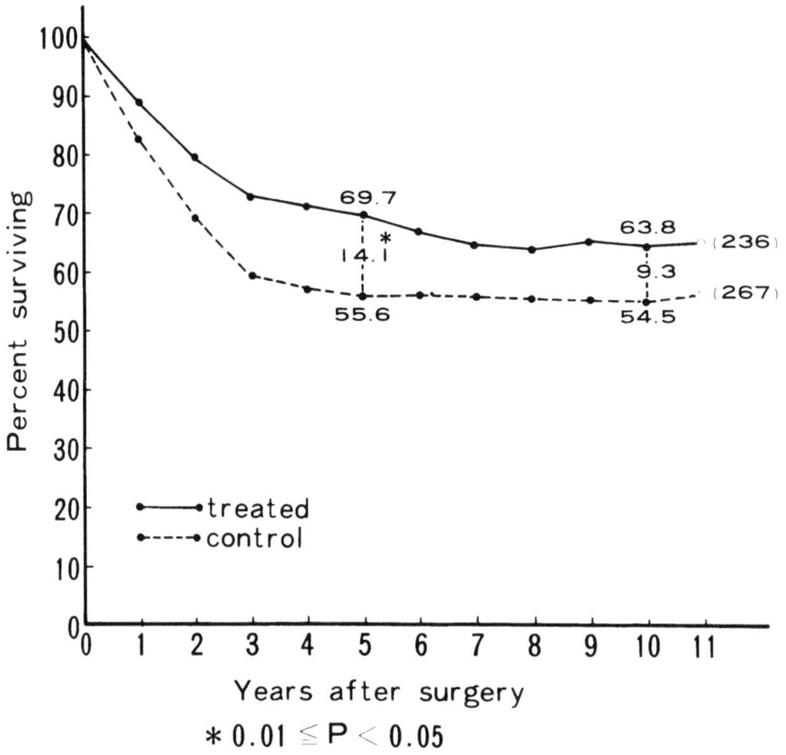

Fig. 4. Survival curves in study I (overall cases) cumulated between Jan. 1965 and June 1966; calculated in Oct. 1977

MMC appeared to be effective in patients without serosal invasion, particularly in preventing hematogenous spread to the liver. This is noteworthy, since this is the form of cancer spread that surgery does not overcome.

The results of study II, in which high-dose MMC was given for 2 days starting with the day of surgery, are shown in Fig. 7. No differences were observed between the treated and control groups in any year. Figure 8 shows the survival curves of the treated and control groups according to the stage of cancer. The difference between them was observed in patients with stage III cancer, but it is not statistically significant. In contrast, the survival rates in stage I cancer were always higher in the control than those in the treated group; they were significant. It may be supposed that when high-dose MMC was given within a short period combined with surgery, the treated patients with stage III cancer were inclined to have higher survival rates than those of the control patients, but in patients with stage 1 cancer, some adverse effects were observed.

Thus, it appears that moderate-dose MMC administered intermittently for several weeks after curative resection of gastric cancer significantly improves the survival of patients whose tumors have not extended to the serosa of the stomach. However, in patients with cancer that invades the serosa, more

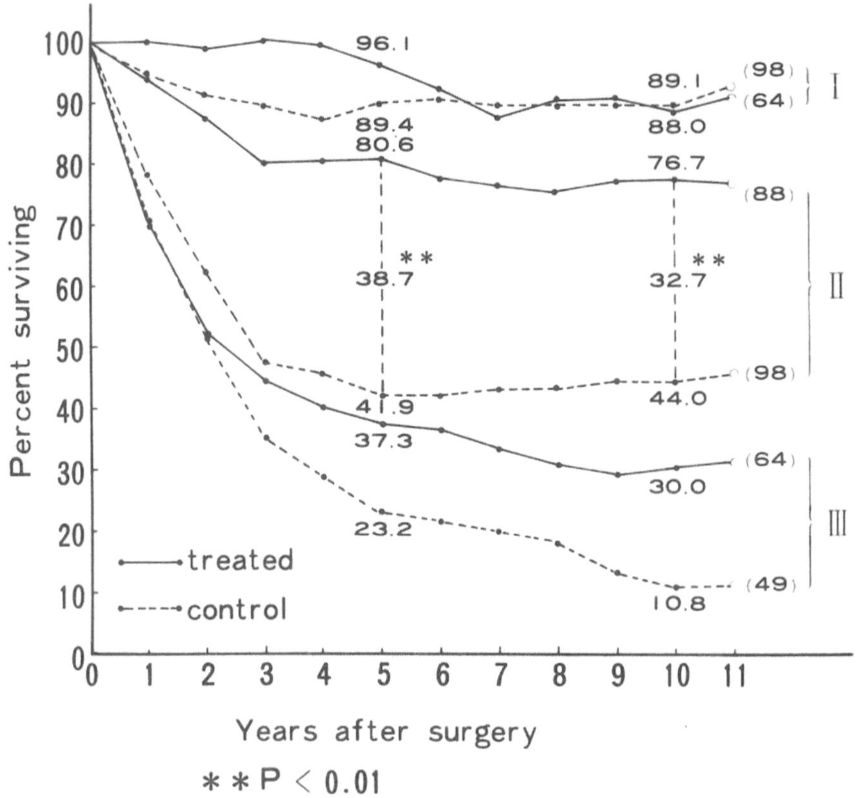

Fig. 5. Survival curves in study I – classified by histological stage. Cumulated between Jan. 1965 and June 1966; calculated in Oct. 1977

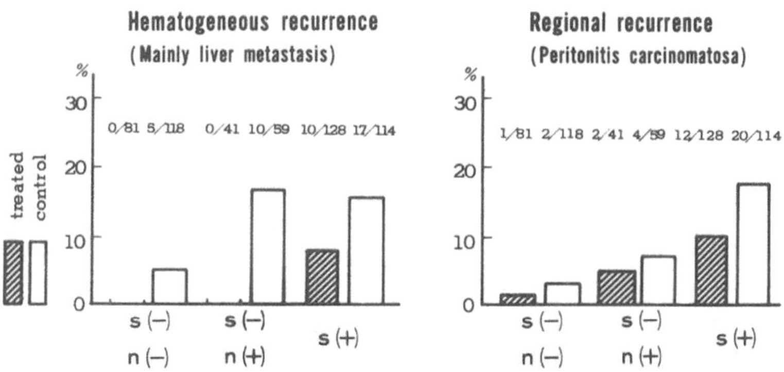

Fig. 6. Effect of MMC on prevention of recurrence (study I)

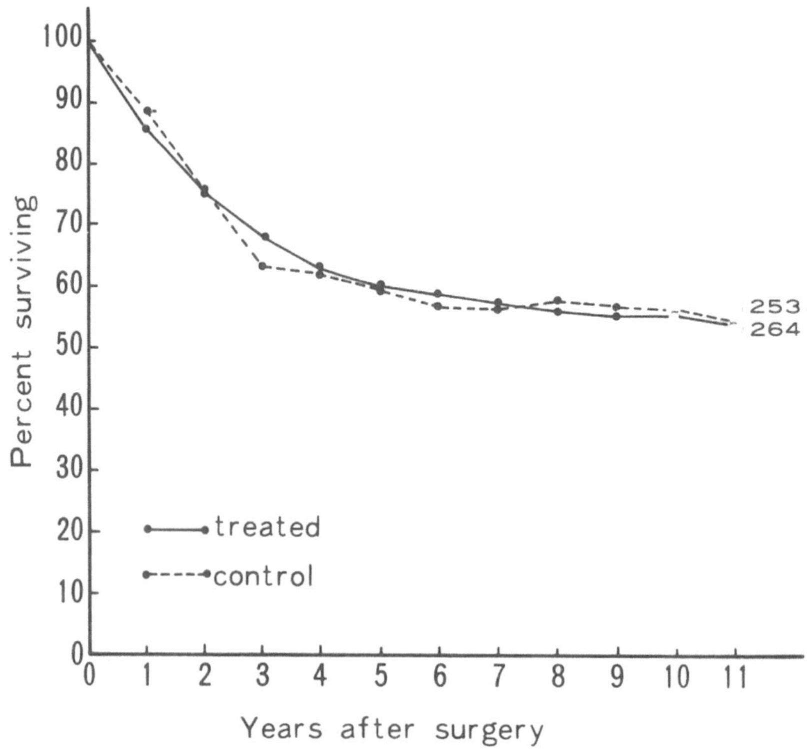

Fig. 7. Survival curves in stage II (overall cases). Cumulated between Jan. 1966 and June 1968; calculated in Oct. 1977

extensive doses of the agent might be administered, but this is not possible because of side effects or adverse effects of such agents. Thus, a different form of adjuvant chemotherapy and combined modalities of other therapies [20] must be found, if survival is to be improved.

Summary

Surgical treatment was evaluated by this study which involved 1628 patients who underwent surgery for gastric cancer between 1964 and 1973. The effect of adjuvant mitomycin C (MMC) therapy was also investigated in four different studies by 19 cooperating hospitals; 2636 patients were involved. These results are summarized as follows:

1) Of the 995 patients who underwent curative resection, 63.7% survived for 5 years and 58.3% survived for 8 years.

2) Evaluation of the influence on survival of the two major staging criteria showed that serosal invasion by cancer had a substantially greater negative effect on survival than regional lymph node metastases.

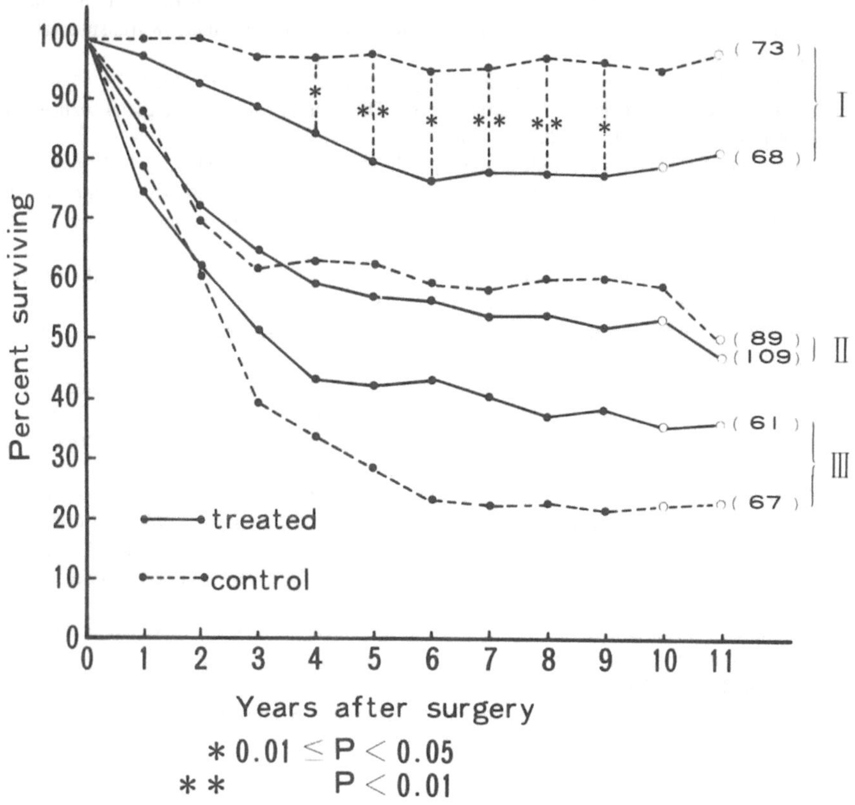

Fig. 8. Survival curves in study II – classified by histological stage. Cumulated between Jan. 1966 and June 1968; calculated in Oct. 1977

3) In the absence of serosal invasion (even when there were regional lymph node metastases), recurrence usually took the form of hematogenous type to the liver than peritoneal disease, indicating that it was possible to eradicate all local disease by surgery, but not in the blood vessels or bloodstream.

4) In the absence of serosal invasion, survival rate was fairly high even in the poorly differentiated type, and a high survival rate in the presence of serosal invasion was only observed in the few cases of the well-differentiated type.

5) Administration of MMC twice weekly for 5 weeks after curative resection increased the overall 5-year survival rate by 13.5% and produced a highly significant 36.6% increase in 5-year survival in patients with stage II cancer. Mitomycin C was particularly effective in preventing hematogenous metastases to the liver in patients who did not have serosal invasion, but it was not effective when the cancer invaded the serosa.

References

1. Everson, T. C., Cole, W. H.: Spontaneous regression of cancer, p. 473. Philadelphia: Saunders 1966

2. Hattori, T., Mori, A., Hirata, K., Ito, I.: Five year survival rate of gastric cancer patients treated by gastrectomy, large dose of mitomycin C and/or allogenic bone marrow transplantation. Jpn. J. Cancer Clin. *19*, 241 (1973)
3. Imanaga, H., Nakazato, H.: Therapy of gastric cancer. Jpn. J. Clin. Med. *28*, 1756 (1960)
4. Japanese Research Society for Gastric Cancer: The general rules for the gastric cancer study in surgery and pathology, 9th edition. 1974
5. Jinnai, D.: Surgical adjuvant chemotherapy. J. Jpn. Soc. Cancer Ther. *1*, 12 (1966)
6. Karrer, K.: Adjuvant Chemotherapy in early cases of cancer, partly with high-dosed therapy under the protection of autologous frozen-stored bone marrow. Gann. Monogr. 2. Cancer Chemother. pp. 235. 1968
7. Kato, K.: Long Term Results of Surgical Treatment of Stomach Cancer. 12th International Cancer Congress, Abstracts. Panel *12*, 135 (1978)
8. Kimura, T.: Chemotherapy as an adjuvant to surgery in gastric carcinoma. Cancer Chemother. *2*, 391 (1975)
9. Kito, T., Imanaga, H., Yamada, E., Miyaishi, S., Nakazato, H., Kato, K., Takagi, H., Yasue, M., Watanabe, T., Kato, T., Morimoto, T., Yamazaki, M., Suchi, T., Sato, T., Suzuki, R.: Studies on the gastric cancer confined to the proper muscle layer. Jpn. J. Cancer Clin. *22*, 15 (1976)
10. Longmire, W. P., Jr., Kuzma, J. W., Dixon, W. J.: The use of triethylenethiophosphoramide as an adjuvant to the surgical treatment of gastric carcinoma. Ann. Surg. *167*, 293 (1968)
11. Moore, G. E.: Introduction to Second Conference on Experimental Clinical Cancer Chemotherapy. Part II. Surgical Adjuvant Session. A. University studies. Cancer Chemother. Rep. *16*, 121 (1962)
12. Nakajima, T., Kajitani, T., Fukami, A., Ohashi, I.: Prognostic study of adjuvant chemotherapy with mitomycin C for gastric cancer after radical surgery. Result of short intensive course regimen. Jpn. J. Cancer Clin. *22*, 15 (1976)
13. National Cancer Institute Monograph 15: International Symposium on End Results of Cancer Therapy. Washington. D.C., U.S. Public Health Service, 1964
14. Shiba, S.: Surgical adjuvant chemotherapy. Jpn. J. Cancer Clin. *14*, 200 (1968)
15. Shiba, S., Taguchi, T.: Clinical and experimental studies for cancer therapy. Chemotherapy *10*, 293 (1962)
16. Tokai Cooperative Study Group of Adjuvant Immuno-chemotherapy of the Stomach Cancer: Study on adjuvant immunochemotherapy of the stomach cancer. Cancer Chemother. *3*, 127, 1976
17. Tokuyama, H.: Adjuvant chemotherapy. Surg. Ther. *6*, 558 (1962)
18. Tsukamoto, K., Gaitán-Yongus, M.: A system for registration and classification of the stomach cancer for WHO International Reference Center. Jpn. J. Clin. Oncol. *12*, 117 (1973)
19. V. A. Cooperative Surgical Adjuvant Study Group: Use of thio-TEPA as an adjuvant to the surgical management of carcinoma of the stomach. Cancer *18*, 291 (1965)
20. Yamada, E.: Clinical studies of recurrent gastric cancer (in Japanese). Saishin Igaku *29*, 325 (1974)

A Controlled Prospective Study of Adjuvant 5-Fluorouracil and BCNU Therapy in Stomach Carcinoma

M. Mayer, M. Linder, W. Schreml, P. Schlag, and W. Queißer

Radical surgical treatment of gastric carcinoma resulted in a 5-year survival rate of only 30%, with the exception of "early cancer," which showed a much better long-term survival. The prognosis depends mainly on location and size of the primary tumor, pathological findings, and on lymph node involvement.

Adjuvant chemotherapy in curative operated stomach cancer with fluorodeoxyuridine [9], thioTEPA [10, 3], or cyclophosphamide [2, 5] did not significantly prolong survival. However, the above mentioned adjuvant studies applied single agent chemotherapy of moderate intensity and of only short-term application. Other studies showed a significant increase in long-term survival after prolonged chemotherapy for up to 3 years [4]. As in advanced stomach cancer high response rates could be obtained with combination chemotherapy [1, 6, 7, 8], it seemed to be useful to apply an intensive long-term schedule for adjuvant chemotherapy. The combination of 5-fluorouracil and BCNU showed a benefit in 41% of advanced gastric carcinomas [6] and may be used for adjuvant chemotherapy. In 1976, a cooperative study was started to study the influence of adjuvant chemotherapy on duration of tumor-free time, survival time, and on side effects of therapy of curative operated patients with tumor stage II and III.

Patients and Method

Stratification of the patients was done according to the TNM classification of the UICC into two risk categories (Fig. 1). For Randomization, patients were chosen

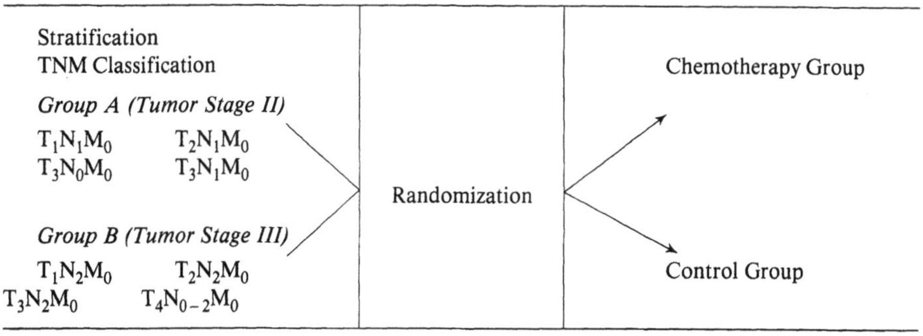

Fig. 1. Stratification and randomization of patients for the trial

for adjuvant chemotherapy or control. Chemotherapy: 5-fluorouracil was given 10 mg/kg/day intravenously and BCNU 40 mg/kg/day intravenously on day 1 – 5 of each therapy course. The first course was started between day 42 and 56, postoperatively. The therapy was restarted every 8 weeks. A total of eight courses were given within $1^1/_2$ years. If granulocytopenia $<2500/mm^3$ or thrombocytopenia $<130\,000/mm^3$ developed, the next therapy was given 2 weeks later. Persistant granulocytopenia or thrombocytopenia caused a dose reduction of two-thirds. For follow-up, the patients entering the study were examined every 2 months in both the control and the chemotherapy group. Endoscopic examination, sonographic check-up, and chest X-ray was performed routinely every 6 months.

Results

During 24 months, 68 patients entered the study. Thirty-one patients were randomly chosen for chemotherapy and 37 for control (Table 1). The age distribution was similar in all groups, ranging from 44 to 69 years when entering the study. The median time after surgery in the chemotherapy or control group was 10 and 10.5 months, respectively, ranging from 1 – 24 months. In nine cases, chemotherapy was discontinued, and 5 of 22 treated patients have already finished eight therapy cycles.

In the control group, two deaths were due to complications unrelated to the tumor. Among those patients chosen for chemotherapy, but refusing treatment, two deaths unrelated to the tumor occurred. The number of tumor recurrences differed distinctly between chemotherapy and control group. One treated patient relapsed after completion of eight therapy cycles compared to nine relapses in the control group. Eight deaths were due to tumor growth. Seven of these eight patients belonged to the high risk group B (tumor stage III), whereas the relapsed treated patient was stratified into group A (tumor stage II).

Neurotoxic side effects or skin manifestations of chemotherapy did not occur. An increase of hepatic enzymes was observed in one patient and it is uncertain whether this was due to therapy. Cholestasis may be related to drug administration and was seen in 3 of 22 cases. Hemopoiesis, however, showed a marked depression in 9 of 22 patients involving granulopoiesis and to a lesser

Table 1. Comparison of chemotherapy and control groups

	Chemotherapy	Control group
Number of Patients	31	37
Treatment discontinued	9/31	–
Average age (years)	60	56
Median time after surgery (months)	10	10.5
Relapses certified	1/22	9/36
Deaths (tumor related)	0	8/36
Deaths (not tumor related)	2/31	2/37

Table 2. Side effects of adjuvant chemotherapy (5-FU and BCNU) in gastric cancer

Granulocytopenia $<1\,500/mm^3$	9/22
Thrombocytopenia $<80\,000/mm^3$	2/22
Hepatotoxic effects	1/22
Cholestasis	3/22
Emesis/Diarrhea/Dumping	11/22

degree, thrombopoiesis. Persistant granulocytopenia with hypoplastic bone marrow granulopoiesis was seen in one case and made the reduction of cytostatic dose necessary (Table 2). Gastrointestinal toxicity was present in 11 of 22 patients, symptoms such as emesis and diarrhea were frequently observed and in 4 of 31 cases, chemotherapy was interrupted because of growing dislike for the therapy.

Conclusion

1) Adjuvant chemotherapy of curatively operated gastric carcinoma with 5-fluorouracil and BCNU was followed by one relapse in 22 patients compared to 9 of 36 patients without treatment.
2) Chemotherapy was not discontinued because of hematological side effects.
3) In 4 of 31 cases, chemotherapy was interrupted because of nausea, emesis, or diarrhea.
4) Neurotoxic effects were not seen.

References

1. Al-Sarraf, M., Vaughn, C. B., Reed, M. L., Vaitkevicius, V. K.: Combined 5-fluorouracil and vinblastine therapy for gastrointestinal and other solid tumors. Oncology *26*, 99 (1972)
2. Blixenkrone-Møller, N.: Long-term results of chemotherapy of operable cancer of the gastro-intestinal tract. Acta Chir. Scand. *133*, 157 (1967)
3. Dixon, W. J., Longmire, W. P., Jr., Holden, W. D.: Use of triethylenethiophosphoramide as an adjuvant to the surgical treatment of gastric and colorectal cancer: Ten year follow-up. Ann. Surg. *173*, 26 (1971)
4. Fujimoto, S., Akao, T., Itoh, B., Koshizuka, I., Koyano, K., Kitsukawa, Y., Takahashi, M., Minami, T., Ishigami, H., Miyazaki, M., Amamiya, K., Ohyama, Y., Ono, K., Kure, M., Itoh, K., Hikosaka, T.: Protracted oral chemotherapy with fluorinated pyrimidines as an adjuvant to surgical treatment for stomach cancer. Ann. Surg. *185*, 462 (1977)
5. Karrer, K.: Adjuvant chemotherapy in early cases of cancer; partly with high-dosed therapy under the protection of autologous frozen-stored bone marrow. Gann Monographs *2*. Cancer Chemotherapy *235* (1968)
6. Kovach, J. S., Moertel, C. G., Schutt, A. J., Hahn, R. G., Reitemeier, R. J.: A controlled study of combined 1,3-bis-(2-chloroethyl)-1-nitrosourea and 5-fluorouracil therapy for advanced gastric and pancreatic cancer. Cancer *33*, 563 (1974)
7. Macdonald, J., Schein, P., Ueno, W., Woolley, P.: 5-fluorouracil, mitomycin-C and adriamycin (FAM): A new combination chemotherapy program for advanced gastric carcinoma. Proc. Am. Soc. Clin. Oncol. *17*, 264 (1976)

8. Moertel, C. G., Hanley, J. A.: Phase II – III studies in chemotherapy of advanced gastric cancer. Proc. Am. Soc. Clin. Oncol. *16*, 260 (1975)
9. Serlin, O., Wolkoff, J. S., Amadeo, J. M., Keehn, R. J.: Use of 5-fluorodeoxyuridine (FUDR) as an adjuvant to the surgical management of carcinoma of the stomach. Cancer *24*, 223 (1969)
10. V. A. Cooperative surgical adjuvant group: Use of thio TEPA as an adjuvant to the surgical management of carcinoma of the stomach. Cancer *18*, 291 (1965)

Chemotherapy in Advanced Gastric Cancer

George A. Higgins

Introduction

The incidence of gastric cancer in the United States has declined at a steady rate for the past 4 decades. Nevertheless, there will be an estimated 23 000 new cases in 1978 with approximately 14 600 deaths from gastric malignancy, making this a still formidable oncologic problem. Worldwide incidence rates, as compiled by the World Health Statistics Manual, show a highly variable incidence rate, the most prevalent areas being in geographically widely separated countries such as Japan, Chile, Costa Rica, and Hungary, with the United States now ranking in the lowest segment of the 44 nations where statistics are available. In all countries surveyed, the incidence is substantially higher in males than in females. The overall adjusted 5-year survival rates in the United States remain at a discouragingly low 12% – 14%, although when still localized to the stomach, and hence favorable for surgical resection, the 5-year survival jumps to a more acceptable rate of approximately 40%. Unfortunately, the symptoms of gastric cancer are nonspecific and all too often appear late in the course of the disease, so that the number of patients on whom surgical resection can be accomplished with any hope of cure remains discouragingly low [3]. It is quite understandable, therefore, that gastric cancer has occupied a prominant position in the massive effort both in the United States and worldwide to search for treatment modalities other than surgery in an effort to improve this dismal picture. This presentation will review pertinent chemotherapy studies in gastric cancer and also discuss ongoing trials.

Review of Chemotherapy in Advanced Gastric Cancer

In numerous studies evaluating single drug therapy in patients with advanced cancer, a number of single agents have demonstrated substantial response rates. The most widely studied single drug has been 5-fluorouracil which has shown an overall response rate of approximately 20%. In addition, adriamycin, mitomycin C and the nitrosoureas have shown substantial activity when used as single agents, with reported objective response rates ranging from 7% to 50%. In an effort to find a more effective treatment, multiple drug combinations have been studied, mostly combining 5-fluorouracil with drugs that have shown activity when used as a single agent. Table 1 summarizes data on two and more combinations compiled from the literature by Bunn and associates [1]. As can be noted,

Table 1. Summary of results from ten studies from the literature of various drug combinations used in patients with advanced gastric cancer compiled by Bunn et al. [1].

Drug regimen	No of patients	Response rate (%)	Median survival (weeks)
5-FU + BCNU	34	41	33
5-FU + methyl-CCNU	30	40	20
5-FU + methyl-CCNU	29	21	~20
5-FU + streptozotocin	12	33	–
5-FU + MMC	15	47	–
5-FU + MMC + adriamycin	18	50	~32
5-FU + MMC + adriamycin	42	24	~23
5-FU + MMC + cytosine arabinoside	32	31	–
5-FU + MMC + cytosine arabinoside	27	55	–
5-FU + methyl-CCNU + MMC + adriamycin	18	11	27

response rates varying from 21% – 55% are reported; however, for the most part, response duration was relatively short. Median survival in patients with nonresectable disease and no additional therapy has generally been in the range of 16 weeks, while most of the various drug combination studies have reported a median survival rate approximately twice that duration (20 – 33 weeks). These investigators report a study combining the four most effective agents, 5-fluorouracil, methyl-CCNU, adriamycin, and mitomycin C. Because of the myelosuppressive properties of each of these agents, the dosage regimen selected was alternating two drug combinations, given at full dose. Only two of 18 patients had objective partial responses, although 11 had stable disease at the completion of one chemotherapy cycle and the median survival period of 27 weeks was essentially the same as reported for the various other drug combinations.

Current Chemotherapy-Trials in Advanced Gastric Cancer

At the 12th International Cancer Congress held in Buenos Aires in October 1978, studies on chemotherapy of advanced gastric cancer were presented by a number of authors from throughout the world, and a summary of data collected from abstracts of these proceedings is shown in Table 2 [7]. As can readily be seen, the response rates generally reported as a combination of complete and partial responses vary markedly, with some reported as high as 62%. Further investigation of these various drug combinations is obviously indicated.

In addition to the above noted reports, there are numerous other studies under way on the chemotherapy of advanced gastric cancer. The International Union Against Cancer (UICC) project on controlled therapeutic trials in cancer has maintained an information office where ongoing trials are registered [2]. It is quite obvious that a wide variety of drug combinations are being investigated for their effectiveness and for the most part, the studies listed are still in progress or have not been reported in full detail.

Table 2. Summary of seven abstracts on treatment of advanced gastric cancer presented at the XII International Cancer Congress in Buenos Aires, October 1978. The wide variety of combinations reported as well as the wide range of response is indicative of the multiplicity and variety of worldwide investigation in the treatment of gastric cancer

		Response
Kurihara (Tokyo)	FU, Endoxan, Mitomycin C	28%
	FU, Endoxan, Cyt. Arab.	29.4%
	Futraful (Cap)	21.8%
	Futraful, Mitomycin C (1 shot)	26.7%
	Futraful, Mitomycin C (weekly)	40%
	Futraful (Suppos)	17.6%
	FU (dry syrup)	26.5%
Minoru (Nagoya)	Mitomycin C FU Cyto. Arab.	44%
Botelli (Buenos Aires)	FU TSPA Methyl Pred	50%
Sakata (Hirosaki)	Mitomycin C Carboquon FU (dry syrup) OK-432	62%
Levi (Sydney)	FU Adriamycin BCNU	Over 50%
Dent (Capetown)	Rad. (2000 r/10 days) vs. FU (Pre- and post-rad) vs. Control	No treatment benefit
Dent (Capetown)	Rad. + FU (as above) vs. Thiotepa vs. Control	

Recent, encouraging results have been reported from investigators at the Lombardi Cancer Center of Georgetown University in Washington, D. C., using multidrug combinations [4]. In a group of 36 patients with advanced gastric cancer treated with the FAM combination (5-fluorouracil, adriamycin, and mitomycin C), a 50% partial response rate was observed. The median duration of remission was approximately 39 weeks; however, in the patients who exhibited response, the median survival was 13 months. These investigators believe that the FAM combination represents the most effective known drug therapy for advanced gastric cancer and note that this combination along with others is under further study by the Gastrointestinal Tumor Study Group. The Southwestern Oncology Group is currently evaluating intensity of dosage and duration of administration of the FAM regimen. In a second trial, the 5-fluorouracil analog Ftorafur was introduced into the regimen in place of 5-fluorouracil. A dosage schema for the FAM and FAM II drug regimens is shown in Table 3.

Table 3. Treatment regimens in the FAM and FAM II combinations as used by Macdonald et al. [4] and Woolley et al. [8]. Results in patients with advanced gastric cancer treated with the FAM combinations have been encouraging as measured by a median duration of remission of approximately 39 weeks and median survival of 13 months in those patients who exhibited response

FAM Combination									
Week	1	2	3	4	5	6	7	8	9
5-Fluorouracil 600 mg/m^2 IV × 1	×	×			×	×			Repeat
Adriamycin 30 mg/m^2 IV × 1	×				×				Cycle
Mitomycin C 10 mg/m^2 IV × 1	×								
FAM II Combination									
Week	1	2	3	4	5	6	7	8	9
Ftorafur 1.5 g/m^2/day IV × 5 days	×				×				Repeat
Adriamycin 40 mg/m^2 IV × 1	×				×				Cycle
Mitomycin 10 mg/m^2 IV × 1	×								

This second combination was discontinued after a trial in 15 patients because of toxicity and its apparent failure to produce responses comparable to the previous combination [8]. This group is also studying an additional nitrosourea drug, chlorozotocin, and have added it to the FAM combination.

In a recently summarized, but as yet unpublished report by Moertel [55] for the Eastern Cancer Oncology Group, various single and multiple drug combinations were evaluated in patients with advanced gastric cancer. The combination of 5-fluorouracil and methyl-CCNU appeared to be superior to methyl-CCNU alone. However, 5-fluorouracil and methyl-CCNU in combination showed no superiority over 5-fluorouracil when used as a single drug. Fluorouracil when combined with either methyl-CCNU or mitomycin C and compared with adriamycin alone showed much the same response and median survival rates.

The Gastrointestinal Tumor Study Group has recently completed a series of trials using three-drug combinations [5]. Fluorouracil combined with methyl-CCNU and adriamycin or combined with mitomycin C and cytosine arabinoside showed superiority to adriamycin when used as a single drug. Similarly, 5-FU combined with adriamycin and methyl-CCNU or combined with adriamycin and mitomycin C demonstrated superiority over a combination of 5-fluorouracil and methyl-CCNU. Using the three-drug combinations, median survival in advanced gastric cancer was approximately 26 – 27 weeks; however, there was a substantial percentage of patients (up to 30%) alive at 1 year. At the present time, the group is comparing these combinations of 5-fluorouracil with adriamycin and mitomycin C or combined with adriamycin and methyl-CCNU with a two-drug combination of 5-fluorouracil and adriamycin. These well-controlled studies along with those reported by Macdonald and associates [4], on the effectiveness of the FAM regimen would indicate that a three-drug combination may well prove to be sufficiently effective and have a tolerable toxicity to warrant extensive trial as a surgical adjuvant. The negative report by Bunn on the four-drug combination may well be due to dosage limitations imposed by the hematotoxicity observed.

In a current overview of chemotherapy for advanced stomach cancer in Japan by Ogawa [6], results with multidrug therapy similar to those outlined above in the United States are reported. In addition to the agents previously mentioned, he reports activity against gastric cancer from carbazilquinone recently developed in Japan, as well as chromomycin A_3, and the still experimental drugs neocarzinostatin, an antibiotic, a water-soluble nitrosourea (ACNU) and an anthracycline compound, aclacinomycin A. For the most part, the MFC regimen combining mitomycin C, 5-fluorouracil, and cytosine arabinoside has been studied most extensively in gastric cancer in Japan with reported response rates varying from 20% – 42%.

In its current trial, the Veterans Administration Surgical Oncology Group is using a combination of 5-fluorouracil and methyl-CCNU. Survival data for patients undergoing "curative" resection in which there is no proven residual disease is shown in Fig. 1. At 20 months, survival in those patients receiving the drug combination is 63.2% compared with 53.6% in patients treated by surgery alone; however, the number of patients randomized is too small and the period of observation too short for this difference to have any significant meaning.

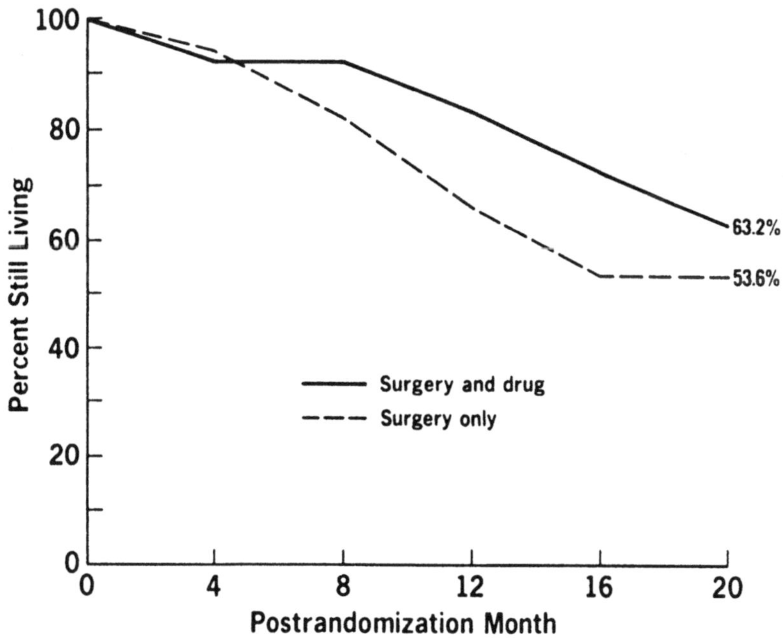

Fig. 1. Survival curves of patients in the current Veterans Administration Surgical Oncology Group Trial comparing surgery alone with a combination of fluorouracil and methyl-CCNU. Although results are thus far encouraging, much additional follow-up is necessary

Conclusion

It can be stated that therapeutic activity against advanced gastric cancer has been demonstrated by at least four cytotoxic drugs when used singly and the degree of effectiveness can be substantially increased when using these substances in varying combination. In addition, other agents are under study and there is increasing evidence for optimism that the use of these drugs, particularly in conjunction with surgical excision of gastric cancer can improve the expectation for survival of these patients.

References

1. Bunn, P. A., Nugent, J. L., Ihde, D. C., Cohen, M. H., Eddy, J. L., Minna, J. D.: 5-Fluorouracil, methyl-CCNU, adriamycin and mitomycin C in the treatment of advanced gastric cancer. Cancer Treat. Rep. *62*, 1287 – 1293 (1978)
2. Flamant, R., Fohanno, C. (eds.): Controlled therapeutic trials in cancer. Vol. 22. Geneva: UICC Tech. Report Series 1978
3. Higgins, G. A., Serlin, O., Amadeo, J. H., McElhinney, J., Keehn, J.: Gastric cancer: Factors in survival. Chir. Gastroenterol. (Surg. Gastroenterol.) *10,* 393 – 398 (1976)
4. Macdonald, J. S., Woolley, P. V., Smythe, T., Ueno, W., Hoth, D., Schein, P. S.: 5-Fluorouracil, adriamycin and mitomycin-C (FAM) combination chemotherapy in the treatment of advanced gastric cancer. Cancer (1979) In press
5. Moertel, C. G.: Personal communication
6. Ogawa, M.: A recent overview of chemotherapy for advanced stomach cancer in Japan. Antibiot. Chemother. *24*, 149 – 159 (1978)
7. 12th International Cancer Congress. Buenos Aires, October 1978, Vol. 2, Abstracts 23/43, pp. 225 – 252.
8. Woolley, P. V., Macdonald, J. S., Smithe, T., Haller, D. G., Hoth, D. F., Rosenoff, S., Schein, P. S.: A phase II trial of ftorafur, adriamycin and mitomycin C (FAM II) in advanced gastric adenocarcinoma. Cancer (1979) In press

Combination of Radio-Chemotherapy in Patients with Advanced Gastric Cancer

E. Hassenstein and V. Diehl

Radiotherapy alone is not able to improve survival time in patients with gastric cancer. Encouraged by the results of Falkson et al. [1], Moertel et al. [3], and Nordman et al. [4], we treated some patients with a combination of radiotherapy and chemotherapy in the last years.

There are many problems in radiation therapy of gastrointestinal tumors. The situation might be defined as a dilemma. On the one hand, patients with advanced gastric cancer are greatly reduced in their general condition and on the other hand, high doses should be applied because of low radiosensitivity of adenocarcinomas. In addition, we point to the fact, that high doses are not possible in all tumors of the gastrointestinal tract. These thin tubular organs have only poor reserves of connective tissue necessary for a cicatrization and a complete restitution. Because of advanced regional lymph node metastases, many patients need a large irradiation volume. In consequence, the rate of complications and side effects, such as nausea and vomiting, is increased.

In the last years, 31 patients with malignant diseases of the stomach were send to us. Eleven of them had Non-Hodgkin-lymphomas and 20 epithelial tumors. Three patients with carcinoma were greatly reduced in their general condition so that only a symptomatic therapy was applied. Bone metastases of four patients were treated with radiotherapy alone.

In 13 patients, a combined treatment with radiotherapy and chemotherapy, simultanously, was practiced. Irradiation was administered to a total tumor dose of 3000 – 4000 rad, 5-fluorouracil (5-FU) was injected once a week in a dosage of 400 mg/m^2.

In some patients, chemotherapy was continued for 3 – 4 weeks after the irradiation period.

Indications for this combined treatment modality were pain, hemorrhage, and obstructive symptoms. These criteria were as well our parameters for the success of this treatment procedure.

Two patients had no lymph node metastases, four others had distant metastases already. Before our therapy, seven patients had undergone surgical palliative resections as BI-, BII-, or fundus resections, whereas the six remaining patients had an exploratory laparatomy only.

An objective response of tumor symptoms was observed in 3 of 13 patients, however, most patients experienced symptomatic relief.

We cannot confirm the optimistic results of Moertel et al. [3], who observed in a study of 48 patients, a significant better survival rate in those patients treated with 5-FU versus a placebo.

Our results were nearly the same as those of Ammon [1], who added vincristine to his treatment regimen.

This type of combination therapy might serve as a less toxic alternative for severely diseased gastric cancer patients to more aggressive modalities.

References

1. Ammon, J.: Möglichkeiten der Kombination von Strahlentherapie und Chemotherapie bei Magenkarzinomen. 10th International Symposion of the stomach. Berlin, 10–12 May 1978
2. Falkson, G., Sandison, A. G., Jacobs, E. L., Richardt, T.: S. Afr. Med. J. *37*, 712 (1963)
3. Moertel, C. G., Childs, D. S., Reitemeier, R. J., Colby, M. Y., Holbrock, M. A.: Combined 5-fluorouracil and supervoltage radiation therapy of locally unresectable gastrointestinal cancer. Lancet *1969 2,* 865
4. Nordman, E., Kauppinen, C.: The value of megavoltage therapy in carcinoma of the stomach. Strahlentherapie *144*, 635 (1972)

Summary: Additional Therapy in Gastric Cancer

The meagre effectiveness of cytostatica and radiotherapy in the treatment of gastric cancer has been disappointing. This is founded on the one hand in the relatively slow cycle of cell division typical of gastric cancer, and on the other hand in the frequently advanced stage of the tumor. An aggressive chemotherapy is therefore partially contraindicated by the poor general condition of many patients with gastric cancer. Significant remissions of tumors (20–25%) in monotherapy were achieved only with 5-fluorouracil or Mitomycin C. The survival time of the patients could not be influenced, however. A certain progress in the cytostatic treatment of gastric cancer was made over the last few years with a combination therapy, particularly with 5-fluorouracil combined with nitrosourea or adriamycin and mitomycin C (FAM). The rate of remission is 40%. Significantly, the survival time of the patients was simultaneously increased. The first results of investigations now in progress are promising.

Some effectiveness of an adjuvant chemotherapy can be demonstrated for part of the patients with gastric cancer. Those patients, whose tumor has not infiltrated the serosa seem to profit most by this. Only a restricted target group of all patients with gastric carcinoma can be considered for an adjuvant therapy. Due to their very favorable prognosis, cases with early cancer are not in need of adjuvant therapy. A relatively large portion of gastric cancer patients, on whom radical surgery was performed, cannot be considered for such therapy because of their age. Only the remaining, relatively small portion of curatively operated patients can potentially derive a profit from adjuvant therapy. Since in a part of the investigations know to date, some patients' prognoses had changed to the worse after treatment with adjuvants, note should be taken of the special responsibility resting in the performance of this therapy, which can only be warranted under the auspices of a prospective, controlled and randomized study.

Pre- and post-operative parenteral nutrition and hyperalimentation is gaining importance as a supporting factor in the therapy of gastric cancer. By compensating an existing malnutrition, the subjective wellbeing of the patients can at least be improved. Perhaps a cytostatic therapy can be better tolerated with this treatment. An especially developed catheter science serves to keep the complication of long-term parenteral nourishment at a minimum for months. How much the survival times of the tumor patients can really be improved by this method, remains to be seen. Whether oral hyperalimentation is the equal of the parenteral form also remains to be investigated.

Subject Index

MIX
Papier aus verantwortungsvollen Quellen
Paper from responsible sources
FSC® C105338

If you have any concerns about our products,
you can contact us on
ProductSafety@springernature.com

In case Publisher is established outside the EU,
the EU authorized representative is:
Springer Nature Customer Service Center GmbH
Europaplatz 3, 69115 Heidelberg, Germany

Printed by Libri Plureos GmbH
in Hamburg, Germany